Principles and Practices
of INHALATIONAL THERAPY

PRINCIPLES AND PRACTICES OF

Inhalational Therapy

BY

ALVAN L. BARACH, M.D.

Associate Professor of Clinical Medicine,
Columbia College of Physicians and Surgeons;
Assistant Attending Physician, Presbyterian Hospital

59 Illustrations

Philadelphia   London   Montreal
J. B. LIPPINCOTT COMPANY

TO

A. R. DOCHEZ

AND

WALTER W. PALMER

Preface

This book is intended for physicians who wish to understand the physiologic basis as well as the technics of inhalational therapy. Numerous studies have been made on the pathologic physiology of respiration, but they are not readily available as a background for the administration of oxygen, helium, carbon dioxide, positive pressure, alternating and equalizing pressure, and the vaporized solutions of various drugs such as epinephrine, neosynephrin, and some of the sulfonamides. It must also be admitted that the advantage of understanding disturbances in respiratory function is not brought to the patient unless the technical procedures employed are carried out by an informed and practiced personnel.

During recent years the practice of inhalational therapy has become so widespread as to call forth the following statement of the Committee on Public Health Relations of the New York Academy of Medicine: "The importance of inhalational therapy in modern medical practice is shown by its use in cardiac failure, coronary artery disease, post-operative atelectasis, atelectasis of the lungs of the newborn, pneumonia, pulmonary edema, emphysema, and cerebral thrombosis. A proper understanding of the technique of application is especially necessary at this time because of its value in the treatment of war gas poisoning, severe hemorrhage, acute altitude sickness and shock."[1]

A handbook on inhalational therapy is therefore presented in the belief that it may prove useful to those who are responsible for the therapeutic use of gases in clinical medicine, and in many phases of war medicine as well.

The pathologic physiology of the clinical entities considered will serve as a guide both to the specific indication for treatment as well as the method of inhalational therapy selected. In a survey of the application of the therapeutic use of gases, a wide range of subjects was inevitably encountered. Greater emphasis was given to those

[1] Standards of effective administration of inhalational therapy, Jour. Amer. Med. Asso., **121**:755, 1943.

syndromes in which inhalational therapy itself played an important rôle, or in which the pathologic physiology of the condition was especially illuminated by the inhalation of the various gases employed. A complete program of treatment for each disease was naturally not intended. The present and future state of the therapeutic use of gases in clinical medicine is described more fully in Chapter 33, Some Considerations Concerning Research in Respiratory Function and Inhalational Therapy.

The methods of inhalational therapy are presented in considerable detail in order to afford the physician in charge the opportunity of making an intelligent selection of apparatus and to understand the most efficient method of using it, as well as to provide those who are actually engaged in carrying out the various technics in inhalational therapy with a practical guide to the operation of the equipment. Technicians and nurses trained in inhalational therapy may also wish to read the clinical chapters to acquaint themselves with the physiologic basis on which the treatment depends. A knowledge of the principles as well as the practice of inhalational therapy may, on this account, be found useful both to physicians and to technical personnel.

A. L. B.

Acknowledgments

I wish to thank Dr. James Howard Means for the encouragement and aid which he generously gave me at the beginning of my studies on inhalational therapy. The clinical investigations on which many of the chapters in this book are based, and such medical training as I have had, were made possible by Dr. Walter W. Palmer, to whom I am deeply grateful.

I wish to acknowledge my appreciation of Mr. Max Soroka's seventeen years of devoted and skillful service as oxygen technician and research assistant, and of the aid given me by Mr. Morris Eckman, not simply as a technical assistant of remarkable ingenuity but also as a comrade in investigation who never withheld valuable criticism.

It is my desire also to express a sincere appreciation to Mr. G. O. Carter, who has for many years contributed an imaginative insight into many phases of the development of oxygen therapy. For their cooperation in technical matters relating to oxygen therapy, my gratitude is due Mr. Jack McKernon and Mr. James Banash.

For gifts of oxygen I am indebted to the Linde Air Products Company, who, by their generosity, made possible many of the studies referred to in this book; for gifts from the Mary W. Harriman Fund, to Mr. W. Averell Harriman and to Mr. E. Roland Harriman.

The pleasure in writing this book was in large measure due to my wife, Frederica, who contributed my Sundays. I wish also to extend my thanks to my secretary, Miss Sylvia Betron, for the care with which she prepared the manuscript.

LIST OF MANUFACTURERS

Acknowledgment is made to the manufacturers listed below for their courtesy in supplying us with photographs or cuts of the apparatus illustrated in the book. This listing does not constitute a recommendation of any particular manufacturer's products, but is inserted here for the convenience of the users of this book who may wish to obtain literature concerning various types of apparatus available for inhalational therapy, nor is it a complete listing of all manufacturers of inhalational equipment.

NAME	ADDRESS
American Hospital Supply Corporation	Merchandise Mart, Chicago, Ill.
Davidson Gas Therapy Company	230th Street & Kingsbridge Avenue, New York, N. Y.
Frederick Stearns and Company	Detroit, Mich.
General Hospital Supply Service, Inc.	256 West 69th Street, New York 23, N. Y.
J. H. Emerson Company	22 Cottage Park Avenue, Cambridge, Mass.
The Linde Air Products Company	30 East 42nd Street, New York, N. Y.
McKesson Appliance Company	Toledo, Ohio
Ohio Chemical and Manufacturing Company	Cleveland, Ohio
Oxygen Equipment Manufacturing Company	405 East 62nd Street, New York, N. Y.
Vaponefrin Company	6812 Market Street, Upper Darby, Pa.
Warren E. Collins, Inc.	555 Huntington Avenue, Boston, Mass.

Contents

1

Historical and Physiologic Background of Inhalational Therapy

In the normal man breathing takes place with so little conscious effort that he is generally unaware that the body mechanism is more thirsty for a precious molecule called oxygen than it is for any other element, nor is he apt to remember that complete deprivation of oxygen results in unconsciousness within 60 seconds and death in less than ten minutes. There are times, however, when breathing is conducted with great difficulty, in which the individual may describe his sensation by saying he is "short of breath." Our first challenge at birth is the attempt to breathe, and the most manifest sign of death is the cessation of respiratory movement. Perhaps no malady fills the human being with alarm so much as that which interferes with comfort in breathing.

A brief history of discoveries in the field of respiration is offered at the beginning of this volume in the belief that it will add to our understanding of the aims and methods of inhalational therapy itself. Our main concern will be to inquire how the various gases in the air were found out, what their function was, and how they were eventually made use of in the relief of suffering and in the saving of life.

In the early history of the human race, air was regarded as one of the four chief elements of which the earth was composed. Fire, earth, and water were the other three. As a child of today thinks of air as a thing in itself, an indivisible entity, so the ancients conceived it, believing that air was in essence a spirit. In 350 B.C. Aristotle conducted the first recorded experiment in respiratory physiology. He kept animals in air-tight boxes until they died, observed their panting for breath, and concluded that their death was due to the inability to cool themselves. Although it is true that one of the results of breathing is the elimination of heat by evaporation of water from the lungs, the

1

primary reason that caused man to breathe was not discovered for the following 2,000 years. Although it had been recognized that air was necessary for life, as in the Bible story in which Elisha restored to life the son of a Shunammite woman by breathing into the mouth of the child, scientists continued to agree with Aristotle that the object of breathing was to cool the inside of the body.

It was not until 1666 that a young Englishman, Robert Boyle, made the following revolutionary statement: "The schools teach the air to be a warm and moist element and consequently a simple and homogeneous body. Our atmosphere, in my opinion, consists not wholly of pure aether . . . but of numberless exhalations of the terraqueous globe . . . the difficulty we find in keeping flame and fire alive . . . without air renders it suspicious that there may be dispersed through the rest of the atmosphere some odd substance, either of a solar, astral, or other foreign nature; on account of whereof the air is so necessary to flame."

Boyle determined the reciprocal relation between volume and pressure of air, and conducted experiments in a decompression chamber in which he demonstrated that aero-embolism could take place in a rarefied atmosphere, and surmised that lack of oxygen was also a destructive factor. Medical history affords no better testimony of profound genius than his note in the *Philosophical Transactions* for September 12, 1670:

"Note, that the two foregoing Experiments were made with an Eye cast upon the inquiry, that I thought might be made; Whether, and how far the destructive operation of our Engin upon the included Animal, might be imputed to this, that upon the withdrawing of the Air, besides the removal of what the Airs presence contributes to life, the little Bubbles generated upon the absence of the Air in the Bloud, juyces, and soft parts of the Body, may by their vast number, and their conspiring distention, variously streighten in some places, and stretch in others, the Vessels, especially the smaller ones, that convey the Bloud and Nourishment; and so by choaking up some passages, and vitiating the figure of others, disturbe or hinder the due circulation of the Bloud? Not to mention the pains that such distensions may cause in some Nerves, and membraneous parts, which by irritating some of them into Convulsions may hasten the death of Animals, and destroy them sooner by occasion of that irritation, than they would be destroyed by the bare absence or loss of what the air is necessary to supply them with, and to shew how this production of Bubbles reaches even to very minute parts of the Body, I shall add on this occasion (hoping that I have not prevented myself on any other,) what may seem somewhat strange, what I once observed in a Viper, furiously tortured in our Exhausted Receiver, namely that it had manifestly a conspicuous Bubble moving to and fro in the waterish humour of one of its Eyes."

In 1628, William Harvey showed that the heart circulated blood, and in 1670 Mayo found that the dark blue blood in the veins became changed into a scarlet red blood in the arteries. He guessed that something of a precious nature was taken up in the lungs which he called the nitro-aerial spirit, and finally in 1775 oxygen was discovered by Joseph Priestley. Having heated the red oxide of mercury, he noticed that a substance (oxygen) came off which was of special value. His subsequent remarks concerning his new gas which he then called dephlogisticated air are characteristic of his engaging personality:

"My reader will not wonder that, having ascertained the superior goodness of dephlogisticated air by mice living in it, and the other tests mentioned above, I should have the curiosity to taste it myself. . . . I have gratified that curiosity by breathing it, drawing it through a glass siphon, and by this means I reduced a large jar full of it to the standard of common air, but I fancied that my breath felt peculiarly light and easy for some time afterwards. Who can tell but that in time this pure air may become a fashionable article in luxury. Hitherto, only two mice and myself have had the privilege of breathing it."

However, Priestley failed to understand the significance of what he had found. He believed that the newly isolated gas, "dephlogisticated air," was air in which the phlogiston, or the spark which was thought necessary for combustion, had been removed. In the meantime, another Englishman, Joseph Black, had mentioned carbon dioxide, but it was the brilliant French scientist Lavoisier who, during the years 1775 to 1794, laid down the fundamental principles of breathing. He demonstrated that oxygen is absorbed through the lungs, carbon dioxide and water are given off during expiration, and that an inert substance, nitrogen, is left. He proclaimed that oxygen is burned in the body in a manner similar to the way fire burns material substances outside the body. Lavoisier was studying an accessory form of respiration, namely perspiration, when he was guillotined in 1794. It is of some interest to realize that Priestley's discovery was what stimulated Lavoisier to clarify the chemistry of breathing. Priestley made the following remarks:

"Having made the discovery some time before I was in Paris in the year 1774, I mentioned it at the table of Mr. Lavoisier, when most of the philosophical people of the city were present, saying that it was a kind of air in which a candle burned much better than in common air, but I had not then given it any name. At this all the company, and Mr. and Mrs. Lavoisier as much as any, expressed great surprise."

The discovery of oxygen excited physicians everywhere, and in 1800 Thomas Beddoes established a pneumatic institute at Bristol where he gave inhalational treatments of oxygen for heart disease and asthma. He made breathing bags and face-pieces of oiled silk, but the technic of administering oxygen was far from adequate to give him the success that he hoped for.

In 1862 Glaisher and Coxwell made a balloon ascent to an altitude of about 29,000 feet. Glaisher noticed a series of untoward symptoms such as loss of vision, paralysis of the legs, and finally unconsciousness; his report of this flight stimulated the great French physiologist, Paul Bert, to study the effects of decreased and increased pressures on the human organism. As a result of his famous "La Pression Barometrique," a book consisting of 1,168 pages, it was shown that the principal effect of high altitude was due to the decreased partial pressure of oxygen, and that the loss of both mental and physical powers was due to lack of oxygen in the blood and tissues of the body.

Since that time many investigators have studied the rôle of oxygen and carbon dioxide in animal and human organisms. Zuntz, Haldane, Barcroft, Krogh, Bohr, Van Slyke, Henderson, Campbell, Poulton— these names represent but a few of the many scientists who provided additional insight into the mechanism of breathing. A crucial experiment was made by Barcroft in 1920 when he lived for five days in a chamber in which the oxygen percentage of the inside air was reduced from 21 to 15 per cent, thus simulating a condition on the tops of high mountains where the pressure of oxygen is diminished because of the rarefied atmosphere. He became sick with nausea, headache, visual disturbances, rapid pulse, and lassitude. Haldane exposed himself to an even more severe deprivation of oxygen with the result that his mind became completely disoriented. The directions to his assistant, had they been followed, would have ended in his death.

These experiences of the harmful effects of a deficiency of oxygen in normal individuals were now seen to occur in the illnesses from which patients suffered. In pneumonia, heart failure, asphyxia of the newborn, and a variety of other diseases it was found that the capacity of the lung to diffuse oxygen or of the heart to circulate blood became damaged to such an extent that individuals suffered from a serious degree of oxygen-want. The term for a lowered pressure of oxygen in the tissues insufficient for normal function was called anoxia, and, more recently, hypoxia.

THE THERAPEUTIC USE OF OXYGEN

The physiologic basis for the therapeutic use of oxygen was put on a more solid basis by the demonstration that the pressure of oxygen in the arterial blood might be critically diminished, and by studies which revealed that the inhalation of oxygen-enriched atmospheres, containing 40 to 60 per cent oxygen, raised the oxygen saturation of arterial blood to or near the normal value in patients with pneumonia and cardiac insufficiency.

The gasometric methods developed by Van Slyke and by Haldane were of great importance in conducting these physiologic studies in clinical disturbances of respiration, and were used by Stadie, Meakins, Barach, and Binger to appraise the results of oxygen therapy. The development of efficient methods of administering oxygen was required for the further advance of inhalational therapy.

An efficient mask was devised by Haldane, and a rubber catheter inserted in the nostril was used by Captain Stokes in the treatment of pulmonary edema due to gas poisoning in the First World War.

Oxygen chambers in which the patient could reside without any appliance to his face were devised by Barcroft in England and Stadie at the Rockefeller Institute; in these chambers air circulation was accomplished by motor-driven blowers. At the Presbyterian Hospital in New York, Barach developed rooms in which the oxygen-enriched atmosphere was circulated by the use of pipes containing circulating ice water or brine on one side of the room and a steam radiator on the other. This ventilation by thermal means accomplished cooling and drying of the atmosphere and air movement without noise, motors, or any electrical contacts. Oxygen chambers were built by Boothby and by Bullowa, both of whom carried out important investigations on the clinical use of oxygen.

In 1920 an oxygen tent was made by Leonard Hill which fitted over the patient in bed, but it contained no provision for eliminating the heat and moisture given off by the patient. Attempts to add efficient cooling mechanisms were made by Barach and Binger and by Roth, and in 1926 a practical method of accomplishing this was described by Barach, in which the oxygen-enriched air was blown in direct contact with chunks of ice contained in a refrigerating cabinet. Due to the large surface area of ice in this form, instantaneous cooling and drying of the tent atmosphere was achieved, and patients were thus provided with effective and comfortable oxygen therapy in a hygienic atmosphere in respect to temperature and humidity.

Other types of oxygen tents have been since developed, including thermal-circulation tents employing ice (Taylor), carbon-dioxide ice (Cohn), and liquid oxygen (Hartman) as refrigerating mediums, and an open-top hood tent (Burgess). In recent years an effective mask apparatus was devised by Boothby, Lovelace, and Bulbulian for the administration of oxygen in concentrations up to 100 per cent. This consists of a comfortably fitting mask, a small rebreathing bag, and sponge-rubber disks through which air is drawn when the bag is collapsed during inspiration, and through which air is expelled during expiration when the rebreathing bag is distended. Barach and Eckman described an injector-mask apparatus (the Meter mask) in which instantaneous and accurate provision of the oxygen concentration desired was made possible, without rebreathing and with little resistance in the operation of the valves in the mask.

Although oxygen therapy was at first used in acute disturbances of lung function such as pneumonia, atelectasis of the lungs of the newborn, massive collapse of the lungs, and asthma, the extension of its use to other conditions was soon put on a firm basis. Boothby established its importance in postoperative conditions, especially bronchopneumonia. Barach, Richards, and Levy described the specific value of continuous inhalation of oxygen in congestive heart failure and coronary thrombosis. Poulton called attention to the vital rôle which inhalation of oxygen may play in cerebral thrombosis, preventing impairment of cerebral function and perhaps brain damage by increase of the oxygen pressure in the collateral blood supply. Richards and Cournand developed accurate methods of determining lung function in pulmonary emphysema and pulmonary tuberculosis.

Recent studies on the dosage of oxygen therapy have a direct bearing on current medical practice. In order to raise the concentration of oxygen in the arterial blood to a level near that of the normal, the percentage of oxygen generally required has been found to be 50 per cent. However, in certain patients who suffer from severe anoxia, such as shock, higher concentrations have a definite advantage. Although continuous inhalation of pure oxygen has been known to produce edema of the lungs of small animals exposed to it for periods of three to five days, it has become evident, largely as a result of the investigations of Evans and of Boothby, that the human being may tolerate for at least two days and probably for four days the inhalation of pure oxygen without harmful effects. It must be stated that the administration of these high concentrations of oxygen has been made by the mask method, in which there is a certain amount of interruption of therapy for feeding and washing. Uninterrupted inhalation of 90 to 100 per cent oxygen for more than one or two days may, however, result in oxygen poisoning.

A fundamental rule in the therapeutic application of oxygen, based on the fact that any abrupt decrease in the pressure of oxygen in the tissues of the body produces harmful consequences, is the administration of oxygen-enriched atmospheres in such concentrations as will overcome the anoxic state. The value, indications, and choice of the various procedures employed in oxygen therapy will be presented under the clinical entities for which its use is intended and in the description of technical methods in the latter half of the book.

THE THERAPEUTIC USE OF CARBON DIOXIDE

The history of the therapeutic use of carbon dioxide has been marked by considerable controversy. In 1885 Miescher showed by experiments on man that a small increase in the percentage of carbon dioxide in the air increased the volume of breathing considerably. Haldane then proved that the volume of breathing was precisely regulated by the pressure of carbon dioxide in the alveolar air of the lungs. It had long been known that lack of oxygen stimulated breathing, and in recent years this has been shown to be largely due to the stimulation of a nerve center near the carotid artery, the carotid sinus in the neck. Carbon dioxide, however, stimulates breathing through a center in the brain, the respiratory center. It is now believed that it is because of its acid nature that the volume of breathing is augmented by inhalation of carbon dioxide. The acid-base equilibrium in the blood under conditions of health and disease was clarified by studies by Gesell, L. J.

Henderson, Means, Van Slyke, Peters, Bock, Yandell Henderson and Haggard, Krogh, Lindhard, and many others.

Although Paul Bert convincingly proved that the symptoms which occurred after residence in high mountains were the result of the decreased pressure of oxygen in the rarefied atmosphere, Mosso still maintained that mountain sickness was due to a loss of carbon dioxide from the blood, as a direct result of the diminished air pressure; he termed this condition *acapnea*. Although the increased breathing which oxygen-want produces is followed by a diminution in the carbon-dioxide content of the blood, it is the result of anoxia and not a primary condition caused by the lowered barometric pressure itself. Some years later Yandell Henderson stressed the importance of the loss of carbon dioxide from the blood which might take place in various conditions in which increased breathing occurred, not only anoxia but the induction phase of anesthesia and mental excitement. When it was found that the lowered carbon dioxide was followed by an approximately proportional decrease in the alkaline bicarbonate in the blood, importance was attached to the loss of bicarbonate which was called *acarbia*.

Oxygen-want was considered by Henderson and Haggard as the first stage of asphyxia. This was followed by an increased volume of breathing which lowered the carbon-dioxide content of the blood, and finally by a compensatory decrease in the blood bicarbonates which migrated to the tissues. Henderson and Haggard believed that it was valuable to inhale mixtures containing 5 to 10 per cent carbon dioxide in order to recall alkali from the tissues into the blood. They showed that animals which had been previously exposed to anesthesia were benefited by this type of therapy. However, Van Slyke, Peters, Austin, Cullen, and others revealed the mechanism of the acid-base equilibrium of the blood in anesthesia in such a way as to cast considerable doubt on the theoretical concept of carbon-dioxide deficiency as a frequent or significant occurrence in clinical illness.

In respect to the effect of anesthesia, the fall in bicarbonate was found to be due not to overventilation but rather to acidosis in which the bicarbonate in the blood was displaced from combination with base by other acids.

In certain clinical conditions a slight lowering of the carbon-dioxide content of the arterial blood may take place due to oxygen deficiency or as a result of disturbed proprioceptive reflexes from the lung. However, oxygen therapy is indicated for the treatment of anoxemic dyspnea, since the carbon dioxide of the blood is generally promptly elevated as the pulmonary ventilation decreases. Barach and Richards have shown that a characteristic, and at times marked, elevation of the carbon-dioxide content of arterial blood takes place in patients with congestive heart failure and pulmonary emphysema treated with oxygen, and that this retention of carbon dioxide represents a homeostatic mechanism. There is, therefore, no secure argument for the administration of carbon dioxide in the dyspnea of either respiratory or cardiac disease, except as shall be referred to later.

In the treatment of babies born in asphyxia, the inhalation of carbon-dioxide–oxygen mixtures has been opposed by Eastman, who found an increased carbon-dioxide content in the blood as well as a more acid shift in the hydrogen-ion concentration in these conditions. Although inhalation of carbon dioxide has been advocated in atelectasis of the lungs of the newborn, this investigator and Kane and Kreiselman regarded the use of carbon dioxide in asphyxia neonatorum as not only superfluous but probably harmful, and recommended simply oxygen-enriched atmospheres and the establishment of a patent airway.

The most evident response to the inhalation of 5 to 10 per cent carbon dioxide is the increased volume of breathing. As was originally shown by Haldane, Priestley, and Douglas, the volume of breathing in the normal man is controlled in a precise way by the percentage of carbon dioxide in the air within the lungs, the so-called alveolar air. Whenever there is good reason to increase the depth of breathing, carbon-dioxide inhalation in the concentrations referred to may be employed, such as in postoperative atelectasis, hiccough, and accidental asphyxia.

In the treatment of carbon-monoxide poisoning Henderson and Haggard have shown that there is a swifter elimination of carbon monoxide from the blood when the ventilation is increased by the stimulating effect of carbon dioxide on the respiratory center. Although Sayers and Yant are of the opinion that the inhalation of 100 per cent oxygen is preferable, the work of Haldane and Stadie showed that the affinity of hemoglobin for carbon monoxide is decreased by carbon dioxide.

The unquestionable value of carbon-dioxide–oxygen mixtures in the treatment of hiccough will be discussed later. Henderson also stated that inhalation of carbon dioxide after operations is followed by an improvement in vitality, in the circulation, and in muscle tonus, increasing the venous return to the heart, but that its main value is in increasing ventilation of the lower lobes of the lungs, tending to prevent atelectasis. Deep-breathing exercises or inhalation of carbon dioxide are now frequently employed to stretch the bronchial tubes and to stimulate cough and the expectoration of mucus, as prophylactic therapy for postoperative atelectasis.

RARE GASES IN THE ATMOSPHERE

Until 46 years ago the world believed that the atmosphere consisted only of 21 per cent oxygen and 79 per cent nitrogen with a trace, 0.03 per cent, carbon dioxide. In 1896 two English scientists, Lord Raleigh and Lord Ramsay, announced to an almost incredulous world that they had found a new gas in the air which amounted to almost 1 per cent by volume. The discovery came about after pondering over a very simple fact; namely, that when nitrogen was prepared from air it was distinctly heavier than a similar volume of this gas produced from ammonia or any other chemical. Since chemically prepared nitrogen was lighter than the same substance isolated from air, it seemed to them that nitrogen must be contaminated by another gas which was heavy. Because the new gas would not go into chemical union with any other substance, they called it argon, meaning idle.

On March 24 of the same year Ramsay wrote to his wife that he had isolated from the mineral cleavite another new gas which was exceptionally light, to which he gave the name "helium." His letter contained the following remarks: "I bottled the new gas in a vacuum tube and arranged it so I could see its spectrum and that of argon in the same spectroscope at the same time. There is argon in the gas; but there was a magnificent yellow line, brilliantly bright, not coincident with but very close to the sodium yellow line . . . You may wonder what it means. Helium is the name given to a line in the solar spectrum, known to belong to an element, but that element has hitherto been unknown to earth."

Three years later Ramsay and Travers discovered three other inert rare gases in the atmosphere: krypton, neon, and xenon. The five rare gases discovered within a period of four years are a monument to the genius of Ramsay, whose imaginative mind was able to grasp, from relatively simple facts, deductions of profound significance. These gases are inert—that is, they do not under ordinary circumstances make combinations with other elements, such as oxygen, carbon, or hydrogen. For that reason they were not thought to have significance as far as animal existence was concerned.

The further developments of Ramsay's work were of great significance. With Dr. Frederick Shoddy he showed that the emanation from the radium salts discovered by Madame Curie contained helium. Ramsay speaks of this production of helium from radium emanation as the first observed case of "transmutation," for radium and its emanation as well as helium must be considered among the substances known as "elements." Ramsay concluded in a memoir on the subject that four atoms of helium separate from one atom of radium.

In 1926 Sayers and Yant made use of the fact that helium has a coefficient of solubility in blood approximately half and a diffusibility approximately twice that of nitrogen in the decompression of animals from ten atmospheres, demonstrating that animals could be released from helium-oxygen mixtures in from one-third to one-fourth the time necessary for nitrogen-oxygen mixtures. In 1938 Behnke and Yarbrough pointed out that the remarkable stupefaction experienced by deep-sea divers at depths below 100 feet could be eliminated by substituting helium for atmospheric nitrogen in the diver's air supply. It was shown that narcosis at high pressures was due to the nitrogen molecule, and that a smaller atom, less soluble in fatty tissue, namely helium, prevented this unusual type of mental impairment.

In 1929 Hershey reported that animals did not survive in atmospheres in which the rare gases were excluded and considered that they were essential to the proper biologic functioning of the organism. However, in careful testing of this hypothesis, in which rigid exclusion of all rare gases was accomplished, Barach showed that animals were in no way influenced by living in an atmosphere of 21 per cent pure oxygen and 79 per cent pure nitrogen for periods as long as 42 days. Furthermore, mice lived for two months in chambers containing 21 per cent oxygen and 79 per cent helium without noticeable change in their condition. Following this confirmation of the biologic inertness of the rare gases, the conception of employing helium as a vehicle for oxygen in the treatment of obstructive dyspnea was advanced.

THE THERAPEUTIC USE OF HELIUM

The introduction of helium as a therapeutic gas was made by Barach in 1934. Since helium is the lightest of all the elements except hydrogen and has a specific gravity one-seventh that of nitrogen, a respirable gas mixture of 20 per cent oxygen and 80 per cent helium was made which had a specific gravity approximately one-third that of air or oxygen. Since movement of a gas past a constricted orifice is inversely proportional to the square root of its molecular weight, the inhalation of helium-oxygen mixtures decreased the physical effort and therefore the dyspnea of patients with severe asthma and those with obstructive lesions in the larynx and trachea. Helium-oxygen therapy was then shown to be at times a life-saving measure in the treatment of status asthmaticus, and also a valuable therapeutic procedure in a program of repeated bronchial relaxation used in cases of intractable asthma. The beneficial effects of helium in patients with severe asthma have been confirmed by Maytum, Prickman and Boothby, Schwartz, Metz, Wearner and Evans, and in obstructive conditions encountered in anesthesia by Eversole.

Although helium-oxygen therapy may be given by a mask, the oxygen tent cannot be employed for this purpose since the mixture leaks out too readily. Barach and Eckman developed a helmet hood which surrounds the head and makes closure at the neck; they also found that greater benefit was obtained if the helium-oxygen mixture was administered under a positive pressure of 2 to 6 cm. of water. Barach and Swenson then demonstrated that the small bronchi showed less constriction in expiration during an attack of asthma when patients breathed under positive pressure. Studies of Barach, Eckman, and Martin revealed the fact that pathologically elevated negative pressures in obstructive dyspnea were diminished by positive-pressure respiration, and a special use of this form of inhalational therapy was established; namely, for the treatment of severe asthma, obstructive dyspnea, and pulmonary edema, in which oxygen-air as well as helium-oxygen mixtures could be employed.

THE THERAPEUTIC USE OF POSITIVE PRESSURE

The administration of gases under positive pressure has a long although neglected history. In 1878 Oertel employed 100 inspirations of air compressed to $\frac{1}{50}$ of an atmosphere excess pressure in the treatment of severe asthma. Haven Emerson in 1909 demonstrated that artificial respiration under pressure was capable of abolishing edema of the lungs when it had been previously produced in rabbits by the intravenous administration of adrenalin. These results were confirmed and amplified by Auer and Gates in 1917, and by Johnson. Both Loeb and Plesch believed that an increased pressure in the air passages of the lungs would be valuable in the treatment of pulmonary edema. Poulton reported beneficial results in the use of positive pressure in some cases of cardiac and bronchial asthma. Barach employed positive pressure in the treatment of patients with severe asthma in combination with helium-oxygen mixtures and very shortly thereafter found that the inhalation of either helium-oxygen mixtures or pure oxygen under a pressure of approximately 5 cm. of water produced a remarkable clearing of edema in certain patients with edema of the lungs, occurring as a consequence of either cardiac or respiratory failure.

A study of the physiologic effects of positive pressure made by Barach, Martin, and Eckman indicated that inhalation of oxygen under positive pressure resulted in a decrease in the heightened negative pressure during the inspiratory cycle, and consequently a cessation of the suction action which like dry cupping tended to cause exudation of serum from the capillaries in the alveolar wall. The administration of positive pressure exerted a direct opposing pressure on the outside walls of the pulmonary capillaries, and thereby counteracted the internal hydrostatic pressure which is partly responsible for serous exudation. In addition positive pressure within the lung retards the entrance of blood into the right heart in cardiac patients, manifested by a rise in venous pressure and a prolongation of the circulation time.

Carlisle has recently treated a series of patients with varying degrees of pulmonary edema due to the inhalation of the fumes of chlorine and nitric acid, with a remarkable clearing of the pulmonary edema in each case. The importance of this procedure in the prevention and treatment of those war gases that are apt to create irritant pulmonary edema is evident.

It is interesting to note that Norton in 1897 had reported a case of advanced edema of the lungs due to carbolic-acid poisoning (fumes) in which rapid clearing of the edema and prompt recovery took place with the use of the Fell-O'Dwyer respiration apparatus, which made possible breathing under positive pressure.

A simple mask apparatus that provides positive pressure in expiration has been developed by Barach, Eckman, and Molomut, which may be used with the inhalation of either oxygen or air.

THE THERAPEUTIC USE OF RESPIRATORS

In patients with paralysis of the respiratory musculature, the artificial maintenance of respiratory function has been employed in the hope that recovery of function of the impaired organ will ultimately take place. In 1926 Thunberg devised a mechanically controlled apparatus for artificial respiration which consisted of a box in which the entire patient was enclosed. The pressure within this chamber, called the barospirator, was alternately raised and lowered one-twelfth of an atmosphere, namely 55 mm. Hg, above and below the atmospheric pressure 25 times a minute. This variation in pressure was found to be adequate to result in the removal of carbon dioxide and the provision of oxygen to the alveoli in the lung. In a series of cases of respiratory paralysis due to drug poisoning and infantile paralysis the function of the lung appeared to be reasonably maintained by this method. (For contrary experimental results, see page 184.)

In 1929 Drinker and his collaborators developed an apparatus in which the patient's body was enclosed in an air-tight chamber but the head extended into the atmosphere through an air-tight rubber collar which fitted around the neck. When the pressure within the box is alternately lowered and restored to that of the atmosphere by means of an electrically driven suction blower or motor-driven bellows, the chest is expanded and the diaphragm lowered, thus causing an inspiration of air. With restoration of pressure to that of the atmosphere, expiration takes place.

More portable types of apparatus have been developed recently in which the suction pressure is applied directly to the chest wall by a metal encasing that surrounds the anterior chest, without the patient being totally enclosed within a box.

An apparatus originally called the pulmotor employed positive and negative pressure to the lung by means of a mask attached to the face and a motor-blower connecting unit. Excessive pressures, during both artificially induced inspiration and expiration, have now been prevented by suitable valves in the newer types of apparatus of this kind, called resuscitators.

In the treatment of various types of asphyxia due to accidental causes or illness, the artificial maintenance of respiration may be of life-saving value.

THE THERAPEUTIC USE OF EQUALIZING CHEST-PRESSURE THERAPY

The use of a room in which alternating pressure was applied to patients with chronic pulmonary disease revealed that an initial compression of the chest wall took place during the positive phase and an expansion of the chest at the start of the negative cycle. Barach found this to be due to the resistance interposed by the tracheobronchial tree to the passage of air in and out of the lungs. To overcome the constricting effect of the tracheobronchial tree, a similar resistance to the air pressure applied to the chest wall was produced, so that the pressure on the inner and outer surface of the thorax was made approximately equal, as well as on the upper and lower surfaces of the diaphragm. Under these circumstances patients with pulmonary tuberculosis were able to suspend completely voluntary breathing and to achieve a degree of local lung rest not hitherto possible.

Although an adequate pulmonary ventilation is maintained by this type of equalizing-pressure therapy, no discernible movement of the ribs or diaphragm can be detected by direct observation or by fluoroscopic or roentgenographic examination. The beneficial effects of physical immobilization of the lung for a period of three to four months in patients with advanced pulmonary tuberculosis have been sufficiently striking to lead to the view that the healing process may be initiated and accelerated by this therapy in patients previously unresponsive to other treatment. The future of this kind of inhalational therapy, which depends upon a supply of a normal volume of breathing without lung movement, cannot be accurately foretold at this time, but the early results are decidedly favorable.

THE THERAPEUTIC USE OF VAPORIZED SOLUTIONS OF EPINEPHRINE AND NEOSYNEPHRIN

Although inhalation of various solutions has been known for a long time through the studies of Hüber and Lageder, an important advance in practical therapy was made by Graeser and Rowe in 1935 with the introduction of a more concentrated 1 : 100 solution of epinephrine. This was recommended for use in patients with asthma, employed with a hand-bulb nebulizer that produced a fine vapor suitable for inhalation. For the majority of cases employment of a hand-bulb nebulizer is of great value and enables many patients with severe asthma to do without hypodermic injection of adrenalin.

For patients with severe intractable asthma, Richards, Barach, and Cromwell advocated the continuous administration of vaporized solutions of 1 : 100 epinephrine and 1 per cent neosynephrin, employing a pressure tank of oxygen with the usual reducing valve to regulate the flow, instead of the hand bulb attached to the nebulizer. In this way 0.5 cc. of the epinephrine solution may be vaporized in a period of 10 to 15 minutes, the patient holding the nozzle of the nebulizer in the open mouth. The value of nebulizing chemotherapeutic drugs in the lungs, such as a 25 per cent solution of promin and the 2.5 per cent sulfadiazine in ethanolamine solution, the former in pulmonary tuberculosis and the latter in nontuberculous infections of the bronchi and lungs, is now under investigation (Barach).

BIBLIOGRAPHY

Barach, A. L.: The therapeutic use of oxygen, Jour. Amer. Med. Asso., 79:693, 1922.

Barach, A. L.: Diseases of the Lungs, Practitioners Library of Medicine and Surgery, New York, D. Appleton & Co., 3:943, 1933.

Barach, A. L.: Rare gases not essential to life, Science, 80:593, 1934.

Barach, A. L.: The gases of the air in medicine, Hygeia, 14:620, 1936.

Barach, A. L.: The therapeutic use of helium, Jour. Amer. Med. Asso., 105:1273, 1936.

Barach, A. L.: Immobilization of lungs through pressure, Amer. Rev. Tuberc., 42:5, 1940.

Barach, A. L.: The therapeutic use of gases, in Modern Medical Therapy in General Practice, 1:199, 1940. Edited by D. P. Barr, Baltimore, Williams & Wilkins Co.

Barach, A. L.: The Therapeutic Use of Gases; The Therapeutics of Internal Diseases. Edited by George Blumer. Vol. I, New York, D. Appleton-Century Co., 1940-1941.

Barach, A. L.: The gases in the atmosphere as therapeutic agents, South. Med. and Surg., 104:2, 1942.

Barach, A. L., Lt. Robert Brookes, Morris Eckman, Emanuel Ginsburg, and Artell Johnson: Appraisal of tests of altitude tolerance: II. Impairment of emotional control as a test of altitude anoxia, Jour. Aviation Med., 14:52, 1943.

Barach, A. L., J. Martin, and M. Eckman: Positive pressure respiration and its application to the treatment of acute pulmonary edema, Ann. Int. Med., 12: 754, 1938.

Barach, A. L., and D. W. Richards, Jr.: Effects of oxygen therapy in congestive heart failure, Arch. Int. Med., 48:325, 1931.

Barach, A. L., and M. N. Woodwell: Studies in oxygen therapy with determination of the blood gases, etc.: I. In cardiac insufficiency and related conditions, Arch. Int. Med., 28:367, 1921. II. In pneumonia and its complications, Arch.

Int. Med., **28**:394, 1921. III. In an extreme type of shallow breathing occurring in encephalitis, Arch. Int. Med., **28**:421, 1921.

Barcroft, J.: Anoxemia, Lancet, **2**:485, 1920.

Barcroft, J.: Oxygen Therapy, Brit. Med. Jour., **1**:150, 1920.

Barcroft, J.: The Respiratory Function of the Blood, Cambridge University Press, Vol. I, 1925; Vol. 2, 1928.

Barcroft, J.: The Architecture of Physiological Function, Cambridge University Press, 1934.

Barcroft, J., A. Cooke, H. Harbridge, T. R. Parsons, and W. Parsons: Flow of oxygen through pulmonary epithelium, Jour. Physiol., **53**:45, 1920.

Barker, M. H.: The broad field of anoxia and advances in treatment, Anesth. and Analg., **17**:21, 1938.

Behnke, A. R., Jr.: Certain physiologic principles underlying resuscitation and oxygen therapy, Anesthesiol., **2**:245, 1941.

Behnke, A. R., and O. D. Yarbrough: Physiologic study of helium, U. S. Nav. Med. Bull., **36**:542, 1938.

Behnke, A. R., and O. D. Yarbrough: Respiratory resistance, oil-water solubility and mental effects of argon, compared with helium and nitrogen, Amer. Jour. Physiol., **126**:409, 1939.

Bert, P.: La Pression Barométrique, Recherches de Physiologie Expérimentale, Paris, Masson et Cie, 1878.

Binet, L., M. Bochet, and M. V. Strumza: L'anoxémie: ses effets—son traitement, L'oxygénothérapie, Paris, Masson et Cie, 1939.

Binger, C. A. L.: Anoxemia in pneumonia and its relief by oxygen inhalation, Jour. Clin. Invest., **6**:203, 1928.

Bohr, C., K. Hasselbalch, and A. Krogh: Ueber einen in biologischer Beziehung wichtigen Einfluss den die Kohlensäurespannung des Blutes auf dessen Sauerstoffbindung übt, Skandinav. Arch. f. Physiol., **16**:402, 1904.

Boothby, W. M.: Oxygen therapy—council on physical therapy, Jour. Amer. Med. Asso., **99**:2026, 1932; **99**:2106, 1932.

Boothby, W. M., W. R. Lovelace, and A. H. Bulbulian: Oxygen administration and therapeutic use: I. Value of high concentration of oxygen for therapy; II Oxygen for therapy and aviation and an apparatus for the administration of oxygen and oxygen-helium by inhalation; III. Design and construction of the masks for oxygen inhalation apparatus, Proc. Staff Meet., Mayo Clin., **13**:641 1938.

Campbell, J. A.: Hypertrophy of heart in acclimatization to chronic carbon monox ide poisoning, Jour. Physiol., **77**:8, 1932.

Campbell, J. M. H.: The effect on breathless subjects of residence in an oxygen chamber, Quart. Jour. Med., **20**:144, 1926.

Campbell, J. M. H., G. G. Douglas, J. S. Haldane, and F. G. Hobson: The response of the respiratory center to carbonic acid, oxygen, and hydrogen ion concentration, Jour. Physiol., **46**:301, 1913.

Campbell, J. M. H., and E. P. Poulton: The effect on breathless subjects of residence in an oxygen chamber, Quart. Jour. Med., **20**:121, 1926.

Campbell, J. M. H., and E. P. Poulton: Oxygen and carbon dioxide therapy, Oxford University Press, 1934.

Dautrebande, L.: Oxygénothérapie et Carbothérapie: Bases Physiologiques, Applications Cliniques, Techniques; Paris, Masson et Cie, 1937.

Dill, D. B., E. H. Christensen, and H. T. Edwards: Gas equilibrium in lungs at high altitudes, Amer. Jour. Physiol., **115**:530, 1936.

Dill, D. B.: Life, Heat, and Altitude, Cambridge, Harvard University Press, 1938.

DuBois, E.: Metabolism in Health and Disease, 2nd Ed., Philadelphia, Lea & Febiger, 1927.

Dumke, R. R., C. F. Schmidt, and H. P. Chiodi: Part played by carotid body reflexes in respiratory response of dog to anoxemia with and without simultaneous hypercapnia, Amer. Jour. Physiol., 133:1, 1941.

Gessell, R.: Respiration and its adjustments, Ann. Rev. Physiol., 1:1, 1939.

Gessell, R., and A. B. Hertzman: The regulation of respiration: XVII. Effects of intravenous injection of sodium cyanide on the acidity of the arterial and venous blood, Amer. Jour. Physiol., 83:420, 1928.

Grollman, A.: The Cardiac Output of Man in Health and Disease, Springfield, Ill., Charles C. Thomas, Publisher, 1932.

Haldane, J. S.: The administration of oxygen, Brit. Med. Jour., 2:517, 1918.

Haldane, J. S.: Recent developments in the therapeutical uses of oxygen, contributions Medic. and Biolog. Research. Dedicated to Sir W. Osler. New York, Paul B. Hoeber, Inc., 1:549, 1919.

Haldane, J. S., J. C. Meakins, and J. G. Priestley: The effects of shallow breathing, Jour. Physiol., 52:432, 1918.

Henderson, L. J.: The principles controlling respiration in health and disease, Practitioners Library of Medicine and Surgery, New York, D. Appleton-Century Co., 1935.

Henderson, Y.: Adventures in Respiration: Modes of Asphyxiation and Methods of Resuscitation, Baltimore, Williams & Wilkins Co., 1938; Anesth. and Analg., 18:532, 1939.

Henderson, Y., and H. W. Haggard: The reversible alterations of the H_2CO_3· $NaHCO_3$ equilibrium in blood and plasma under variations in CO_2 tension and their mechanism, Jour. Biol. and Chem., 45:189, 1920.

Hershey, J. W.: Components of the atmosphere and synthetic gases in relation to animal life, Anesth. and Analg., 13:107, 1934.

Heymans, C., and J. J. Bouckaert: Ergebn. d. Physiol. biol. Chem. u. exper. Pharmakol., 41:29, 1938.

Hilderbrand, J. H., R. R. Sayers, and W. P. Yant: Possibilities in the use of helium-oxygen mixtures as a mitigation of caisson disease, U. S. Bureau of Mines, Report of Investigation No. 2670, 1925.

Hill, L.: A simple oxygen bed tent and its use in a case of edema and chronic ulcer of the leg, Jour. Physiol., Proc. Physiol. Soc., 55:20, 1921.

Krogh, A.: Comparative Physiology of Respiratory Mechanisms, Philadelphia, University of Pennsylvania Press, 1941.

Lovelace, W. R., Jr., W. M. Boothby, and O. O. Benson: Aeroembolism: A Medical Problem in Aviation at High Altitude, Scient. Monthly, 53:30, 1941.

Meakins, J. C.: Gases in human arterial blood in certain pathological pulmonary conditions and their treatment with oxygen, Jour. Pathol. and Bacteriol., 24: 79, 1921.

Meakins, J. C.: Oxygen-want: its causes, signs and treatment, Edinburgh Med. Jour., 29:142, 1922.

Meakins, J. C., and H. W. Davies: Respiratory Function in Disease, London, Oliver & Boyd, 1925.

Means, J. H.: Dyspnea, Medicine, 3:309, 1924.

Means, J. H., and L. H. Newburgh: Studies of the blood flow by the method of Krogh and Lundhard, Trans. Asso. Amer. Physic., 30:51, 1915.

Meltzer, S. J.: Observations on the gases in human arterial blood in certain path ological conditions and their treatment with oxygen, Jour. Pathol. and Bacteriol., 24:79, 1921.

Miller, A. H.: The pneumatic institution of Thomas Beddoes at Clifton, 1798, Ann. Med. Hist., 3:253, 1931.

Priestley: Experiments and Observations on Different Kinds of Air, Londres, 1775-1777.

Richards, D. W., Jr., and A. L. Barach: Prolonged residence in high oxygen atmosphere: effects on normal individuals and on patients with chronic cardiac and pulmonary insufficiency, Quart. Jour. Med., 3:437, 1934.

Sayers, R. R., and W. P. Yant: Value of helium-oxygen atmosphere in diving and caisson operations, Anesth. and Analg., 5:127, 1926.

Schmidt, C. F.: Effect of carotid sinus and carotid body reflexes upon respiration, Anesth. and Analg., 19:261, 1940.

Schmidt, C. F.: Mechanism and probable significance of the convulsions produced by cyanide, Science, 93:465, 1941.

Stadie, W. C.: The oxygen of the arterial and venous blood in pneumonia and its relation to cyanosis, Jour. Exper. Med., 30:215, 1919.

Stadie, W. C.: Treatment of anoxemia in pneumonia in an oxygen chamber, Jour. Exper. Med., 35:337, 1922.

Tovell, R. M., and J. E. Remlinger, Jr.: History and present status of oxygen therapy and resuscitation, Jour. Amer. Med. Asso., 117:1939, 1941.

Van Slyke, D. D., H. Wu, and F. C. McLean: Studies of gas and electrolyte equilibria in the blood: V. Factors controlling the electrolyte and water distribution in the blood, Jour. Biol. Chem., 56:765, 1923.

Waters, J. G., P. R. Dumke, and J. H. Comroe, Jr.: The part played by carotid and aortic body reflexes in respiratory control in unanesthetized dogs, Federation Proc., 1:90, 1942.

Yant, W. P., J. Chornyak, H. H. Schrenk, F. A. Patty, and R. R. Sayers: Studies in asphyxia, Public Health Bull. No. 211, United States Public Health Service, 1934.

2

Acute Altitude Sickness, Acute Anoxia

DEFINITION

Acute altitude sickness is the term employed by Schneider and Armstrong to designate acute oxygen-want occurring in airplane flight at moderate or high altitudes. This syndrome is justifiably differentiated from mountain sickness since physiologic adaptation gradually takes place as a result of continuous exposure to a rarefied atmosphere. No acclimatization has been shown to develop after repeated exposure to short periods of altitude anoxia. This entity is, therefore, a good illustration of the effect of oxygen-want without other complicating features. At extremely high altitudes aero-embolism may take place, but up to a height of 18,000 feet the decreased partial pressure of oxygen in the lungs and consequently in the arterial blood affords an example of what is called anoxic or arterial anoxia or, a more accurate designation recently used, hypoxia. Since many clinical disturbances of respiratory and circulatory function produce acute anoxia, which is the essential indication for oxygen therapy, the syndrome of acute altitude sickness is now presented.

ETIOLOGY

Acute altitude sickness is the result of inspiring air under decreased atmospheric pressures in civil and military aviation. Symptoms of oxygen-want begin at an altitude of 9,000 to 10,000 feet, become more definitely evident at 12,000 feet, and are well marked at 15,000 feet and above. The effects of a decreased partial pressure of oxygen have been observed experimentally by withdrawing air from steel chambers until the pressure within them has been lowered to that which exists at various altitudes. Studies have also been carried out at sea level in which subjects have breathed mixtures containing decreased oxygen concentrations as a result of adding nitrogen to air.

In clinical illness, such as pneumonia and edema of the lungs, the pressure of oxygen in atmospheric air may be insufficient to accomplish diffusion of oxygen through swollen alveolar walls at the normal velocity, with the result that a lowered supply of oxygen is given to the arterial blood passing through the lungs. Acute oxygen-want may also take place as a result of circulatory failure and other conditions which will be described later. Whatever the cause of acute anoxia, the symptomatology is characteristic; it may become the dominating feature in clinical disease or may be added to symptoms that may come from toxemia or infection.

PATHOLOGIC PHYSIOLOGY

The disturbance in the physiology of the human being during ascents to high altitudes is primarily due to the decrease in partial pressure of oxygen as the total barometric pressure is lowered. At an altitude of 18,000 feet the atmosphere pressure, 380 mm. Hg, is one-half the sea-level barometric pressure of 760 mm. Hg. At this altitude a liter of gas would have expanded in a free state to two liters of gas, and the expanded volume then hold the same number of oxygen and nitrogen molecules, but each molecule would be separated from each other by a greater distance. Since the volume of the chest is constant, the inspired air would at first glance contain one-half the number of oxygen molecules which were in the inhaled air at sea level. However, the pressure of oxygen in the lungs is somewhat less than one-half the sea-level pressure because of certain additional factors which require consideration. As air is taken into the lung it becomes saturated with water vapor which has a pressure of 47 mm. Hg at body temperature. There is also a constant evolution of carbon dioxide in the alveoli from the pulmonary capillaries. The pressure of carbon dioxide under normal circumstances is 40 mm. Hg. In order to determine accurately the pressure of oxygen in the lungs at 18,000 feet, i.e., 380 mm. Hg, the following calculation is undertaken: $(380 - 47) \times .209$, the percentage of oxygen in a saturated atmosphere, -40 or 29.6 mm. Hg, the alveolar oxygen pressure. Subtraction of 47 mm. Hg represents the pressure contributed by water vapor, and 40 mm. Hg that of carbon dioxide. Since an individual at 18,000 feet would greatly increase the volume of breathing due to want of oxygen, the carbon dioxide in the lungs would be blown off to a variable extent and the pressure of carbon dioxide would be replaced by an equivalent pressure of oxygen.   The actual alveolar oxygen pressure might then be [(380 — 47) × .209] — 30 (the lowered carbon-dioxide pressure) or 39.6 mm. Hg.   In these calculations the respiratory quotient of 1 is assumed.

In the normal individual at sea level the alveolar oxygen pressure is about 108 mm. Hg.   This is sufficient to saturate the hemoglobin in the red cells to 95 per cent of its potential saturation.   Arterial

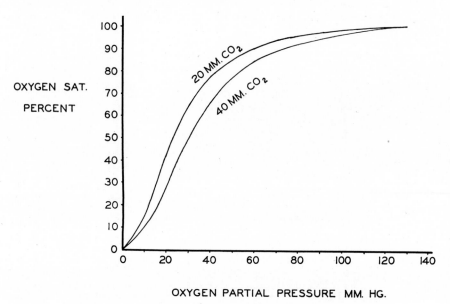

OXYGEN PARTIAL PRESSURE MM. HG.

FIG. 1.   Per cent saturation of hemoglobin with oxygen with different partial pressures of oxygen and carbon dioxide.

blood is thus 95 per cent saturated with oxygen under normal conditions.   It will be readily seen that a pressure of 39.6 mm. Hg of oxygen will not adequately saturate the hemoglobin in the red corpuscles. The blood then passes to the tissues with a deficient content as well as pressure of oxygen, and it is because of this circumstance that the normal function of the various organs is not preserved.   The characteristic decrease in the oxygen saturation of arterial blood with decreasing pressure of oxygen in the atmosphere, and therefore in the lungs, is illustrated in the accompanying charts.   These two curves illustrate the reason the hemoglobin in red blood cells at high altitudes is supplied with oxygen at a lower pressure, with the consequence that the arterial blood carries oxygen at a lower pressure to the various organs and therefore the condition of oxygen-want in the tissues, or anoxia,

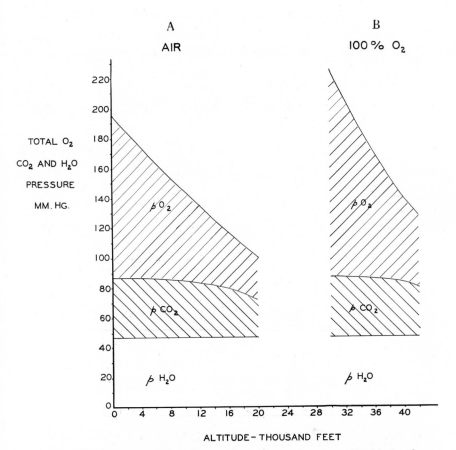

$$A \qquad\qquad B$$

AIR   100 % O_2

FIG. 2. Fall in partial pressure of oxygen and carbon dioxide in the lungs at increasing altitudes. A, Breathing air, B, breathing 100 per cent oxygen.

A. During ascent to an altitude of 20,000 feet there is a progressive fall in the pressure of nitrogen and oxygen in the alveolar air, whereas the carbon-dioxide pressure is only slightly lowered and the pressure of water vapor remains constant.

B. Although 100 per cent oxygen is breathed during ascent from 30,000 to 42,000 feet, the alveolar oxygen pressure is reduced to that which occurs in a subject breathing air at 14,500 feet. The sum of water vapor and carbon-dioxide pressure, 83 mm. Hg, constitutes at an altitude of 42,000 feet a far larger proportion of the total barometric pressure, 128 mm. Hg, than at the lower altitudes. Thus, the necessitous evolution of carbon dioxide and water vapor from the lungs limits more and more the quantity of oxygen that can be inhaled as progressively higher altitudes are reached.

takes place. The higher pressure of oxygen in blood exposed to increasing carbon-dioxide pressure will be discussed below.

Inhalation of oxygen-enriched atmospheres up to 100 per cent oxygen will compensate for the diminished partial pressure of oxygen in the atmosphere until an altitude of 34,000 feet is obtained. At this altitude, corresponding to a barometric pressure of 187 mm. Hg, the arterial blood of a man breathing pure oxygen is saturated with oxygen in the same degree that takes place in a normal individual at sea

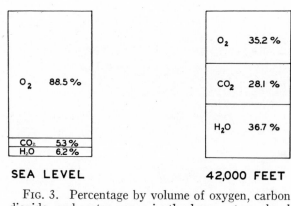

SEA LEVEL   42,000 FEET

Fig. 3. Percentage by volume of oxygen, carbon dioxide, and water vapor in the lungs, at sea level (760 mm. Hg) and at 42,000 feet (128 mm. Hg), when breathing 100 per cent oxygen.

level breathing air, namely 95 per cent oxygen saturation. At an altitude of 42,000 feet, 128 mm. Hg, the blood has become markedly less saturated even during the inhalation of pure oxygen. Reference to the accompanying chart will illustrate the mechanism of this. A barometric pressure of 128 mm. Hg must have subtracted from it the pressure of water vapor (47) and carbon dioxide (40 mm. Hg), to obtain the pressure of oxygen in the lungs during the inhalation of pure oxygen. Although some hyperventilation takes place, lowering the alveolar carbon-dioxide pressure to 36 mm. Hg, there still must be subtracted the sum of 47 plus 36 mm. from 128, or 45 mm. Hg, which does not provide an adequate oxygen saturation of the arterial blood.

The situation may be expressed differently by remembering that the *percentage by volume* of carbon dioxide and water vapor in the lungs is much greater at 42,000 feet than at sea level since these gases have expanded many times their sea-level volume, inasmuch as the pressure at this altitude is one-sixth the barometric pressure of 760 mm. Hg, as seen in the illustration on p. 24. The oxygen concentration of the alveolar air during the inhalation of 100 per cent oxygen is thus reduced because of the increasing percentage of lung volume occupied by carbon dioxide and water vapor at 42,000 feet.

The fact that water vapor is present in the lungs in such an increased percentage is illustrated by measuring the volume of the gases in the

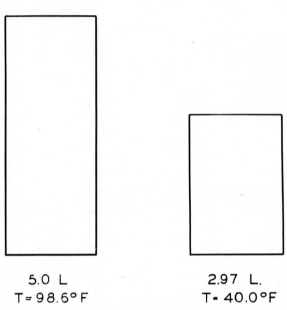

5.0 L
T = 98.6° F

2.97 L.
T = 40.0 °F

Fig. 4. Decrease in volume of gases of the lung when collected in a gasometer at 40° F. at an altitude of 42,000 feet. 75 per cent of the decrease is due to precipitation of moisture.

lung when collected in a gasometer at 40° F. at an altitude of 42,000 feet. As seen in Fig. 4, the apparent vital capacity has diminished from 5.0 to 2.97 liters, due in large part (75 per cent) to precipitation of moisture as the expired air is transported from a temperature of 99° F. to 40° F. No true loss in vital capacity has occurred.

The early signs of disturbance in the physiology of the human organism begin at an altitude of 10,000 feet. This corresponds to an oxygen concentration in the inspired air of slightly below 14 per cent. The arterial oxygen saturation at this degree of anoxia is approximately 88 to 90 per cent, only slightly lower than the usual normal level of 95 per cent saturation. The cyanotic color which individuals exposed to high altitudes or patients suffering from disturbances in cardiorespiratory function frequently show is due to the reduced hemoglobin, and is not generally observed until the arterial oxygen saturation has fallen below 85 per cent, which would be produced at an altitude of 12,000 feet. It should be borne in mind that the bluish color is furnished by the amount of reduced hemoglobin and not by the degree of saturation of the hemoglobin with oxygen. In other words, an anemic patient who has only 5 Gm. of hemoglobin may not reveal a cyanotic color even if he suffers from a very serious decrease in arterial oxygen saturation; on the other hand, a patient with polycythemia who has seven million red blood cells instead of five million may have an arterial oxygen saturation of 93 per cent and yet look definitely bluish, since 7 per cent of his relatively larger total hemoglobin is in a reduced state. However, in patients with pneumonia who are not anemic the degree of cyanosis frequently parallels the extent of lowering of the arterial oxygen saturation. Exceptions to this are (1) shock, in which a grayish pallor is present with serious anoxia, (2) local tissue anoxia, due to thrombosis of an artery, (3) histotoxic anoxia, due to agents which impair the oxidative enzymes, and (4) hyperventilation, which results in alkalotic constriction of the cerebral and coronary circulation.

The first effects noted at an altitude of 10,000 feet are an increase in the volume of breathing and a more rapid pulse rate. The increase in pulmonary ventilation, more pronounced above 12,000 feet, results in a blowing off of carbon dioxide from the blood. The alkalosis which is produced by exposure to high altitude is gradually compensated for by a corresponding reduction in the sodium-bicarbonate level of the blood, a lessened excretion of acid in the urine, and a compensatory increase of chloride ions in the blood.

When normal individuals or patients are exposed to acute severe anoxia, such as occurs during the inhalation of 10 per cent oxygen for a period of 20 minutes or abrupt ascent to an altitude of 18,000 feet, an actual shift in acid-base equilibrium toward the alkaline side takes place which may amount to as much as a change from a pH of 7.42 to 7.52. This is due to a relatively more rapid elimination of carbon dioxide in proportion to the adaptive reduction in the total base ions in the blood. However, in extreme severe experimental oxygen-want an acidosis takes place, with low carbon-dioxide content and capacity. Hyperventilation accentuates the anoxia, and acid products, due to deficient oxidation, shift the pH to the acid side.

In prolonged exposure to low oxygen pressures, which occurs during residence in mountainous regions or in chronic clinical anoxia, an increase in the hemoglobin and in the red cells takes place. The initial response of this nature is due to diminution of the plasma blood volume and also to contraction of the spleen, which sends red cells into active circulation. At the end of six days, the blood volume returns to normal and there is then an actual increase in the total number of red corpuscles in the circulating blood due to stimulation of the bone marrow. Another compensation to acute oxygen-want is the increase in the amount of blood delivered by the heart. It appears that this increase in cardiac output takes place when the anoxia is of such a degree as to be represented by an arterial oxygen saturation of 82 per cent or below. Apparently mild degrees of oxygen-want do not result in an increase in cardiac output although an increase in pulse rate takes place. When anoxia has persisted for a relatively long time, excessive carbon-dioxide elimination from the blood is compensated for by such a decrease in basic ions as to result in no change in the acid-base equilibrium in the blood.

The undue loss of carbon dioxide which occurs as a result of initial anoxia has been discussed by many physiologists, at times with the suggestion that carbon dioxide be administered to overcome this condition. It has become increasingly clear that the best physiologic approach to treatment of increased excretion of carbon dioxide is the inhalation of oxygen-enriched atmospheres, in order to overcome the anoxia. By restoring the oxygen saturation of the arterial blood to the normal range, the stimulus for an increased pulmonary ventilation and therefore the loss of carbon dioxide is prevented. There is at the present time no valid reason for the administration of carbon dioxide either to aviators or to most patients suffering from dyspnea in clinical medicine. It should always be borne in mind that continuous inhalation of increased percentages of carbon dioxide may result in fatigue of the respiratory musculature.

It has been indicated that inhalation of oxygen-enriched atmospheres up to 100 per cent oxygen will overcome the anoxia of increasing altitude up to 34,000 feet, and that above this level the oxygen percentage of the arterial blood progressively falls. At an altitude of 42,000 feet, 128 mm. Hg, the increased volume of breathing lowers the carbon-dioxide pressure in the lung from 40 to 36 mm. Hg, and the actual oxygen pressure to which the capillaries of the lungs are exposed is decreased, as discussed above, by the sum of water-vapor pressure and carbon-dioxide pressure $(47 + 36)$ subtracted from 128 mm. Hg, or 45 mm. Hg.

As will be observed in the accompanying table the average arterial oxygen saturation at 42,000 feet is 80.6 per cent, which is slightly

TABLE I

ALVEOLAR AND ARTERIAL pCO_2 AND pO_2 AND ARTERIAL OXYGEN SATURATION OF SUBJECTS BREATHING AIR OR OXYGEN AT VARIOUS ALTITUDES

Alti-tude Feet	Gas Breathed	Alveolar		Arterial			Remarks
		pCO_2	pO_2	pCO_2	pO_2	O_2 Sat	
0	Air	40.4	102.4				88 tests on 17 subjects
15,000	"	34.4	41.0	33.6	40.6	78.6	Alv.—92 " " 18 " Art.—36 " " 10 "
40,000	100% O_2	36.3	54.5	39.4	60.2	89.8	Alv.— 4 " " 4 " Art.— 5 " " 5 "
42,000	"	36.6	43.1	36.6	44.1	80.6	Alv.—10 " " 5 " Art.—11 " " 5 "

higher than the arterial oxygen saturation at 15,000 feet in a subject breathing air; namely, 78.6 per cent. The lowered oxygen pressures available at an altitude of 15,000 feet in the absence of oxygen and at an altitude of 42,000 feet during the inhalation of pure oxygen are both apt to result in serious disturbance in the physiology of the organism.

Oxygen is present in the blood mainly in loose chemical combination with hemoglobin, but a small amount, namely 1/20 of the total content, exists in physical solution in the plasma. After oxygen enters the pulmonary capillaries from lung air it is delivered by arteries and capillaries to the tissues which first take up the physically dissolved oxygen and then additional oxygen derived from the hemoglobin, which speedily increases its supply to the plasma as the oxygen is consumed by the cells. The carbon dioxide produced in the tissues passes into the capillary blood and because of its acid nature facilitates the un-loading of oxygen from the hemoglobin. The return venous blood is exposed to a high concentration of oxygen in the alveolar air and the hemoglobin in red corpuscles then becomes 95 per cent saturated with oxygen. The carbon dioxide which has been taken up in the venous blood passes outward into the alveolar air because of the relatively small tension of carbon dioxide in the atmosphere, i.e., 0.03 per cent. Since hemoglobin when combined with oxygen is a stronger acid than when it is in the reduced state it aids in the elimination of carbon dioxide as the blood is exposed to a higher oxygen concentration in the lungs.

Carbon dioxide is itself transported partly by hemoglobin but its function in causing an increased delivery of oxygen to the tissue is important, as shown in the oxygen dissociation curves of Fig. 1. It will be seen that at a given saturation of hemoglobin, such as 60 per cent, a greater pressure of oxygen exists if the blood is in contact with 40 mm. carbon dioxide, than with 20 mm. carbon dioxide; namely, approximately 9 mm. It is also true that a more acid blood will take up less oxygen in the lung but the actual diffusion of oxygen into the tissues as a result of an increased carbon-dioxide tension (or a more acid state of the blood) is more significant in the physiologic behavior of oxygen. The effect of a marked increase in the alkalinity of the blood is that the hemoglobin holds on to oxygen more tightly as it passes through the tissues, and thus under certain circumstances aggravates anoxia. It may be pointed out parenthetically at this point that alkalosis also tends to constrict capillaries, especially in the coronary and cerebral circulation, which still further enhances tissue oxygen-want.

SYMPTOMS

The earliest signs of oxygen-want are, then, an increased volume of breathing and a more rapid beating of the heart, regularly observed at an altitude of 10,000 feet. After several hours of exposure to higher altitudes, such as between 12,000 and 15,000 feet, characteristic symptoms appear; namely, headache, nausea, and lassitude. There is increased difficulty in mental concentration and in more than 50 per cent of normal individuals exposed to these altitudes a definite impairment of emotional control takes place which is very similar to that produced by alcoholic intoxication. Feelings of overconfidence and euphoria are apt to be present, together with inevitable impairment of judgment and reason. In some cases boisterousness is accompanied by irritability and pugnacity. In slightly less than half of the individuals so exposed a depressed state tending toward sleep takes place from the start. This disturbance in affective behavior is the most significant sign of intolerance to altitude anoxia and is of very real importance in both civil and military aviation.

TABLE II

EMOTIONAL REACTIONS TO INHALATION OF 13 PER CENT OXYGEN FOR THREE HOURS

DULLNESS IRRITABILITY LETHARGY FATIGUE	41%	44%	DULLNESS IRRITABILITY DROWSINESS
ELATION OVERCONFIDENCE FOLLOWED BY DULLNESS DROWSINESS HEADACHE	59%	56%	PROLONGED EXCITEMENT, LACK OF INHIBITIONS, OVERACTIVITY HEADACHE

17 MEDICAL STUDENTS   9 PSYCHONEUROTIC PATIENTS

Since mental impairment frequently takes place at an altitude of 12,000 feet when exposure has lasted as long as one to four hours, there is reason to believe that "pilot error" is in part caused by impaired judgment due to oxygen-want when oxygen is not breathed by the pilot at this increased altitude. At the present time the civil aeronautics authority has entered the following amendment in its regulations of May 1, 1941: "Post 61.743. Oxygen Apparatus and Its Use. No air-carrier aircraft shall be operated in scheduled air transportation at an altitude exceeding 10,000 feet above sea level continuously for more than thirty minutes, nor at an altitude exceeding 12,000 feet above sea level for any length of time, unless such aircraft is equipped with an effective oxygen apparatus and an ample supply of oxygen

TABLE III

COMPARISON OF SCORES OF PHYSIOLOGIC TESTS AT A BAROMETRIC PRESSURE OF 429 MM. HG, EQUIVALENT TO 15,000 FEET, ON AN EMOTIONALLY IMPAIRED GROUP AND AN EMOTIONALLY UNIMPAIRED GROUP

Test	Unimpaired Group			Impaired Group			Remarks
	Sea Level	Altitude	Change	Sea Level	Altitude	Change	
Vital Capacity	4.51 L.	4.45	−.06	4.97	4.97	.00	Corrected to 37° C. moist.
Systolic B.P.	112 MM.	113	+1	112	110	−2	Impaired group showed greater fluctuations from group mean
Diastolic B.P.	77 MM.	78	+1	78	78	0	" " "
Pulse	77	85	+8	77	84	+8	
Minute Vent.	9.70 L.	10.98	+1.28	8.09	9.36	+1.25	
Alveolar pCO_2	39.4 MM.	34.3	−5.1	41.0	35.2	−5.8	
Alveolar pO_2	102.6 MM.	418	−60.8	101.2	39.8	−61.4	
Arterial pCO_2		35.6 MM.			34.1		
Arterial pO_2		41.9 MM.			39.9		
Arterial O_2 Sat.		79.3%			77.8		
Arterial pH		7.47			7.48		
E.K.G. T_1	+3.4	+2.6	−0.8	+2.9	+2.3	−0.6	
T_2	+3.0	+2.3	−0.7	+2.6	+2.2	−0.4	
T_3	−0.3	−0.4	+0.1	+0.2	+0.3	+0.1	
T_4	+6.2	+4.5	−1.7	+5.7	+4.9	−0.8	
S-T_1	+0.3	+0.2	−0.1	+0.2	+0.2	0.0	
S-T_2	+0.1	0.0	−0.1	+0.2	+0.2	0.0	
S-T_3	−0.3	−0.3	0.0	0.0	0.0	0.0	
S-T_4	+1.1	+0.9	−0.2	+0.7	+0.7	0.0	

Each figure represents an average of three to five determinations on each of eight subjects.

31

available for the convenient use of the operating crew, and proper use is made of such apparatus."

In many individuals an initial response of exuberant boisterousness and euphoria changes to a state tending toward sleep or depression. When lack of oxygen is very severe, as at extremely high altitudes in the absence of oxygen, the pulse rate becomes rapid and feeble, breathing is greatly accelerated, consciousness is rapidly impaired and finally lost, and death takes place due to excessive damage to the central nervous system, heart, and other organs.

In recent years the appraisal of the effect of anoxia has been clarified by the concept that certain tissues are more sensitive to oxygen-want than others. Thus, the arms or legs may be deprived of oxygen for periods of one and a half hours by complete closure of the arterial blood supply, but may be used thereafter with completely normal function. On the other hand, a guinea pig dropped in an atmosphere of nitrogen dies in convulsions within 60 seconds. Human beings may die when exposed to complete asphyxia for periods of 10 minutes and probably less. The brain is the organ most sensitive to anoxia and pathologic changes appear in the cortical cells accompanied by hemorrhage as a result of asphyxia. The heart is swiftly impaired in its function when the oxygen pressure supplied to it is lowered, and the adrenal glands are also probably quickly impaired by anoxia.

There are other disturbances created by anoxia which are justifiably not emphasized in clinical medicine but which are of great importance in aviation. Thus, at an altitude of 12,000 feet, corresponding to an arterial oxygen saturation of 85 per cent, which is the level at which cyanosis appears, the performance of some of the special senses and neuromuscular efficiency are impaired. Changes in visual function take place, as shown by impairment in dark adaptation and enlargement of the blind spot. One of the most convincing illustrations of the advantage of breathing oxygen for pilots is to expose them to a simulated altitude of 15,000 feet in a low-pressure chamber for one hour and then allow them to breathe pure oxygen through a mask. The subject remarks that the room suddenly becomes light, and notices also that the dizziness from which he was vaguely suffering disappears. Not all the special senses are as sensitive to oxygen-want as vision. Hearing is not disturbed until altitudes are reached which are near those where consciousness is lost; namely, between 18,000 and 20,000 feet. However, there is definite impairment in equilibratory and neuromuscular control at more moderate altitudes, observed by inability to perform the Romberg test or to carry out tests designed to measure this function, such as putting pegs into appropriate holes or piling them up carefully one on top of the other.

Although determination of sensory motor function is of no significance in the anoxia of clinical illness, tests of this character in flying personnel have been employed to determine altitude tolerance. In the attempt to distinguish the safe from the unsafe flyer, it appears, however, that loss of emotional control, difficulty in concentration, and the tendency to sleep are the more important criteria in the attempt to weed out the *unsafe* flyer.

Although the brain is the organ whose function is most significantly impaired by acute anoxia, the effects on the heart are of considerable importance. Although an increase in pulse rate is one of the earlier signs of acute anoxia, produced either in clinical illness or at altitude, it does not necessarily represent an increased blood flow unless the degree of oxygen-want is equivalent to an arterial oxygen saturation of 82 per cent or below, at which time the elevated pulse rate is accompanied by an increase in cardiac output. In normal individuals exposed to an altitude of 15,000 feet or to inhalation of a 12 per cent oxygen mixture, the electrocardiogram frequently shows characteristic changes, such as a depression of the T-wave. In cases with coronary artery disease, the inhalation of low oxygen mixtures, for example 10 to 12 per cent oxygen, has been used as a test of coronary insufficiency. When the electrocardiogram reveals not only depression of the T-wave but depression of the S-T segment, presence of disease in the coronary artery is suggested. In these patients the inhalation of low oxygen mixtures or airplane flights above 12,000 feet may reproduce not only electrocardiographic changes but attacks of anginal pain.

INHALATIONAL THERAPY

The treatment of acute anoxia in disorders of the heart and lungs generally involves the use of oxygen or an allied form of inhalational therapy. It is of primary importance in clinical medicine to maintain the function of respiration in order to offer the patient an additional opportunity to recover from his illness. It is of no importance that his vision or judgment may be transiently impaired. However, acute altitude sickness in civil and military aviation is a condition which should be *prevented,* if possible, because the aviator generally carries the responsibility of piloting a plane in which his own life and the

lives of others may be involved. For this reason diminution in neuromuscular efficiency, vision, emotional control, and mental concentration, as well as the appearance of bodily symptoms of nausea, headache, and lassitude, should be avoided wherever possible. Due to
the circumstance that moderate anoxia, such as occurs between 10,000

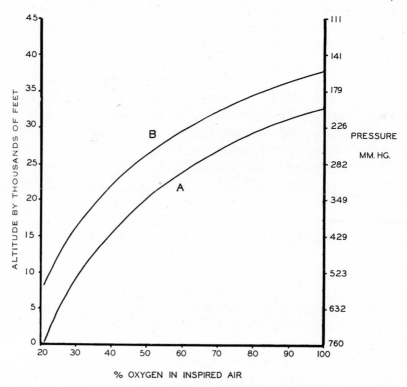

Fig. 5. Per cent oxygen in inspired air required to maintain alveolar
oxygen pressures of: (A) Sea level, and (B) 8,000 feet.

and 15,000 feet, frequently induces a euphoric and overconfident state,
pilots are apt to believe that such relatively low altitudes do not affect
them unfavorably but on the contrary in some instances think that
they feel better than they do at sea level. However, it is now generally recognized that anoxia may be a significant factor in pilot error,
and inhalation of oxygen should in general be recommended at all alti-
tubes above 10,000 feet in civil flying. It also seems desirable to
maintain the combat flyer at the peak of his efficiency by inhaling
oxygen at those altitudes in which mental function begins to become
impaired. In the accompanying illustration, the percentage of oxygen

in the inspired air required to maintain a sea-level oxygen pressure at various altitudes is depicted as well as that necessary to obtain a pressure comparable to an altitude of 8,000 feet, at which the symptoms are slight for most normal young adults.

There is little need for a young man to inhale oxygen because of an increased heart rate. In the absence of coronary disease, no damaging effect is produced on the heart of a young man by moderate anoxia. The aviator is engaged in a sedentary occupation and it is the disturbance in brain function that is of crucial importance. Lack of knowledge of the damaging effect of acute anoxia on brain function is dangerous, since it allows an inexperienced or an overconfident pilot the opportunity of making mistakes in judgment which may be the cause of fatal accidents. When ample opportunity is provided personally to experience the effects of acute altitude sickness, most pilots will be persuaded that decisive advantages follow adequate oxygen inhalation. It should be emphasized that no true acclimatization develops in the aviator as a result of repeated exposures to altitude anoxia. Although the man who has become a resident of a mountainous region as high as 14,000 feet will in a period of a week generally become comfortable as a result of a compensatory increase in red blood cells and hemoglobin, and by other mechanisms of this kind, the aviator is not in the air long enough to develop any of these responses. On the contrary, there is some evidence that repeated exposure to acute anoxia results in fatigue, and at times in a nervous state that tends to unfit him for further flying. Although Van Liere and Emerson showed that red corpuscles and hemoglobin do increase after exposure of six to nine hours each day to simulated altitudes of between 12,000 and 18,000 feet, aviators are not likely to fly daily for such long periods of time. There is good reason, therefore, to insist on the inhalation of oxygen by both the civil and the military flyer whenever it is possible to do so, both to preserve his own health and to ensure the safety of his mission.

The inhalation of 40 per cent oxygen is adequate to overcome altitude anoxia up to approximately 18,000 feet, as seen in Fig. 5. If higher altitudes are reached, the oxygen concentration may be increased to that of 100 per cent, which protects the individual from anoxia up to 34,000 feet. In order to overcome anoxia above this altitude, pressure cabins have been employed in the military services, in which air is admitted to small chambers enclosing the pilot under increased pressure. In civil aviation the pressure of cabin airplanes has been that which corresponds to an altitude of 8,000 feet. Another method is the pressure suit in which oxygen is supplied to the aviator at a pressure approximately two and one-half pounds per square inch in a suit which encloses the entire body.

BIBLIOGRAPHY

Armstrong, H. G.: A special form of functional psychoneuroses appearing in airplane pilots, Jour. Amer. Med. Asso., 106:1347, 1936.

Armstrong, H. G.: Effects of repeated daily exposure to anoxemia, Jour. Aviation Med., 9:92, 1938.

Armstrong, H. G.: Principles and Practice of Aviation Medicine, Baltimore, Williams & Wilkins Co., 1940.

Asmussen, E., and H. P. Chiodi: Effect of hypoxemia on ventilation and circulation in man, Amer. Jour. Physiol., 132:426, 1941.

Barach, A. L.: Pilot error and oxygen want, Jour. Amer. Med. Asso., 108:1868, 1937.

Barach, A. L.: Effect of low and high oxygen tensions on mental functioning, Jour. Aviation Med., 12:30, 1941.

Barach, A. L.: Principles of aviation medicine, Jour. Asso. Amer. Med. Coll., 17: 283, 1942.

Barach, A. L., Lt. Robert Brookes, Morris Eckman, Emanuel Ginsburg, and Artell Johnson: I. Appraisal of tests of altitude tolerance; II. Impairment of emotional control as a test of altitude anoxia, Jour. Aviation Med., 14:52, 1943.

Barach, A. L., M. Eckman, and N. Molomut: Modification of resistance to anoxia with especial reference to high altitude flying, Amer. Jour. Med. Sci., 202:336, 1941.

Barach, A. L., and J. Kagan: Disorders of mental functioning produced by varying the oxygen tension of the atmosphere, Psychosomatic Med., 2:1, 1940

Barach, A. L., R. A. McFarland, and C. P. Seitz: The effects of oxygen deprivation on complex mental functions, Jour. Aviation Med., 8:1, 1937.

Barcroft, J.: The respiratory function of the blood, Cambridge University Press, Vol. I, 1925; Vol. 2, 1928.

Barcroft, J., C. A. L. Binger, A. V. Bock, J. H. Doggart, H. A. Forbes, G. Harrop J. C. Meakins, and A. C. Redfield: Observations upon the effect of high altitude on the physiological processes of the human body, carried out in the Peruvian Andes, chiefly at Cerro de Pasco, Phil. Trans. Roy. Soc. London, ser. B, 211:351, 1923.

Bauer, L. H.: Aviation Medicine, Baltimore, Williams & Wilkins Co., 1926.

Bauer, L. H.: Aviation Medicine, New York, Oxford University Press, 1943.

Behnke, A. R., Jr.: High atmospheric pressures; physiological effects of increased and decreased pressure; application of these findings to clinical medicine, Ann. Int. Med., 13:2217, 1940.

Bert, P.: La Pression Barométrique, Recherches de Physiologie Expérimentale, Paris, Masson et Cie, 1878.

Birley, J.: Report on the medical aspect of high flying, British Privy Council. Special Report Series, 63:5, 1920.

Boothby, W. M., and W. R. Lovelace, II: Oxygen in aviation: the necessity for the use of oxygen and a practical apparatus for its administration to both pilots and passengers, Jour. Aviation Med., 9:172, 1938.

Boothby, W. M., W. R. Lovelace, and O. O. Benson: High altitude and its effect on the human body, Journal of the Aeronautical Sciences, 7:1, 1940.

Boothby, W. M., W. R. Lovelace, and A. H. Bulbulian: Oxygen administration and therapeutic use: I. Value of high concentration of oxygen for therapy; II. Oxygen for therapy and aviation and an apparatus for the administration of oxygen and oxygen-helium by inhalation; III. Design and construction of the masks for oxygen inhalation apparatus, Proc. Staff Meet., Mayo Clin., 13: 641, 646, 654, 1938.

Campbell, J. A.: Further evidence that mammals cannot acclimatize to ten per cent oxygen or 20,000 feet altitude, Brit. Jour. Exper. Pathol., 16:39, 1935.

Chornyak, J.: Structural Changes Produced in the Human Brain by Oxygen Deprivation (Anoxemia) and Their Pathogenesis, Ann Arbor, Mich., Edwards Brothers, 1938.

Cohn, D. J., A. Tannenbaum, W. Thalhimer, and A. B. Hastings: Influence of oxygen and carbon dioxide on the blood of normal and pneumonic dogs, Jour. Biol. Chem., 28:109, 1939.

Dill, D. B.: Life, Heat, and Altitude, Cambridge, Harvard University Press, 1938.

Dill, D. B., E. H. Christensen, and H. T. Edwards: Gas equilibrium in lungs at high altitudes, Amer. Jour. Physiol., 115:530, 1936.

Dill, D. B., and N. Zamcheck: Respiratory adjustments to oxygen lack in presence of carbon dioxide, Amer. Jour. Physiol., 129:47, 1940.

Douglas, E. G., J. S. Haldane, Y. Henderson, and E. C. Schneider: Physiological observations made on Pike's Peak, Colorado, with special reference to low barometric pressures, Phil. Trans. Roy. Soc., B, 103:310, 1913.

Eckman, M., and A. L. Barach: The effect on the vital capacity of a swift ascent to a simulated altitude of 35,000 feet, Jour. Aviation Med., 13:36, 1942.

Evans, J. N., and R. A. McFarland: Alterations in dark adaptation under reduced oxygen tensions, Amer. Jour. Physiol., 127:37, 1939.

Fulton, J. F.: Physiology and high altitude flying with particular reference to air embolism and effects of acceleration, Science, 95:207, 1942.

Gellhorn, E.: The vasomotor system in anoxia and asphyxia, Urbana, University of Illinois Press, 1939.

Gellhorn, E.: Fundamental principles in the adjustment reactions of the organism to anoxia, Ann. Int. Med., 14:1518, 1941.

Gellhorn, E., and A. Joslyn: The influence of oxygen want, hyperpnea and carbon dioxide excess on psychic processes, Jour. Psychol., 3:161, 1936.

Gemmill, C. L.: Physiology in Aviation, Springfield, Ill., Charles C. Thomas, Publisher, 1943.

Gerard, R. W.: Anoxia and neural metabolism, Arch. Neurol. and Psychiat., 40: 985, 1938.

Graybiel, A., V. Missiuro, D. B. Dill, and H. T. Edwards: Experimentally induced asphyxiation in cardiac patients with especial reference to certain hazards in air travel and to use of asphyxiation as cardiac functional test, Jour. Aviation Med., 8:178, 1937.

Greene, C. W., and N. C. Gilbert: Studies on responses of circulation to low oxygen tension: cause of changes observed in heart during extreme anoxemia, Amer. Jour. Physiol., 60:155, 1922.

Grow, M. C.: Effect of cold on oxygen content of blood: preliminary report, Mil. Surgeon, 86:225, 1940; Jour. Amer. Med. Asso., 114:2061, 1940.

Hall, F. G.: The effect of altitude on the affinity of hemoglobin for oxygen, Jour. Biol. Chem., 115:485, 1936.

Himwich, H. E., A. O. Bernistein, H. Herrlich, A. Chester, and J. F. Fazekas: Mechanisms for maintenance of life in newborn during anoxia, Amer. Jour. Physiol., 135:387, 1942.

Himwich, H., J. Fazekas, H. Herrlich, A. E. Johnson, and A. L. Barach: Studies on the effects of adding carbon dioxide to oxygen-enriched atmospheres in low pressure chambers, Jour. Aviation Med., 13:177, 1942.

Hurtado, A.: Studies at high altitude: blood observations on the Indian natives of the Peruvian Andes, Amer. Jour. Physiol., 100:487, 1932.

Johnson, A. E., M. Eckman, C. Rumsey, Jr., and A. L. Barach: Studies on the effects of adding carbon dioxide to oxygen-enriched atmospheres in low pressure chambers, Jour. Aviation Med., 13:130, 1942.

Keys, A., B. H. C. Matthews, W. H. Forbes, and R. A. McFarland: Individual variations in ability to acclimatize to high altitude, Proc. Roy. Soc., London, ser. B, 842:126, 1938.

Lovelace, W. R., C. W. Mayo, and W. M. Boothby: Aero-otitis media: its alleviation or prevention by inhalation of helium and oxygen, Proc. Staff Meet., Mayo Clin., 14:91, 1939.

Lutz, B. R. and Schneider, E. C.: The Reactions of the Cardiac and Respiratory Centers to Changes in Oxygen Tension, Am. J. Physiol., 1:327, 1919-20.

McFarland, R. A.: The psychological effects of oxygen deprivation (anoxemia) on human behavior, Columbia Univ. Arch. Psychol., No. 145, 22:1, 1932.

McFarland, R. A.: Psycho-physiological studies at high altitudes in the Andes: I. The effects of rapid ascents by aeroplane and train; II. Sensory and motor responses during acclimatization; III. Mental and psychosomatic responses during gradual adaptation; IV. Sensory and circulatory responses of the Andean residents at 17,500 feet, Jour. Comp. Psychol., 23:1, 1937; 24:1, 1937.

McFarland, R. A., and A. L. Barach: The response of psychoneurotics to variations in oxygen tension, Amer. Jour. Psychiat., 93:1315, 1937.

McFarland, R. A., and D. B. Dill: A comparative study of the effects of reduced oxygen pressure on man during acclimatization, Jour. Aviation Med., 9:18, 1938.

McFarland, R. A., and H. T. Edwards: The effects of prolonged exposures to altitude of 8,000 to 12,000 feet during trans-Pacific flights, Jour. Aviation Med., 8:4, 1937.

Schneider, E. C.: Physiological effects of altitude, Physiol. Rev., 1:631, 1921.

Schneider, E. C.: A record of experience with certain physical efficiency and low oxygen tests, Amer. Jour. Med. Sci., 161:395, 1921.

Seitz, C. P.: Effects of anoxia on visual function, Arch. Psychol., 257:1, 1940.

Van Liere, E. J.: Anoxia, Its Effect on the Body, Chicago, University of Chicago Press, 1942.

White, M. S.: Effect of anoxia in high altitude flights on the electrocardiogram, Jour. Aviation Med., 2:166, 1940.

3

Pneumonia

DEFINITION

Lobar pneumonia is an inflammation of the lung in which one or more lobes become filled with purulent exudate. The disease is caused by a micro-organism, generally the pneumococcus. The main clinical features are chill, fever, pain in the side, cough, and expectoration of rusty, blood-tinged sputum. In some cases, headache, nausea, vomiting, lassitude, and irrationality are present during the disease.

Bronchopneumonia is an inflammatory disease of the lung which generally begins in the terminal bronchioles and extends to the adjacent alveolar cells. It may be caused by a variety of micro-organisms, and usually follows another disease or occurs after operations. A primary form of bronchopneumonia has been described in recent years, thought to be due to a virus. In the latter condition inflammation and constriction of the small bronchi are characteristic, and constitute a contributing factor to the disturbance in respiratory function which takes place in many patients.

PATHOLOGIC PHYSIOLOGY

In the early stage of lobar pneumonia circulation of blood through the diseased lobe results in unoxygenated blood flowing into the aorta; later, there is little or no circulation of blood through the consolidated lung as the blood vessels to the involved area are closed. In areas of the lung that border on the consolidated region, edema of the alveolar walls prevents the normal rate of diffusion of oxygen through the pulmonary capillaries. Shallow respiration, which is characteristic of pneumonia, accomplishes a washing-out of the dead space between the pharynx and the alveoli but allows a relatively smaller amount of fresh air to be drawn into the alveolar cells themselves. Another factor in the production of anoxia is swelling of the small alveolar ducts and bronchi leading to the air cells, which may intermittently close the passageway to the respiratory epithelium. As a result of inadequately ventilated areas in the lungs, blood in the pulmonary capillaries passes through air cells which have little or no oxygen. Peribronchial swelling is of special significance in bronchopneumonia and in virus pneumonia, in which some of the smaller bronchi may be entirely occluded.

Cyanosis is the outstanding sign of anoxia in pneumonia, occurring when the arterial oxygen saturation falls below 85 per cent. However, it cannot be relied on as a sure guide, as it may be absent in patients with anemia and in those suffering from shock. This is of clinical importance, since many patients who show delirium, tachycardia, dyspnea, or insomnia are benefited by oxygen inhalation even though cyanosis is entirely absent, especially when they present a grayish pallor which is indicative of a grave form of anoxia.

There is no interference in the elimination of carbon dioxide in the majority of cases of lobar or bronchopneumonia. In a few cases with extensive involvement and widespread edema in the lungs the content of carbon dioxide in the blood is elevated. In dyspneic patients the carbon-dioxide tension of the arterial blood may be less than normal and gradually increase as convalescence takes place. There is no significant deviation of the acid-base equilibrium in the blood in most patients with pneumonia.

The circulatory system in the classic case of lobar or bronchopneumonia reveals merely an increase in its function; namely, a swifter circulation velocity of the blood and a compensatory dilatation of the heart. The venous pressure is normal, and, in the absence of pre-existing heart disease, there is no cardiac embarrassment. In certain patients, peripheral circulatory failure takes place, in which the venous return to the heart is markedly diminished without actual impairment of the heart muscle.

The volume of breathing is notably increased, due to toxemia, anoxia, and stimulation of proprioceptive reflexes in the lung. The vital capacity is sharply reduced even at the onset of the disease, and the total lung capacity and the functional residual air are also diminished.

INDICATIONS FOR TREATMENT

From a physiologic point of view the primary purpose of oxygen treatment is to prevent or overcome anoxia. A decreased mortality rate in oxygen-treated cases of pneumonia, as compared to control series, has been shown by several investigators. Furthermore, there is a close relation between mortality rate and a lowered saturation of the arterial blood with oxygen. It has been shown in certain carefully studied individual patients that inhalation of oxygen-enriched atmospheres is responsible for prolonging life, which affords the individual an increased opportunity to develop an immunity to his disease.

The inhalation of atmospheres containing 50 per cent oxygen not only raises the arterial oxygen saturation to or near the normal value in the majority of cases of pneumonia, but accomplishes a clinical improvement characterized by (1) slowing of the pulse rate, (2) disappearance or decrease of cyanosis, (3) diminution of delirium, (4) increased sleep, and (5) a lowered fever in some cases. The dyspnea is frequently lessened, although it is not completely relieved. The rate of breathing is lowered in about one-third the cases, but it is probable that the total volume of ventilation is decreased in almost all instances of anoxemic dyspnea.

The purpose of oxygen treatment in pneumonia is then to maintain function of the lung in respect to absorption of oxygen and in that way prevent damage to the various organ systems, until the patient himself is able to overcome the infection. Although cyanosis itself is the classic sign for beginning treatment, there are other indications which are of greater importance. These are a rapid pulse, especially if it is increased out of proportion to the temperature, delirium, difficult or shallow breathing, abdominal distention, persistent cough, high fever, peripheral circulatory failure, and evidence of widespread moisture in the lungs.

In the presence of massive pulmonary involvement it may be assumed that the patient is in a state of anoxia. After extensive abdominal operations, the prompt institution of oxygen therapy tends to prevent the development of pneumonia. As a result of splinting of the diaphragm after surgery in the upper abdomen, movement of the lower part of the lung may be diminished, absorption of air may take place in the unventilated alveolar cells, and areas of atelectasis develop which become a source of infection.

Certain procedures which aim to ventilate the lower portions of the lungs have been found helpful in preventing postoperative atelectasis and subsequent bronchopneumonia. Avoidance of unnecessarily tight abdominal bandaging allows more excursion of the diaphragm. In-

halations of carbon dioxide or deep-breathing exercise at the end of
the operation and at intervals afterward open the bronchial passageway, promote coughing and expectoration of retained secretions.
Eliminating anesthetic gases and pure oxygen postoperatively by
breathing helium-oxygen mixtures, or carbon dioxide in air, have been
advocated to substitute inert gases for those which are soon absorbed,
in order to prevent localized atelectasis.

INHALATIONAL THERAPY

When the decision to institute inhalational therapy has been made,
the first consideration should be the dosage or concentration of oxygen
in the atmosphere to be provided for the patient. The second is
selection of the method of treatment which will provide the concentration of oxygen desired and be best suited to the individual patient.
Physiologically, the oxygen-enriched atmosphere should contain that
concentration of oxygen which will overcome arterial anoxia. It is
obviously not feasible to check the oxygen saturation of the arterial
blood from day to day and the physician must therefore determine
in his own mind the degree of oxygen-want from the clinical state of
the patient. Studies have been made which are helpful in this respect
since they reveal that arterial anoxemia is overcome in a majority of
patients with pneumonia by the inhalation of an atmosphere containing 50 per cent oxygen. Patients with mild anoxemia may be treated
by lower oxygen concentrations, such as between 40 and 50 per cent
oxygen in the inspired air. In cases that have more serious anoxia
the oxygen saturation in the arterial blood will not be elevated to a
normal level until concentrations between 60 and 100 per cent are
employed. Peripheral circulatory failure and edema of the lungs,
which would benefit from inhalation of the higher oxygen concentrations, will be discussed later under these headings.

When narrowing of the bronchi takes place either as a result of
swelling of the mucous membrane or spasm of the circular bronchial
muscle, inhalation of oxygen under positive pressure or of helium-
oxygen mixtures or both may be indicated, as will be described in the
sections on asthma and obstructive dyspnea. One of the indications
for inhalation of 95 to 100 per cent oxygen is severe distention, since
intestinal gases diffuse into the circulation and are removed through
the lungs by diffusion when the alveolar air contains no nitrogen.
The removal of nitrogen could be secured by inhalation of a mixture

of 50 per cent oxygen and 50 per cent helium, which would avoid the theoretical disadvantage of possible irritative effect taking place in the lung following prolonged administration of pure oxygen.

Although animals regularly develop edema of the lungs after three to four days' inhalation of atmospheres containing 80 to 100 per cent oxygen, human beings *appear* to be able to tolerate these high concentrations without harm for at least two days and possibly for as long as one week. However, the evidence on the administration of 95 to 100 per cent oxygen in patients has been obtained with the employment of the mask method of administering oxygen, in which periodic removal of the mask for eating and bathing the face interrupts the treatment to some extent. The administration of oxygen in concentrations under 70 per cent may be continued indefinitely.

The selection of equipment to be used depends on the preference of the physician, on the training of the personnel in charge of administration, and on the patient himself. A rubber catheter introduced into the nasal pharynx is the simplest and least expensive effective method of providing oxygen-enriched atmospheres in the inspired air. Although the oxygen concentration achieved by this method varies with the total volume of breathing, being less in patients who have a large volume of ventilation due to dilution of oxygen with atmospheric air, a flow of 5 liters per minute of oxygen will provide 35 per cent oxygen in the inspired air in the average adult patient. Slower flows than this are generally not indicated in the treatment of pneumonia. When a flow of 7 liters per minute of oxygen is employed an oxygen concentration of between 40 and 50 per cent is obtained. A double nasal catheter may be used, but is rarely necessary.

If the rubber catheter is placed in the oral pharynx opposite the uvula, higher concentrations of oxygen are obtained for similar rates of flow. More care is necessary in utilizing the oral-pharyngeal position of the catheter in order to prevent gas from going into the stomach. When flows of 7 liters per minute are used with the pharyngeal placement of the catheter, the oxygen concentration of the inspired air is between 55 and 65 per cent. Drying of the back of the throat may be avoided by employing humidified oxygen and maintaining the patency of the small holes in the terminal one inch of the catheter.

The most comfortable method for most patients of administering oxygen concentrations between 40 and 60 per cent is the oxygen tent. When a canopy is largely or entirely composed of transparent pliofilm or plastocele, the patient has no sense of claustrophobia, and the doctor and nurse may readily inspect his condition. One of the disadvantages of the earlier types of canopies was that extensive rubberized canopies created a darkened atmosphere inside the tent which interfered with close observation by the nurse. In patients with fever, especially when the weather is warm or humid, the cool dry atmosphere maintained is a distinct advantage. An atmosphere hygienic in terms of temperature, humidity, and air movement is provided by an oxygen tent with motor-blower circulation and direct passage of the air over chunks of ice the size of a grapefruit. The thermal circulation tent is apt to give a higher oxygen concentration at comparable rates of oxygen flow but it is smaller and does not possess a wide control over temperature, humidity, and air movement. Furthermore, soda-lime must be used at flows below 9 liters per minute, or, preferably, an injector may be attached to the regulator to draw in sufficient air with the oxygen to wash out carbon dioxide. The open-top tent may be used both in adults and in children, but appears to have more advantages in the treatment of infants and small children. It may be employed with a self-contained ice compartment, or used without ice for infants in whom the provision of a high temperature and humidity is desirable. Other methods of refrigerating the tent have been developed, such as the employment of dry ice or liquid oxygen, but for most hospitals these methods are more expensive and less practical than the employment of ice.

The oxygen room has the advantage of comfort and a continuously maintained oxygen-enriched atmosphere even during the carrying-out of complicated procedures and examinations. The initial greater expense as well as the cost of upkeep of oxygen rooms has limited their use to those patients in whom special indications exist. In patients with chronic cardiac or respiratory disease, who are treated over long periods of time, or in whom surgery is conducted during the course of illness, such as an empyema operation, the use of an oxygen room has certain advantages. In very delirious and restless patients nursing attention and medical oversight are obtained with a minimum interruption of oxygen treatment.

The double or forked nasal tube may be employed for conditions similar to those in which the rubber catheter is used, although oxygen concentrations obtained by this method are generally not so high as can be provided by the nasal catheter, especially if inserted into the pharynx. Furthermore, the metal cannula may initiate mouth breathing.

A mask apparatus may be selected for the administration of low, moderate, and high oxygen concentrations up to theoretically 100 per cent oxygen. The mask may fit around the nose (the nasal mask) or it may enclose the nose and mouth (the oronasal mask). Although many patients tolerate a mask without complaint, there are a good number who find the close application of rubber to the face distressing. This is more apt to be evident when long-continued therapy is carried out, or when attempts are made to strap the mask too tightly to the face. If the patient manifests discomfort in wearing the mask and makes frequent attempts to take it off, it is desirable to shift to some other method of treatment, either the nasal catheter, which is generally accepted better when oxygen administration is carried out for long periods of time, or the oxygen tent if it is available. The special advantage of the oxygen mask is its capacity to provide very high concentrations of oxygen, such as 70 to 100 per cent. In the treatment of severe distention, shock, hemorrhage, or cardiac failure, these higher percentages of oxygen are of greater value than the administration of 30 to 50 per cent oxygen.

Two types of masks are available, the B.L.B. and the Meter mask, both of which are comfortable and efficient in supplying an oxygen-enriched atmosphere in the inspired air. In the B.L.B. mask a rebreathing bag allows a certain amount of rebreathing, with the development at low oxygen flows, between 2 and 4 liters per minute, of increased percentages of carbon dioxide in the inspired air, ranging from 2.0 to 2.5 per cent. At the higher oxygen flows between 6 and 10 liters a minute this accumulation of carbon dioxide is washed out. Sponge-rubber disks, creating a slight resistance during inspiration and expiration, serve as valves in expiration and inspiration. In obstructive dyspnea the degree of resistance which is produced by inhalation through the sponge-rubber disks at *low* flows of oxygen is too great to allow its use under these conditions. When high flows of oxygen are admitted into the mask, 6 and 10 liters a minute, this inspiratory resistance is diminished or disappears. The desired concentration of oxygen is obtained by regulating the flow of oxygen from the regulator, but the inspired air may vary as much as 15 per cent in its oxygen percentage at a given flow depending upon the volume of breathing of the patient. It should be borne in mind that a flow of 5 liters per minute in a small child may give a relatively high concentration and in a large man in dyspnea a relatively low oxygen concentration because of the dilution effect of atmospheric air entering the mask through the sponge-rubber valve.

In the Meter mask there is attached to the regulator a hollow cylinder with variable-sized orifices which operates as an injector, like a Bunsen burner. As oxygen passes through the injector into the connecting rubber tubing, a negative pressure is set up which draws in a variable amount of air depending on the size of the orifice. These apertures have been calibrated so that an instantaneous provision of any concentration between 40 and 100 per cent may be provided with an error of approximately —2 per cent. An inspiratory valve at the bottom of the mask prevents rebreathing and accumulation of carbon dioxide, the light latex bag serving simply as an oxygen-collecting bag. In this apparatus various oxygen concentrations may be accurately provided with *minimal* respiratory resistance, both in inspiration and expiration, and with less than 0.2 per cent carbon dioxide under all circumstances. If rebreathing is desired, the inspiratory valve may be removed from the mask. However, it must be pointed out that carbon dioxide in percentages as high as 2 per cent increases the volume of breathing approximately 40 to 50 per cent, which is generally undesirable in dyspnea of cardiorespiratory origin.

In patients who have had operations on the upper respiratory tract or in any patient with a tendency to pulmonary edema or with the slightest degree of obstruction in the respiratory passageway, the volume of breathing should be kept as low as possible and particular care should be exercised to keep the concentration of carbon dioxide below 1 per cent, as both Boothby and Barach have emphasized. The reason for this is that an increase in intrapulmonary negative pressure favors the production of pulmonary edema, as will be discussed in that section. It is therefore necessary to point out that the B.L.B. mask should not be used with any flow of oxygen below 6 liters per minute, and preferably well above this level, if there is any possibility that edema of the lungs may be present or if there is obstruction to breathing.

Since, in the Meter mask, oxygen from the cylinder is diluted with air before it enters the collecting bag, resistance to inspiration is avoided even with low flows of oxygen, provided the bag is not allowed to collapse completely at the end of inspiration. In severe dyspnea, negative pressures are prevented by employing high flows of oxygen-enriched air. For example, when the meter has been set at 40 per cent oxygen with a flow of 3 liters per minute, there will be an intake of air into the rubber tube leading to the mask of approximately 5 liters per minute; when the flow is increased to 6 liters a minute, with the meter still kept at 40 per cent, there will be an intake of twice that amount of air with a provision of 6 liters of oxygen and 10 liters of air; thus, 16 liters of the combined mixture will be offered to the patient during inspiration without resistance. In the B.L.B. apparatus, when 6 liters of oxygen pass through the regulator, the ventilation requirement of the patient above 6 liters per minute is obtained partly from the rebreathing bag and, when it has collapsed, through suction of air through the sponge-rubber disks. Dilution of the oxygen with air is thus carried out by the patient's effort rather than by the pressure of oxygen from the cylinder.

When there is widespread moisture in the lung or when pulmonary edema has actually developed, a high flow of an oxygen-enriched atmosphere into the mask should be used to prevent the slightest degree of negative pressure developing during inspiration. Under these circumstances the Meter mask with the metered *positive-pressure* device may be employed, as will be discussed shortly.

When oxygen treatment has been instituted it is important to maintain the concentration of oxygen prescribed, to determine that the apparatus is functioning efficiently and, finally, to make the patient as comfortable as possible during the treatment. When the oxygen tent is used the concentration of oxygen should be tested at least twice daily and in very ill patients more often.

The duration of oxygen treatment in pneumonia depends on the condition of the individual patient. In general it may be said that when the temperature has returned to normal and the pulse rate has declined, it is safe to terminate oxygen therapy abruptly. However, in patients with widespread consolidation, especially if there is evidence of moisture in the lungs, a gradual lowering of the oxygen concentration is advisable. If interruption of oxygen treatment brings on a state of dyspnea and cyanosis, administration of oxygen is resumed and continued until there is substantial clearing of the disease process in the lung. In patients with peripheral circulatory failure, interruption of oxygen treatment should be undertaken for only very short intervals in order to avoid cardiorespiratory failure as a result of abrupt discontinuance of inhalation of oxygen. There is no indication for gradual reduction of the oxygen percentage in the atmosphere in pneumonia provided that the lungs have substantially cleared. If coexistent congestive cardiac failure should be present, gradual reduction of the oxygen concentration in the atmosphere may be carried out, as will be described in the section on heart disease.

BIBLIOGRAPHY

Barach, A. L.: Methods and results of oxygen treatment in pneumonia, Arch. Int. Med., 37:186, 1926; Med. Clin. N. Amer., 9:471, 1925.

Barach, A. L.: Acute disturbance of lung function in pneumonia; methods of oxygen treatment, Jour. Amer. Med. Asso., 89:1865, 1927.

Barach, A. L.: Oxygen therapy in pneumonia, N. Y. State Jour. Med., 29:985, 1929.

Barach, A. L.: Physiologically directed therapy in pneumonia, Ann. Int. Med., 17: 812, 1942.

Barach, A. L., and N. Molomut: A study of the therapeutic effect of sulfapyridine in pneumococcus infected mice in atmospheres of varying oxygen tension, Jour. Lab. and Clin. Med., 26:1915, 1941.

Barach, A. L., and M. N. Woodwell: Studies in oxygen therapy with determination of the blood gases, etc.: I. In cardiac insufficiency and related conditions, Arch. Int. Med., 28:367, 1921. II. In pneumonia and its complications, Arch. Int. Med., 28:394, 1921. III. In an extreme type of shallow breathing occurring in encephalitis, Arch. Int. Med., 28:421, 1921.

Barker, M. H.: General management of pneumonia, Illinois Med. Jour., 76:416, 1939; Jour. Amer. Med. Asso., 114:356, 1940.

Binger, C. A. L.: Therapeutic value of oxygen in pneumonia, New York State Jour. Med., 25:953, 1925.

Binger, C. A. L., J. M. Faulkner, and R. L. Moore: Oxygen poisoning in mammals, Jour. Exper. Med., 45:849, 1927

Binger, C. A. L.: Anoxemia in pneumonia and its relief by oxygen inhalation, Jour. Clin. Invest., 6:203, 1928.

Binger, C. A. L., and J. A. Davis, Jr.: The relation of anoxemia to the type of breathing in pneumonia: a study of respiration by means of a body plethysmograph, Jour. Clin. Invest., 6:171, 1928.

Binger, M. W., E. S. Judd, A. B. Moore, and R. M. Wieder: Oxygen in the treatment of postoperative broncho-pneumonia, Arch. Surg., 17:1047, 1928.

Blankehorn, M. A.: Oxygen therapy: indications and methods of application; relation to other therapy, Jour. Amer. Med. Asso., 113:1410, 1939.

Boothby, W. M., and Haines, S. F.: Oxygen Therapy, Jour. Amer. Med. Asso., 90:372, 1928.

Bullowa, J. G. M.: Inhalation of oxygen in pneumonia, Jour. Amer. Med. Asso., 102:1870, 1934.

Burgess, A. M.: Oxygen in the treatment of lobar pneumonia, New England Jour. Med., 222:563, 1940.

Campbell, J. A.: Oxygen administration; further observations, Lancet, 1:82, 1937.

Cohn, D. J., A. Tannenbaum, W. Thalhimer, and A. B. Hastings: Influence of oxygen and carbon dioxide on the blood of normal and pneumonic dogs, Jour. Biol. Chem., 28:109, 1939.

Evans, J. H., and C. J. Durshordwe: Indications for oxygen therapy in respiratory diseases, Anesth. and Analg., 14:162, 1935.

Faget, G. H., and W. B. Martin: Oxygen therapy of pneumonia: five years' experience at the U. S. Marine Hospital, Norfolk, Va., Hospital News, 4:20, 1937; Ann. Int. Med., 12:32, 1938.

Haines, S. F., and W. M. Boothby: Oxygen treatment with special reference to treatment of complications incident to goiter, Amer. Jour. Surg., 7:174, 1929.

Haldane, J. S.: The administration of oxygen, Brit. Med. Jour., 2:517, 1918.

Hastings, A. B., J. M. Neill, H. J. Morgan, and C. A. L. Binger: Blood reaction and blood gases in pneumonia, Jour. Clin. Invest., 1:25, 1924.

Kotkis, A. J.: Treating pneumonia early with oxygen therapy, Bull. St. Louis Med. Soc., 33:212, 1939.

Lundsgaard, C.: Anoxemia in lobar pneumonia, Medicine, 4:345, 1925.

Meakins, J. C.: The therapeutic value of oxygen in pulmonary lesions, Brit. Med. Jour., 1:324, 1920.

Meakins, J. C.: Gases in human arterial blood in certain pathological pulmonary conditions and their treatment with oxygen, Jour. Pathol. and Bacteriol., 24: 79, 1921.

Means, J. H., and A. L. Barach: The symptomatic treatment of pneumonia, Jour. Amer. Med. Asso., 77:1217, 1921.

Means, J. H., M. N. Woodwell, and A. L. Barach: Hydrogen ion concentration and bicarbonate level of blood in pneumonia, Jour. Biol. Chem., 50:413, 1922.

Scott, J. R., and J. S. Davis, Jr.: Oxygen therapy, New York State Jour. Med., 28:922, 1928.

Stadie, W. C.: The oxygen of the arterial and venous blood in pneumonia and its relation to cyanosis, Jour. Exper. Med., 30:315, 1919.

Stadie, W. C.: Treatment of anoxemia in pneumonia in an oxygen chamber, Jour. Exper. Med., 35:337, 1922.

4

Edema of the Lungs

DEFINITION

Edema of the lungs produces suffocation as a result of transudation of serous fluid from the pulmonary capillaries into the alveoli of the lungs. It is one of the most frequent and serious causes of anoxic (arterial) anoxia. Pulmonary edema when fully developed presents a characteristic clinical picture manifested by bubbling râles in the lungs and audible gurgling in the throat.

PATHOLOGIC PHYSIOLOGY

Although exudation of serum from the blood in the pulmonary capillaries into the alveoli is characteristic of all types of pulmonary edema, the physiologic factors involved depend on the underlying disease, as will be illustrated below:

1. **Heart Disease.** In this group of cases left ventricular failure is the precipitating cause of the condition, frequently as a result of coronary-artery or hypertensive vascular disease. In attacks of paroxysmal cardiac asthma, which often occur at night, the amount of blood in the lungs is increased, and it has recently been shown that the total blood volume is also increased during sleep. An additional influence is that of the prone position which promotes a freer flow of blood into the right heart. The vital capacity is also less when the patient is lying down and the diaphragm relatively elevated. The combination of these various circumstances may result in left ventricular failure with a damming of blood in the lungs, increased hydrostatic pressure in the pulmonary capillaries, and consequent oozing of serum into the alveoli. The original explanation of Welch was that pulmonary edema occurred when a relative weakness of the left ventricle took place because blood would then accumulate in the lungs under steadily increasing pressure at the same time that the

right ventricle, the function of which was not impaired, continued to pour blood into the pulmonary capillaries.

Experimental investigation has shown that this type of pulmonary edema can be produced in rabbits by the intravenous injection of adrenalin. The left ventricle under these circumstances fails to discharge the customary amount of blood into the aorta and congestion of the lungs takes place, at first with exudation of red blood cells and then with outpouring of fluid into the alveoli. When breathing is conducted under positive pressure, pulmonary edema originating in this way is either prevented or cleared. The mechanism appears to be a direct physical force exerted on the external wall of the capillaries counteracting the increased internal hydrostatic pressure in the capillaries and at the same time the elevated intrapulmonary pressure retards to a variable extent the flow of blood into the lungs.

2. **Lobar and Bronchopneumonia.** The development of pulmonary edema in pneumonia appears to be largely caused by an increase in capillary permeability induced by inflammation, toxemia, anoxia, and, at times, left ventricle insufficiency.

3. **Peripheral Circulatory Failure.** The lungs may swiftly become edematous in both medical and surgical shock. A marked reduction in oxygen consumption is characteristic of the severe anoxia present in this condition. Increase in capillary permeability is undoubtedly involved, but there may also be other etiologic influences, such as efferent impulses from the central nervous system.

4. **War Gas and Industrial Gas Poisoning.** The fumes of chlorine, phosgene, and nitric acid exert an irritant effect on the lungs, directly increasing the permeability of the pulmonary capillaries to serum. The capillary permeability of the lungs may also be altered by severe toxic states, which may occur in glomerulonephritis and other diseases.

5. **Asthma, Obstructive Lesions in the Tracheobronchial Tree, and the Post-tracheotomy State.** During obstructive dyspnea, due to asthma (in the absence of pulmonary emphysema) or to lesions in the upper respiratory passages which produce resistance to the passage of air, a high negative intrapulmonary pressure develops which makes possible the entrance of air past the point of constriction. A direct suction action on the pulmonary capillaries may result in transudation of serum into the alveolar cells as well as production of mucus from the intrathoracic bronchial mucous membrane. The heightened negative pressure during the inspiratory cycle also tends to draw blood into

the right heart and at the same time hinders the passage of blood into the left heart and into the extrathoracic aorta. Experimental studies have demonstrated that prolonged pathologically elevated negative intrapleural pressures are followed by congestion and edema in the lung.

An interesting example of the effect of altered pressures in the mechanism of pulmonary edema is found in the behavior of certain patients who have been subjected to tracheotomy for long-standing laryngeal obstruction. Although no cough or expectoration is generally present prior to tracheotomy, a profuse outpouring of serous and mucous fluid into the bronchial tree often necessitates aspiration after tracheotomy at frequent intervals for days and sometimes weeks. It would seem likely that the pulmonary capillaries, previously accustomed to a positive pressure during expiration against resistance, develop an increase in capillary permeability when positive pressure is suddenly withdrawn. This probably applies to the secreting glands in the tracheobronchial tree as well. The existence within the lung of considerable congestion due to high intrapulmonary negative pressures during the inspiratory cycle prior to tracheotomy probably is an additional factor in predisposing the capillaries to a change in their permeability.

In patients with severe asthma excessive repeated injection of morphine appears to produce a similar result; namely, a sudden outpouring of fluid into the alveolar cells due to abrupt lessening of the effort of breathing which was formerly accompanied by a sustained positive pressure during the expiratory cycle exerted on the pulmonary capillaries. However, moderate doses of morphine are at times very helpful by decreasing the volume of breathing and hence the heightened negative intrathoracic pressure, as well as by lessening spasm of the bronchial constrictor muscles.

A similar sequence of events takes place following the withdrawal of a large amount of fluid from the chest; namely, an altered permeability of the capillaries which were formerly exposed to a pressure very near that of the atmosphere and which suddenly become exposed to a heightened negative pressure during inspiration to which they were not accustomed.

INHALATIONAL THERAPY

The treatment of edema of the lungs depends on the underlying condition, but in so far as the application of inhalational therapy is concerned, the essential basis of treatment is to provide a positive pressure on the walls of the pulmonary capillaries and directly oppose the tendency for serum to leak outward.

In patients who have developed edema during obstruction of the air passages, the inhalation of oxygen-enriched atmospheres under positive pressure is indicated. The effect of positive pressure is to lower the pathologically elevated negative pressure present during the inspiratory cycle, decreasing thereby the suction action on the pulmonary capillaries as well as diminishing the dyspnea. Oxygen itself, by lowering the total volume of air breathed, not only combats anoxia but also decreases the negative intrapleural pressure during inspiration because of the diminished volume of ventilation. In patients with asthma, or with lesions in the respiratory passageway which produce a constricted orifice, the pressure is best administered during both inspiration and expiration. No harmful effects have been noted as far as dyspnea is concerned by breathing out against a positive pressure under these circumstances. In fact, positive-pressure respiration tends to maintain a more patent lumen during expiration in the intrathoracic bronchi.

Positive pressure during the inspiratory cycle gently blows the oxygen-enriched atmosphere into the lungs past the point of obstruction, thereby decreases the effort of breathing, and interrupts the series of pathophysiologic events which were instrumental in causing the edema. In these cases the mixture of helium with oxygen is of special value because the lighter-than-air mixture is itself capable of being breathed with almost one-half the physical effort required for the inhalation of either oxygen or air. However, positive-pressure respiration with pure oxygen considerably decreases the dyspnea. Further discussion of the function of helium will be given under the section on Asthma.

The helium-oxygen hood has been designed to give positive pressure during inspiration and expiration, and may be used with 100 per cent oxygen or a mixture of helium and oxygen. The pressure at first employed is between 4 and 5 cm. of water. After the edema has cleared, which may be in a period of one to four hours, the pressure is gradually lowered, generally 1 cm. every three to four hours. The rapidity with which the pressure is lowered may be varied, depending upon the condition of the individual patient.

In cases who have developed oozing from the tracheobronchial tree after tracheotomy, it is desirable to introduce a special tracheotomy tube which projects ¼″ outward so that a Y-tube may be attached to it, one part connected with an inspiratory valve that allows inspiration to proceed unchanged and the other side connected to a glass tube inserted into an appropriate bottle of water, 1 to 5 cm. as prescribed. The patient exhales at first under a positive pressure of 5 cm. of water, with a gradual 1-cm. lessening of the pressure every three to four hours until it is entirely withdrawn. If a tracheotomy tube of this character is inserted immediately after the operation and expiration conducted under pressure of 3 to 5 cm. of water, there is little likelihood that pulmonary edema will develop or that oozing from the tracheobronchial tree will be as burdensome as it generally is. A special apparatus may be obtained for this purpose in which a motor blower unit maintains the desired pressure.[1]

In cases of pulmonary edema due to increased permeability of the pulmonary capillaries, such as is induced by industrial or war gas poisoning, lobar and bronchopneumonia, the inhalation of 40 to 100 per cent oxygen with a positive pressure of 3 to 6 cm. of water is indicated. Although a positive-pressure helmet hood is the more comfortable and effective method of applying positive pressure, the injector Meter mask metered for positive pressure in expiration has been successfully employed in these conditions. Even advanced cases of pulmonary edema due to inhalation of the fumes of chlorine or nitric acid have shown relatively prompt clearing of edema, and recovery after continuous administration of positive pressure. (See section on War Gas Poisoning.) In these conditions also the pressure is generally begun at a higher level and then gradually lowered to that of the atmosphere. When the pressure mask is employed it is customary to begin with 4 cm. pressure for a brief period of 10 to 15 minutes. If this pressure is uncomfortable to the patient, it may soon be lowered to 3 cm. positive pressure. In actual practice it is probably more desirable to begin with that pressure which the patient will find not too uncomfortable. The positive-pressure meter may, therefore, be set at 3 cm. until the edema is mostly cleared, and then lowered to 2 cm., and at two- to four-hour intervals decreased to that of atmosphere.

In the accompanying illustration, the clinical response of a patient with bronchopneumonia and pulmonary edema is illustrated. The patient was a middle-aged woman with primary atypical bronchopneumonia in whom the development of acute edema of the lung appeared

---

[1] This is made by Pilling and Sons, Philadelphia, Pa.

to indicate a fatal outcome. Gurgling râles were heard in the throat, and there were widespread moist râles throughout both lungs. The pulse was 154 when positive pressure was applied with a helmet-hood apparatus—at first 4 cm. of water, with gradual reduction during the

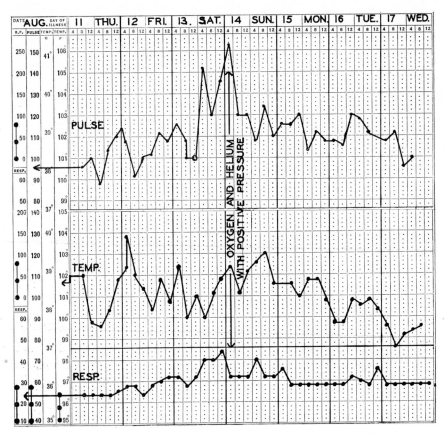

FIG. 6. Effect of positive-pressure respiration in a case of broncho-pneumonia.

following 36 hours to 1 cm. of water, when it was discontinued. Although a mixture of 50 per cent oxygen and 50 per cent helium was employed, the swift and favorable outcome could be traced to the positive pressure rather than to the helium. During the first four hours following the application of the hood a dramatic improvement took place, characterized by a fall in pulse rate with increased volume, a marked lowering of the respiratory rate, and a clearing of the major portion of the signs of pulmonary edema. The betterment in the subjective state of the patient was equally pronounced, dyspnea was relieved, the patient rested during the day, slept soundly at night, and the following day was apparently out of danger.

In patients with pneumonia, clearing of pulmonary edema may be followed by recovery in a period of 12 to 48 hours. In other cases, the toxemia of the disease may result in cardiorespiratory failure even after the lungs have been cleared of moisture. It must be understood that many of the underlying conditions responsible for the development of pulmonary edema are such that a fatal outcome may take place. In this category is the edema which follows severe glomerulo-nephritis, cerebral thrombosis, or injury to the brain.

When acute pulmonary edema occurs as a complication of left ventricular failure, the inhalation of 100 per cent oxygen under a positive pressure of 2 to 4 cm. of water may be followed by disappearance of the condition. The effect of positive pressure in patients of this type is to retard the entrance of blood into the right heart, resulting in a marked increase in systemic venous pressure and a prolongation of the circulation time. The heart thus deals with a smaller volume of blood, and the procedure is comparable to tourniquets applied to the extremities, and to phlebotomy. In addition, the positive pressure exerts a physical effect on the pulmonary capillary wall as it does in the conditions mentioned above. In a normal individual inhalation of gases under the pressure described results in a moderate increase in venous pressure, but in little or no retardation of the circulation velocity.

The development of pulmonary edema in shock is to be treated in a manner different from what has been described up to this point. In peripheral circulatory failure there is already a deficient return of blood to the right heart and the presence within the lung of an increased intrapulmonary pressure may further retard the flow of blood into the right auricle. Although positive pressure has been applied during expiration to a few cases of this type, inspiration being conducted *without* positive pressure, caution must be exerted in the treatment of pulmonary edema in the presence of shock. The blood pressure should be taken at 10-minute intervals in order to be certain that the degree of pressure employed is not such as to cause an aggravation of the circulatory failure already present. Very few cases of pulmonary edema in shock have been treated, but there is sufficient physiologic evidence at hand to warn against its use, except under very carefully controlled conditions and close clinical observation. In these patients the intravenous injection of blood or plasma and the inhalation of 100 per cent oxygen are obviously emergency indications. It may be mentioned that two cases of pulmonary edema following severe hemorrhage from the lung have been successfully treated with positive pressure applied during expiration. When positive pressure is administered in the helmet-hood apparatus, the pressure is exerted during inspiration and expiration. Care should be exercised regularly to determine that the systolic blood pressure does not fall more than 15 mm. Hg as a result of the pressure used. From previous experience it may be said that very small increases in pressure, such as 3 cm. of water, may be followed by clearing of pulmonary edema when used over a longer period of time instead of the application of pressures of 6 cm. of water. When the mask is employed, positive pressure is exerted on the lung only during expiration. During the inspiratory cycle there is therefore a free flow of blood into the lung.

The function of positive pressure in expiration may be compared to the mechanism of the expiratory grunt in lobar pneumonia. Observations made on a tracheotomized subject who simulated grunting respiration revealed that pressures as high as 20 to 40 cm. of water were obtained in a manometer connected to the larynx from the tracheotomy tube. It seems reasonable to accept the hypothesis that there are physiologic advantages to grunting in certain respiratory conditions such as lobar pneumonia, asthma, and emphysema. An additional function of positive pressure during expiration is seen in patients with bronchial asthma in whom it tends to prevent constriction of the intrathoracic bronchi at the end of expiration.

Another form of inhalational therapy that is at times of considerable value in the treatment of pulmonary edema is the inhalation of the vaporized spray of 1 : 100 epinephrine and 1 per cent neosynephrin. Although these substances may be inhaled by squeezing the hand bulb attached to the ordinary nebulizer, a more effective and prolonged effect is obtained by vaporizing the solutions through the passage of a stream of oxygen, 4 liters per minute, from a high-pressure oxygen tank. The end of the nebulizer is held in the open mouth and the nebulin is gradually inhaled over a period of 5 to 15 minutes, depending upon the dose. In patients with bronchial spasm, such as may occur in asthma, in virus pneumonia, or in certain forms of war gas poisoning, the inhalation of the spray of 0.5 cc. of 1 : 100 epinephrine is of considerable value in relieving bronchial spasm. In other cases where there is congestion of the mucous membrane of various parts of the tracheobronchial tree the inhalation of 1 to 2 cc. of 1 per cent neosynephrin is also of help. In some cases a mixture of 1 cc. of each is employed. The patient inhales the vapor of these two substances at intervals of two to four hours, depending upon the individual requirements of his condition. Neosynephrin is an efficient vasoconstrictor, but it is not considered a good bronchodilator.

BIBLIOGRAPHY

Auer, J., and F. L. Gates: Experiments on the causation and amelioration of adrenalin pulmonary edema, Jour. Exper. Med., 26:201, 1917.

Barach, A. L.: Pulmonary edema; Modern Medical Therapy in General Practise, Baltimore, Williams & Wilkins Co., 1940.

Barach, A. L.: Physiologically directed therapy in pneumonia, Ann. Int. Med., 17:812, 1942.

Barach, A. L., J. Martin, and M. Eckman: Positive pressure respiration and its application to the treatment of acute pulmonary edema, Ann. Int. Med., 12: 754, 1938.

Barach, A. L., and P. Swenson: Effect of breathing gases under positive pressure on lumens of small and medium-sized bronchi, Arch. Int. Med., 63:946, 1939.

Boothby, W. M.: Oxygen therapy—council on physical therapy, Jour. Amer. Med. Asso., 99:2026, 1932; 99:2106, 1932.

Boothby, W. M., W. R. Lovelace, and C. W. Mayo: The use of oxygen and oxygen-helium, with special reference to surgery, Surg. Clin. N. Amer., 20:1107, 1940.

Emerson, H.: Artificial respiration in the treatment of edema of the lungs, Arch. Int. Med., 3:368, 1909.

Hoover, C. F.: Moisture in the air spaces of the lungs and oxygen therapy, Jour. Amer. Med. Asso., 71:880, 1918.

Johnson, S.: The experimental production and prevention of acute edema of the lungs in rabbits, Proc. Soc. Exper. Biol. and Med., 25:181, 1927-1928.

Landis, E. M.: Micro-injection studies of capillary permeability: III. The effect of lack of oxygen on the permeability of the capillary wall to fluid and to the plasma proteins, Amer. Jour. Physiol., 83:528, 1928.

Luisada, A.: The pathogenesis of paroxysmal pulmonary edema, Medicine, 19:475, 1940.

Norton, N. R.: Forced respiration in a case of carbolic acid poison, Med. and Surg. Rep. Presbyterian Hosp., N. Y., 1:127, 1896.

Plesch, J.: Funktionelle Gefässdiagnostik: Beziehung zwischen Schlagvolumen und Gefässsystem, Ztschr. f. klin. Med., 123:168, 1933.

Poulton, E. P.: Left-sided heart failure with pulmonary edema treated with the pulmonary plus pressure machine, Lancet, 231:983, 1936.

Richards, D. W., Jr., A. L. Barach, and H. A. Cromwell: Use of vaporized bronchodilator solutions in asthma and emphysema; a continuous inhalation method for severe asthmatic states, Amer. Jour. Med. Sci., 199:225, 1940.

Segal, M. S., and M. Aisner: The management of certain aspects of gas poisoning with particular reference to shock and pulmonary complications, Ann. Int. Med., 20:219, No. 2, 1944.

Welch, W. H.: Zur Pathologie des Lungenödems, Virchows Arch. f. path. Anat., 72:375, 1878.

5

Congestive Heart Failure

DEFINITION

In congestive heart failure there is a damming back or congestion of blood in the lungs, or in the peripheral organs, due to failure of the heart to maintain its normal output of blood. This impairment in the function of the heart may take place as a result of rheumatic fever, syphilis, hypertensive vascular disease, and coronary sclerosis. Cardiac failure may develop as a result of hyperthyroidism, pulmonary emphysema, pericarditis, as well as infections of the heart valve and other diseases. Dyspnea, cough, and edema are the dominant clinical features.

PATHOLOGIC PHYSIOLOGY

If the function of the right ventricle is impaired, there is a damming of blood in the extremities and abdomen, as a result of failure of this organ to discharge its customary allotment of blood into the lung. This may be due to increased resistance in the lungs themselves, for example, by pulmonary fibrosis, or to valvular right heart disease or to a disturbance in the heart muscle itself. In failure of the left ventricle there is a congestion of blood in the lungs, and it is in fact this congestion which results from left ventricular insufficiency that is the most common cause of right ventricular failure, since under these circumstances the right heart is forced to deliver blood into the lungs under increased pressure.

As a result of inefficient contraction of the left ventricle there is an incomplete emptying of this chamber, with residual blood under increased pressure remaining in it. The left auricle then delivers less blood into the ventricle until a new equilibrium is reached at a higher level of auricular pressure. The lungs become engorged with blood as the increased auricular pressure is reflected backward into the pulmonary capillaries. If the pressure of blood in the capillaries becomes

59

sufficiently increased, serum then passes through their walls, as described in the section on pulmonary edema. Since an increased amount of blood is present in the pulmonary capillaries, the volume of the air spaces is correspondingly diminished with the result that the amount of air that can be taken into the lung is decreased. This is determined by measurement of the vital capacity.

The velocity of the circulation through the lungs is also diminished. The oxygen saturation of arterial blood falls below the normal range due to impairment of diffusion through swollen alveolar membrane as well as through an unequal and inefficient distribution of air in the alveoli of the lung. It is probable that small alveolar ducts may be in places markedly swollen so as to prevent entrance of air into the alveoli of some sections of the lung. Blood in the pulmonary capillaries may thus be exposed to a lowered oxygen pressure as it passes through these alveoli and hence become inadequately oxygenated.

As a result of the prolonged time of circulating blood through the tissues, a proportionally large amount of oxygen is taken from the blood by the tissue cells, with a consequent lowering of tissue oxygen pressure. The type of oxygen want due to slowed circulation is termed *stagnant anoxia*. In left ventricular insufficiency, however, the body suffers from a combination of anoxic or arterial anoxia and stagnant anoxia, since pulmonary congestion with at times areas of edema results in a lowered arterial oxygen saturation as well as a lowered venous saturation. The volume of breathing is increased in the presence of impairment of function of both the circulatory and respiratory systems and it is because of the events just related that the symptoms of cough and dyspnea are produced.

When the right ventricle fails to empty itself completely, there is a damming back of blood into the systemic organs, such as the spleen, liver, kidneys, and into the extremities. The velocity of the circulation from the extremities to the lungs is diminished, and the venous oxygen saturation is lowered. Since right-sided heart failure is generally accompanied by some disturbance in lung function, the arterial oxygen saturation is generally lowered also.

The cause of shortness of the breath in congestive heart failure has been extensively studied. The filling of the pulmonary capillaries with blood results in an impairment of the elastic quality of the lung. Expiration becomes in part an active muscular effort, as shown by a positive or nearly positive intrapleural pressure during the expiratory cycle. In addition to impaired diffusion of oxygen through the edematous or congested alveolar wall, the decreased elasticity of the lung results in unequal ventilation of the lung and the peripheral alveoli may be hyperventilated at the expense of those more deeply situated. The diffusion of carbon dioxide is, however, not impaired since this gas is 30 times as soluble in tissue fluid as oxygen. In fact, there is a diminution of the alveolar carbon-dioxide percentage during the stage of congestive heart failure in many cases. This is due to the increase in volume of breathing, which is itself caused partly by anoxia and partly by proprioceptive reflexes that emanate from the engorged lung.

A cause of cardiac dyspnea may be found in the increased breathing requirement, the increased volume of ventilation, which the patient is forced to employ in the presence of an engorged and heavy lung. Although the sensation of dyspnea is transmitted from afferent nerve impulses which lead into the central nervous systems from the air passages, lungs, and moving framework of the chest, the important physiologic factor is contributed by anoxia. The presence of tissue oxygen-want is due in part to a slight or moderate lowering of the arterial oxygen saturation and to a condition of stagnant anoxia in which the partial pressure of oxygen in the cell falls below the normal level. Emphasis on the importance of the respiratory exchange is required since there has been an overevaluation of the factor of pulmonary engorgement in the causation of cardiac dyspnea.

Although it is acknowledged that shortness of breath in heart failure is often proportional to the diminution of vital capacity, the increased volume of breathing is not primarily due to proprioceptive reflexes that emanate from the congested lung but rather to the state of tissue anoxia which engenders an elevated ventilation. This has been conclusively proven in certain cases of congestive heart failure in which the shortness of breath was relieved 48 hours after residence in an oxygen room, at which time the vital capacity was unaltered or lower than it was prior to treatment.

The decreased dyspnea in the presence of either no change or even an increase in congestion of the lungs, furnishes striking evidence of the importance of chemical factors in both the causation and the treatment of cardiac dyspnea, and equally good evidence for the thesis that proprioceptive reflexes play a secondary rôle in the maintenance of dyspnea in those patients in whom inhalation of high concentrations of oxygen is followed by a decrease in the volume of breathing. Patients with left ventricular failure are dyspneic as a result of an increased ventilation which maintains an arterial oxygen saturation that is so near the normal level as to have aroused in some investigators the erroneous opinion that arterial anoxia was too slight to be a factor in the etiology of cardiac dyspnea. It may be mentioned here that a lowered pulmonary ventilation is less apt to result from oxygen inhalation in patients with rheumatic valvular disease than in cardiac failure due to coronary sclerosis or hypertensive vascular disease.

Additional evidence that proprioceptive reflexes have been overemphasized in dyspneic states has been submitted in connection with the increase in breathing produced by exercise in men and animals. Although the heightened pulmonary ventilation after exercise had been ascribed to reflex causes, studies on normal men have proven that the effective stimulus was chemical and not reflex. When subjects walked on a treadmill, total ischemia of both legs resulted in a marked fall in pulmonary ventilation, even though the nervous pathways were intact. Release of the ischemia was followed at once by a marked hyperventilation.

The complete cessation of voluntary breathing with arrest of lung movement produced in the equalizing-pressure chamber is additional testimony toward the importance of the chemical regulation of breathing, as opposed to the emphasis on proprioceptive reflexes streaming from the lungs.

Even the presence of a normal arterial oxygen saturation does not indicate that the patient is not suffering from anoxia. In a reported case of congestive heart failure due to hypertensive vascular disease the arterial oxygen saturation was found to be 96 per cent. This patient nevertheless regained compensation as a result of continuous oxygen therapy for a period of four weeks, although previously employed bed rest and routine measures had accomplished little or no improvement. It must be remembered that during the drawing of arterial blood patients frequently hyperventilate to such an extent as to increase the oxygen concentration of alveolar air. This temporary elevation in the oxygen concentration of the alveolar air may be responsible for a rise of the oxygen saturation of arterial blood as much as 10 per cent above the patient's basal level. Excitement and a transient stimulation of the respiratory center account for some of the high observations reported on the arterial oxygen saturation in patients with heart disease, but they do not reflect in many instances the degree of anoxia present when the patient is resting quietly.

The response of the patient referred to above will illustrate a recently discovered physiologic mechanism involved in cardiac dyspnea. On the tenth day following inhalation of 45 per cent oxygen the arterial oxygen saturation had risen from 96 to 99 per cent with *an increase in the carbon-dioxide content* of the arterial blood from 46 to 57 volumes per cent. The oxygen capacity decreased from 18.6 to 15.6 volumes per cent. The drop in hemoglobin was larger than that usually found as a result of inhalation of oxygen.

The behavior of carbon dioxide in the blood is one of the most interesting physiologic consequences of oxygen therapy in patients with chronic anoxemic dyspnea, and will be additionally discussed in the chapter on Pulmonary Emphysema. The immediate cause of the increase in carbon-dioxide content in the blood is the lowered pulmonary ventilation which is initiated by inhaling a high oxygen percentage in the atmosphere. The resultant higher pressure of carbon dioxide in the blood accomplishes a faster rate of diffusion through the pulmonary capillaries into the alveolar air, and therefore a corresponding increase in the elimination of carbon dioxide per unit of air breathed. A gradual replacement of chlorine ions in the blood by carbon dioxide occurs which ultimately maintains the acid-base equilibrium of the blood within the normal range.

The increased blood content of carbon dioxide during oxygen treatment continues as long as the lungs are congested with blood and edema. Despite the high carbon-dioxide pressure, the dyspnea is progressively relieved. In fact, the increase in carbon-dioxide content in the blood during the early stages of oxygen therapy makes possible an efficient excretion of carbon dioxide in the presence of a lower volume of breathing. Thus, when the pulmonary ventilation falls from 12 to 6 liters per minute at the end of the first two weeks of oxygen treatment, the elimination of carbon dioxide continues in the same *quantity* because there has been an increased percentage of carbon dioxide in the expired air. When the lungs finally clear, the carbon-dioxide content of the blood and of the alveolar air returns to normal even during continued residence in a high oxygen atmosphere, since free diffusion of carbon dioxide is now possible through unimpaired pulmonary capillaries.

In Fig. 7, the effect of inhalation of 50 per cent oxygen for a two-week period is illustrated in a patient with congestive heart failure. The fall in pulmonary ventilation from 11.9 to 6.2 liters per minute was accompanied by a decrease in basal metabolic rate from $+29$ to

+4 per cent. The elevated oxygen consumption was probably due to the increased work on the part of the respiratory musculature during severe dyspnea. The vital capacity rose during this time from 1,500 to 2,200 cc.

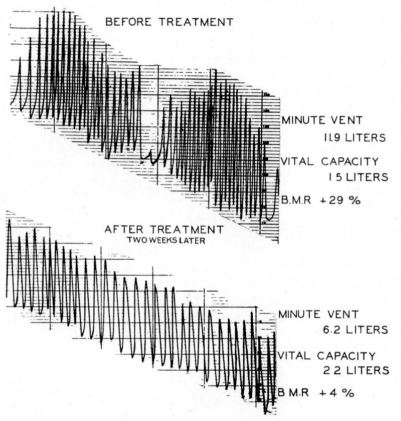

FIG. 7. Effects of 50 per cent oxygen inhalation in congestive heart failure.

In Fig. 8, the onset of diuresis is shown in another patient with congestive failure, in whom an increase in arterial oxygen saturation was followed by an elevation in arterial carbon-dioxide content, increased urinary output, and marked loss of body edema. The rise in the content of carbon dioxide in the blood is accompanied by a fall in blood chlorides, which is a factor in the diuresis that generally sets in between the fourth and sixth days after oxygen treatment is begun.

The crucial rôle played by anoxia in the causation of cardiac dyspnea is therefore revealed by the favorable response to inhalational therapy in some patients. This includes, in summary, progressive relief of dyspnea during the first three days of oxygen treatment accompanied by a rise in arterial oxygen saturation and a progressive

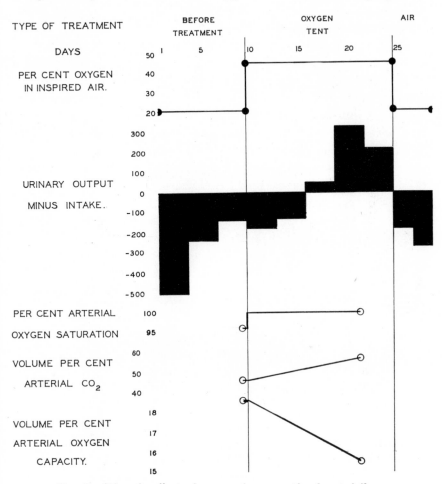

Fig. 8. Diuretic effect of oxygen in congestive heart failure.

increase in the carbon-dioxide tension in the blood and alveolar air. The increased elimination of carbon dioxide per unit of air breathed makes it possible for the pulmonary ventilation to be lowered as a consequence of breathing an increased oxygen percentage in the atmosphere. During this time the vital capacity, representing the degree of pulmonary congestion, may show little or no change, which is clear evidence of the priority of the respiratory exchange and not proprioceptive reflexes in maintaining cardiac dyspnea. In other words, when the volume of breathing is lowered *toward* the normal level, there is relief of dyspnea, and at the same time a lessened stimulus to the afferent nerve endings in the lungs and moving framework of the chest wall.

The explanation of the diuresis that develops in patients who respond favorably to oxygen treatment is at least in part due to more efficient functioning of the heart muscle. The fact that there is a fall in blood chloride suggests that this may play some part in facilitating the increased urinary output. That the diuresis is specifically due to the inhalation of oxygen has been repeatedly shown by the withdrawal of oxygen during the early stage of treatment, and the demonstration that urinary output then promptly falls.

Another instance of the effect of anoxia in maintaining cardiac dyspnea occurs in Cheyne-Stokes dyspnea in which inhalation of 100 per cent oxygen generally terminates periodic breathing immediately, whereas inhalation of 50 per cent oxygen relieves the dyspnea more gradually, as compensation is regained.

INHALATIONAL THERAPY

In *acute* cardiac insufficiency, the inhalation of oxygen-enriched atmospheres between 50 and 100 per cent is indicated, irrespective of the cause. Oxygen therapy should be continued until the patient is no longer suffering from acute anoxia.

In patients with *chronic* cardiac insufficiency, the decision to employ oxygen therapy depends on the cause. In cases with valvular heart disease with evidence of rheumatic activity, inhalation of oxygen does not generally produce a striking result. The relief of dyspnea and the betterment of cardiac function are apt to be temporary. However, in patients with arteriosclerotic heart disease, coronary sclerosis, and hypertensive vascular disease, continuous inhalation of 50 per cent oxygen may restore compensation when other measures have proved unavailing. In carrying out a program of oxygen therapy, routine procedures should also be employed. It is of especial importance to restrict sodium chloride and sodium bicarbonate since it has been found that the ingestion of salt will prevent the diuresis which would otherwise take place as a result of oxygen therapy. Intake of fluids without sodium need not be diminished. When oxygen therapy has been decided upon in the treatment of congestive heart failure, the aim should be complete restoration of cardiac function. A program which will consume between three and six weeks may be described as follows:

The oxygen concentration in the atmosphere provided the patient should be not less than 50 per cent since it has been found that lower concentrations may be insufficient to achieve the improvement desired. There is reason to believe as a result of clinical studies that higher oxygen concentrations of between 60 and 70 per cent may be additionally valuable, because of the increase in physically dissolved oxygen. The patient will then inhale as continuously as possible an oxygen-enriched atmosphere consisting of 50 to 70 per cent oxygen. During the first three days, dyspnea, restlessness, and apprehension generally show a marked improvement. During the following three days, increasing relief of dyspnea and orthopnea occur, and the diuresis begins. The increased output of fluid is generally manifested in a rise in urinary output, although the total decrease in body weight is frequently much larger than can be accounted for by the difference between intake and output of fluid. The output of salt in the urine increases to a maximum and then is gradually lowered, paralleling the urinary secretion.

The carbon-dioxide content in the arterial blood is apt to reach its height at the peak of diuresis and gradually fall as the lungs become less congested. During the second and third week of inhalation of 50 per cent oxygen, there is additional improvement, manifested by an elevation in the vital capacity and decrease in edema of the extremities. When the signs of congestive failure have disappeared or have notably decreased, the patient is prepared to breathe atmospheric air. Gradual lowering of the oxygen concentration during the following week is desirable in order to prevent the possibility of recurrence of cardiac failure. The oxygen concentration is therefore lowered to 40 per cent for two days and 35 per cent for three days. When the percentage of oxygen has been reduced to this level, the nasal catheter may be employed for an additional two to five days, a flow of 5 liters per minute being gradually lowered to 2 liters per minute, followed by complete cessation of oxygen treatment. An alternate procedure is to dispense with oxygen completely when the concentration has been lowered to between 30 and 35 per cent one week after the signs of dyspnea and edema have disappeared.

In selecting the *method* of treatment, comfort of the patient should be considered since the duration of oxygen inhalation is a longer one than that employed in pneumonia. Although the oxygen room possesses real advantages in this respect, because of its roominess and absence from any appliance to the face, a large well-ventilated oxygen tent with a completely transparent pliofilm or plastocele canopy causes no feeling of claustrophobia and appears to be the most comfortable method. In cases in which adequate technical supervision is not available or in which expense of treatment is a consideration, the simpler appliances to the face may be employed. The rubber catheter with placement in the nasal or oral pharynx or an oxygen mask may be used. If the B.L.B. apparatus is employed, oxygen should be administered at a flow of not less than 6 liters per minute and preferably 7 or 8 liters in order to avoid accumulation of carbon dioxide.

If the injector Meter mask is used the flow of oxygen may be adjusted to that which is required to keep the collecting bag from completely collapsing at the end of inspiration. The meter should be set at the oxygen concentration desired. If the dyspnea is not excessive, 5 to 6 liters per minute of oxygen administered from the regulator will keep the collecting bag sufficiently full, and also provide a concentration of 50 per cent oxygen. The carbon-dioxide percentage is always 0.2 per cent or lower, due to absence of rebreathing. In regulating the flow of oxygen from the regulator it is important to spend a few minutes at the start of treatment to determine the effect of the oxygen-enriched atmosphere on the pulmonary ventilation. A patient may at first require 8 to 10 liters per minute to fulfill the requirement of his ventilation. After he accustoms himself to the apparatus, the volume of breathing will decrease, in part due to lessened stimulation of the respiratory center because of excitement and also because of the relief of anoxia. At the end of two to three minutes it may be found that a flow of 5 to 6 liters per minute is adequate, i.e., to prevent the collecting bag from collapsing at the end of inspiration.

During the period of oxygen treatment it should be remembered that digitalis and the mercurial diuretics should be employed in the same manner as would be indicated in the absence of oxygen treatment. There is little or no indication for restriction of fluid but complete elimination of sodium in the form of salt and sodium bicarbonate is essential for restoration of compensation in cases of chronic congestive heart failure treated with oxygen. The duration of improvement depends upon the condition of the individual patient and the local environment to which he returns, but in some instances of this type of therapy compensation has lasted for periods in excess of one to two years. In other patients, recurrence of cardiac insufficiency has taken place at a shorter interval and necessitated another course of oxygen therapy.

BIBLIOGRAPHY

Barach, A. L.: The therapeutic use of oxygen in heart disease, Ann. Int. Med., 5:428, 1931.

Barach, A. L.: Treatment of asphyxia in clinical disease, with especial reference to recent developments in the use of oxygen in heart disease, N. Y. State Jour. Med., 34:672, 1934.

Barach, A. L., and D. W. Richards, Jr.: Effects of oxygen therapy in congestive heart failure, Arch. Int. Med., 48:325, 1931.

Barach, A. L., D. W. Richards, Jr., A. T. Milhorat, and R. L. Levy: Effects of oxygen therapy on patients with congestive heart failure, Proc. Soc. Exper. Biol. and Med., 27:308, 1929.

Barach, A. L., D. W. Richards, Jr., and W. B. Parsons: Oxygen treatment and thyroid ablation in treatment of heart disease, Ann. Int. Med., 9:1513, 1936.

Barach, A. L., and Woodwell, M. N.: Studies in oxygen therapy with determination of the blood gases, etc.: I: In cardiac insufficiency and related conditions, Arch. Int. Med., 28:367, 1921. II. In pneumonia and its complications, Arch. Int. Med., 28:394, 1921. III. In an extreme type of shallow breathing occurring in encephalitis, Arch. Int. Med., 28:421, 1921.

Barman, J. M., M. F. Moreira, and F. Consolazio: The effective stimulus for increased pulmonary ventilation during muscular exertion, Jour. Clin. Invest., 22:53, 1943.

Campbell, J. M. H.: The effect on breathless subjects of residence in an oxygen chamber, Quart. Jour. Med., 20:144, 1926.

Campbell, J. M. H., and E. P. Poulton: The effect on breathless subjects of residence in an oxygen chamber, Quart. Jour. Med., 20:121, 1926.

Cohn, D. J., L. N. Katz, S. Soskin, and W. W. Hamburger: Observations on the effects of oxygen therapy: III. Blood chemical changes, Amer. Jour. Med. Sci., 184:818, 1932.

Harrison, T. R.: Failure of the Circulation, Baltimore, Williams & Wilkins Co. 1935.

Harrop, G. A., Jr.: The oxygen and carbon dioxide content of arterial and of venous blood in normal individuals and in patients with anemia and heart disease, Jour. Exper. Med., 30:241, 1919.

Knipping, H. W., and G. Zimmerman: Oxygen therapy in patients with cardiac and pulmonary disease, Ztschr. f. klin. Med., 124:435, 1933.

Meakins, J. C.: Modern muscle physiology and circulatory failure, Ann. Int. Med., 6:506, 1932.

Means, J. H., and L. H. Newburgh: Studies of the blood flow by the method of Krogh and Lundhard, Trans. Asso. Amer. Physic., 30:51, 1915.

Richards, D. W., Jr., and A. L. Barach: Prolonged residence in high oxygen atmosphere: effects on normal individuals and on patients with chronic cardiac and pulmonary insufficiency, Quart. Jour. Med., 3:437, 1934.

6

Coronary Thrombosis and Coronary Sclerosis

DEFINITION

In coronary thrombosis an acute obstruction of a branch of one of the coronary arteries takes place, generally due to the development of a thrombus which results in infarction or death of the heart muscle supplied by the occluded artery. It occurs most frequently in cases of hypertension and arteriosclerosis, especially in patients who have previously suffered from the syndrome called angina pectoris. The outstanding symptoms are severe pain, over the heart or in the upper abdomen, followed by shock and at times collapse, in some cases by congestive failure.

Coronary sclerosis is generally manifested by periodic attacks of pain in the region of the heart or epigastrium with or without radiation to the arm or the jaw. Pain of a similar nature may be due to aortic stenosis or to syphilitic aortitis, in which there is an obstruction to the flow of blood at the mouth of the coronary artery. When the coronary artery has been narrowed by plaques of sclerosis, a resistance to the flow of blood is present which is apt to produce cardiac pain under conditions of exertion; sclerosis is also a predisposing cause of thrombotic occlusion of the affected vessel.

PATHOLOGIC PHYSIOLOGY

In patients with narrowing of the coronary artery due to sclerosis or spasm, cardiac pain is generally produced by circumstances which increase the oxygen consumption. Physical exercise, eating, and emotional excitement are frequent causes of pain over the precordium. The concept that anoxia of the heart muscle is responsible for cardiac pain has been strengthened by studies made in recent years in which

70

it has been found that inhalation of 10 to 12 per cent oxygen for a period of 20 minutes will frequently result in pain over the chest, as well as a characteristic alteration in the electrocardiogram, especially depression of the T-wave and the S-T segment. Conversely, the relief of precordial pain by inhaling high concentrations of oxygen is also evidence that the precipitating cause of angina is anoxia, and the resultant metabolic products of deficient oxidation in cardiac muscle. In many patients inhalation of 100 per cent oxygen results in an elevation of the T-wave in one or more leads. In many cases of coronary thrombosis inhalation of 100 per cent oxygen results in prompt relief of severe pain even when previous injection of morphine and aminophyllin have not relieved the condition.

The severity of coronary thrombosis depends upon the diameter of the obstructed artery. Although agonizing pain is characteristic, there are other patients who complain of only moderate distress. In some patients a state of profound shock develops quickly, characterized by a progressive fall in blood pressure, a cold, clammy skin, and marked anxiety. If a large area of the heart muscle has been affected, congestive heart failure may take place as a result of the inability of the heart to deliver its customary volume of blood. At times, edema of the lungs follows with even more severe generalized anoxia. The heart muscle is not only deprived of oxygen in the infarcted area but may also show impairment in its function as a result of a lowered arterial oxygen saturation due to pulmonary congestion or edema in the lungs.

Inhalation of 10 per cent oxygen has been employed as a test of coronary insufficiency, since it frequently produces pain in patients with coronary sclerosis and shows electrocardiographic changes qualitatively and quantitatively different from those which are seen in normal individuals during inhalation of low oxygen mixtures. Physiologic studies made during the inhalation of a 10 per cent oxygen mixture have revealed that the heightened volume of breathing induced by anoxia is followed by a marked loss in carbon dioxide, with a shift in the acid-base equilibrium to the alkaline side. When the alkaline shift has been prevented by inhaling 10 per cent oxygen with 2 or 3 per cent carbon dioxide, there is generally absence both of the symptoms of anginal pain and of the electrocardiographic changes said to be characteristic of anoxia, except in patients with narrowing of the mouth of the coronary artery, such as in luetic aortitis. This finding indicates that alkalosis is significantly involved in the production of cardiac pain, resulting in spasm of the coronary artery and probably also in ischemic contraction of the smaller blood vessels in the coronary circulation. The result of alkalosis is increased tissue anoxia; in addition oxygen is more firmly bound to hemoglobin when it is alkaline. The inhalation of low oxygen mixtures does not generally produce the signs of coronary insufficiency when alkalosis has been prevented by the simultaneous inhalation of small percentages of carbon dioxide, which admittedly also diminishes anoxia.

INHALATIONAL THERAPY

In the treatment of patients with coronary sclerosis who have repeated attacks of anginal pain, the inhalation of pure oxygen is a measure of considerable value. It may be used not only for the relief of pain in those patients in whom nitroglycerine produces headache but it also may be employed as a measure which diminishes the frequency of attacks. In patients who have two to ten attacks of anginal pain daily the inhalation of 100 per cent oxygen for a period of 30 minutes twice a day at times results in a striking decrease in the number of attacks of anginal pain and an increase in exercise tolerance. However, this improvement does not take place in cases of luetic aortitis or aortic stenosis.[1]

When patients with coronary occlusion reveal either the symptoms of shock or cardiac failure, the inhalation of oxygen in concentrations between 50 and 100 per cent is urgently indicated. Even in cases in which relatively few symptoms are present, the provision of oxygen therapy at the bedside should be instituted immediately, since a progression of the thrombus may result in shock, aggravation of anoxia and in death due to cardiac insufficiency. Rest in bed, warmth and morphine are inadequate therapy in the majority of cases of coronary occlusion. The results of continuous oxygen treatment, described in a sufficiently large series of cases, reveals unmistakable improvement beginning within one to three hours after the administration of oxygen. Relief of pain is striking, the breathing is less labored, restlessness is diminished, cyanosis is decreased or abolished. Other manifestations of the value of oxygen treatment are the disappearance of Cheyne-Stokes breathing, if present, a slower heart rate, and an increase in the volume of the pulse. When oxygen treatment is discontinued be-

---

[1] Unpublished observations of Barach, A. L., and Steiner, Alfred.

fore an adequate readjustment of the circulation has taken place, there may be a recurrence of the symptoms of the condition.

Although the injury to the heart muscle may be so extensive as to make recovery impossible, it has been decisively demonstrated that the inhalation of high concentrations of oxygen is responsible for the saving of life when no other measure could accomplish the same result. Even though the oxygen saturation of the arterial blood may be normal, it should be borne in mind that the inhalation of 100 per cent oxygen is accompanied by a significant increase in the physically dissolved oxygen of the arterial blood leading to the collaterals of the occluded blood vessel. This results in a substantial increase in the pressure of oxygen available to the heart muscle, which may maintain the function of the circulation as a whole, even in the presence of a considerable area of infarcted and functionless cardiac muscle. In severe cases, oxygen treatment should be continued for approximately five days after onset of the attack.

Although the oxygen tent is generally the most comfortable method of providing concentrations of oxygen of 50 to 60 per cent, the catheter inserted in the oral pharynx may be employed to achieve a similar result. When the condition of the patient is grave, with shock or congestive failure, an oxygen concentration of 100 per cent is desirable. A mask oxygen apparatus may therefore be employed with a high flow of oxygen, in excess of the pulmonary ventilation of the patient, namely, between 12 and 15 liters per minute. If the condition of the patient shows improvement after the first day or two, the oxygen percentage may be gradually lowered to that of 50 per cent and finally discontinued after a period of 4 to 6 days, depending upon the clinical state of the patient.

BIBLIOGRAPHY

Barach, A. L.: The therapeutic use of oxygen in heart disease, Ann. Int. Med., 5:428, 1931.

Barach, A. L., and R. L. Levy: Oxygen in the treatment of acute coronary occlusions, Jour. Amer. Med. Asso., 103:1690, 1934.

Barach, A. L., D. W. Richards, Jr., and W. B. Parson: Oxygen treatment and thyroid ablation in treatment of heart disease, Ann. Int. Med., 9:1513, 1936.

Barach, A. L., and A. Steiner: Effect of inhalation of high oxygen concentrations, with and without carbon dioxide, on the electrocardiogram, Proc. Soc. Exper. Biol. and Med., 45:175, 1940.

Barach, A. L., A. Steiner, M. Eckman, and N. Molomut: The physiologic action of oxygen and carbon dioxide on the coronary circulation, as shown by blood gas and electrocardiographic studies, Amer. Heart Jour., 22:13, 1941.

Boland, E. W.: Oxygen in high concentration for relief of pain in coronary thrombosis and severe angina pectoris, Jour. Amer. Med. Asso., 114:1512, 1940.

Burgess, A. M., and F. H. Chafee: Oxygen in the treatment of coronary occlusion in the home, New England Jour. Med., 216:203, 1937.

Greene, C. W., and N. C. Gilbert: Studies on responses of circulation to low oxygen tension: cause of changes observed in heart during extreme anoxemia, Amer. Jour. Physiol., 60:155, 1922.

Hensel, C. N.: Treatment of acute coronary occlusion by long continued use of oxygen therapy, Minnesota Med., 24:61, 1941.

Katz, L. N., W. W. Hamburger, and W. J. Schultz: The effect of generalized anoxemia on the electrocardiogram of normal subjects; its bearing on the mechanism of attacks of angina pectoris, Amer. Heart Jour., 9:771, 1934.

Keefer, C. S., and W. H. Resnik: Angina pectoris: a syndrome caused by anoxemia of the myocardium, Arch. Int. Med., 41:769, 1928.

Kilgore, E. S.: The treatment of acute coronary occlusion, Jour. Amer. Med. Asso., 100:315, 1933.

Kissin, M.: Production of pain in exercising skeletal muscle during induced anoxemia, Jour. Amer. Med. Asso., 103:1336, 1934.

Kountz, W. B., and Hammouda, M.: The effect of asphyxia and of anoxemia on the electrocardiogram, Amer. Heart Jour., 8:259, 1932.

Levy, R. L.: Diseases of the Coronary Arteries and Cardiac Pain, New York, The Macmillan Co., 1936.

Levy, R. L., and A. L. Barach: The therapeutic use of oxygen in coronary thrombosis, Jour. Amer. Med. Asso., 94:1363, 1930.

Levy, R. L., A. L. Barach, and H. G. Bruenn: Effects of induced oxygen want in patients with cardiac pain, Amer. Heart Jour., 15:187, 1938.

Levy, R. L., N. E. Williams, H. G. Bruenn, and H. A. Carr: Anoxemia test in diagnosis of coronary insufficiency, Amer. Heart Jour., 21:634, 1941.

Resnik, W. H.: Observations on the effect of anoxemia on the heart: I. Auriculoventricular conduction, Jour. Clin. Invest., 2:93, 1925.

Riseman, J. E. F., and M. G. Brown: The effect of oxygen on the exercise tolerance of patients with angina pectoris, Amer. Heart Jour., 18:159, 1939.

Rizer, R. I.: Oxygen treatment of coronary occlusion, Minnesota Med., 12:506, 1929.

7

Shock

DEFINITION

The term shock is commonly used to describe failure of the circulation which is not caused by cardiac insufficiency but primarily due to failure of the peripheral circulation. Primary shock designates the state of circulatory failure which immediately follows an injury. Secondary shock refers to that type of failure of the circulation in which there is a more prolonged interval between the injury and the development of symptoms. Primary shock is predominately of reflex origin and secondary shock includes in addition the injurious consequences of chemical as well as physical mechanisms such as trauma and hemorrhage. The clinical state is characterized by a rapid, feeble pulse, shallow breathing, collapse of the superficial veins, a marked decrease in arterial and auricular blood pressures, cold and pale extremities, sweating, and apprehension followed by a depressed sensorium.

PATHOLOGIC PHYSIOLOGY

Although the clinical manifestations of well-developed shock are characteristic, the pathogenesis of the condition varies widely and it is altogether probable that the physiologic state itself is subject to considerable differences in individual patients. Despite many divergent theories of the origin and nature of shock, there is agreement concerning the fact that a decreased return of venous blood to the right heart takes place. In well-developed shock there is in most instances a decrease in the volume of circulating blood. A marked decrease in cardiac output results from the diminished entrance of blood into the heart, producing a profound stagnant anoxia in the tissue cells. This is also portrayed by the severe lowering of the total oxygen consumption.

The marked tissue anoxia results in increased capillary permeability, with exudation of serum into the tissue spaces, in some cases manifested by the development of pulmonary edema. In some patients the kidneys are no longer able to excrete waste products adequately, with the result that the acid-base balance in the blood is not maintained and the nonprotein nitrogen in the serum is increased. The functions of all the organs in the body are undoubtedly impaired to a variable degree.

In appraising the pathologic physiology of shock, two main characteristics of the condition should be kept in mind: (1) A persistent progressive state of low blood pressure, which may be around 70 mm. Hg or lower, and (2) a persistent decrease in cardiac output. In most patients with shock the volume capacity of the vascular system is relatively larger than the circulating blood volume. Whether the blood vessels themselves are relaxed, or whether there is a total decrease in the absolute circulating blood volume, or both, are questions that cannot be decided at this time.[1] However, the result is a diminished venous pressure, a decreased filling of the right heart, and an inevitable reduction in cardiac output accompanied by a decline in arterial blood pressure and a diminished volume of circulation to all organs. Attempts to compensate for the diminished effective circulating blood volume are (1) an increased rate of the heart and (2) a reduction in the volume of the blood reservoirs such as the spleen and probably also the liver. As these mechanisms fail to compensate for the condition and the arterial blood pressure continues to decline, varying degrees of compensatory vasoconstriction occur in parts of the body which are relatively less sensitive to anoxia, such as the skin, connective tissue, abdominal viscera, and voluntary muscle; this per-

---

[1] Since this chapter was written an illuminating study of the circulation in human shock (Cournand, et al.) has revealed that cases of shock due to skeletal trauma and hemorrhage show hemodilution rather than hemoconcentration, whereas hemoconcentration takes place in cases of shock due to burns and abdominal injuries. The total blood volume is reduced 40 per cent, and the cardiac output lowered one-third, as determined by the direct Fick technic. The blood lactic acid is markedly increased, and the pH is shifted in the acid direction. The oxygen saturation of the mixed venous blood, withdrawn by catheter from the right heart, shows a fall from a normal level of 65 to 35 per cent, and in some cases to 15 per cent. This exceedingly low value for oxygen saturation of right heart blood is evidence of the most severe type of tissue anoxia, and is manifestly the explanation for the lactic-acid accumulation and the acidosis, which is more marked in mixed venous than in arterial blood. Conclusive evidence for increasing the physically dissolved oxygen in arterial blood by inhaling 70 to 100 per cent oxygen is thus provided by this investigation.

mits the available circulation being continued to a larger extent to the brain and the heart, organs which are most sensitive to anoxia.

As the volume of circulation becomes progressively diminished, there are areas of relative ischemia which produce an increase in the permeability of the capillaries with the consequence that the serum and proteins of the plasma pass into the extravascular tissues and red cells accumulate in the dilated capillaries. A decrease of the metabolism of the tissues and organs so affected takes place, with a marked total lowering of the oxygen consumption and consequent increase in tissue anoxia. A vicious cycle is then set up because the discrepancy between the circulating blood volume and the vascular volume is exaggerated by the absolute decrease in the circulating blood, as well as the increase in the vascular capacity due to relaxation of the capillaries. The return of blood to the heart is thus additionally decreased, with a lowering in cardiac output and arterial blood pressure; the total minute volume of the circulation to the tissues is further reduced. In the end, there is more marked depression of capillary and tissue function, a final diminution in the effectiveness of cardiac emptying and more severe tissue anoxia ending in death.

In experimental observations on shock produced by long-continued hemorrhage, reduction of cardiac output and of blood volume frequently does not take place during the initial stage of shock. It may be that compensatory processes take place in response to the diminution of blood volume by hemorrhage, such as a reduction in the capacity of the blood reservoirs, the spleen, and the liver, and in addition absorption of fluid from the tissues, which thus may maintain a relatively normal cardiac output. Finally, however, as the systolic blood pressure drops a fall in cardiac output does take place. During the stage in which the aortic pressure is declining as a result of continued hemorrhage, the blood flow to the skin and muscles is decreased more rapidly than is explained by the fall in aortic pressure. Although vasoconstriction may be a factor in explaining this phenomenon, it does not appear to be the only influence at work. The brain and heart do not show so great a reduction of blood flow during shock as do the skin and muscles. In burn shock determination of the hematocrit reveals a concentration of red blood cells either during the initial or later stages of shock, which suggests that a loss of plasma takes place. Contraction of the spleen may be the cause of some of the increase in red corpuscles in the circulating blood, but hemoconcentration may also occur at the end phase of shock when the spleen has already become fully contracted.

Accompanying a marked drop in systolic blood pressure the metabolic rate of the experimental animal invariably begins to fall. When the systolic blood pressure reaches 70 mm. Hg the decrease in oxygen consumption is considerable, and is associated with a lowering of body temperature. This is in all probability explained by the fact that the flow of blood through some tissues is decreased or absent so that no oxygen is consumed in the cells of many organs. Decreased reactivity of the experimental animal as well as the patient is generally observed, which also contributes to the lowered basal metabolism.

A few instances of the precipitating cause of shock may be mentioned: Shock may be caused by burns, with a consequent loss of plasma from the blood, by injuries in which there may be a local loss of fluid in the traumatized area and in which nervous reflexes may play an important part. Other mechanisms have been described, such as impairment of capillary function caused by histamine, the potassium ion, or some other product of tissue necrosis. Prolonged and severe hemorrhage is a common cause of shock, and clinical diseases, such as coronary occlusion, intestinal obstruction, Addison's disease, cholera, prolonged anesthesia, severe dehydration, and pneumonia.

In the treatment of shock the administration of intravenous fluid to overcome the discrepancy between the diminished circulating blood volume and the relatively larger vascular bed is the most common procedure. The introduction of plasma or whole blood is frequently followed by beneficial results and until the phase is reached in which heart failure itself takes place, this appears to be the procedure of choice. Since the condition is primarily a diminution in the volume of circulation to the various organs in the body, and because it is progressive, accompanied by local ischemia and severe lowering of the oxygen consumption, inhalation of 100 per cent oxygen should be employed in order to combat the profound cell anoxia.

The fact that immediate clinical improvement may not in some cases follow oxygen inhalation is not an argument against its critical value. The symptoms of altitude anoxia may persist for 12 to 24 hours after the blood oxygen saturation has been restored to normal as is shown by the experience of men suffering from mountain sickness who may remain ill for many hours after return to a sea-level atmosphere. There is no justification in allowing such a severe form of anoxia to go untreated, since physiologic studies have shown it is possible to raise the tissue oxygen tension substantially through increase in the physically dissolved oxygen. The damaging effect of anoxia (to the extent present in shock) is no longer open to question, in respect to central nervous system and cardiac function. In both clinical and experimental investigations, inhalation of oxygen has been found beneficial. Although oxygen administration does not restore the circulation to normal functioning, it may prevent the consequences of anoxia to a degree that will aid in the recovery of the patient. The dramatic improvement in patients with shock after coronary occlusion is evidence that inhalation of oxygen is at times of lifesaving value in this type of peripheral circulatory failure.

Some observers have found that adrenal cortical extract diminishes capillary permeability and elevates blood pressure in experimental and clinical shock, especially that caused by burns. Neosynephrin hydrochloride has also been used since it is followed by an elevation in systolic pressure and a decrease in heart rate.

That inhalation of pure oxygen under three atmospheres' pressure has not been found valuable in experimental shock in dogs cannot be accepted as evidence that 100 per cent oxygen is not therapeutically advantageous in human shock. Oxygen under three atmospheres causes an accumulation of carbon dioxide in the tissues, thus *increasing* the acidosis in shock, and adding an additional toxic factor, i.e., oxygen poisoning. Inhalation of 100 per cent oxygen at atmospheric pressure has on the contrary been found to be helpful in experimental shock in dogs.

From the point of view of anoxia it may be said in summary that inhalation of pure oxygen has been followed by clinical improvement in both experimental and human shock; the content of oxygen in arterial, femoral vein, and right heart blood has been shown to be substantially increased when 100 per cent oxygen was breathed, i.e., from 1.0 to 2.5 cc. of oxygen per 100 cc. of circulating blood.

INHALATIONAL THERAPY

Each case of shock must be treated individually, depending upon the special circumstances which were responsible for development of the condition. The restoration of an effective circulatory blood volume by appropriate introduction of fluid is in most instances an important part of the treatment. However, *excessive* injection of normal or hypertonic solutions may be followed by cardiac failure.

In respect to inhalational therapy the highest concentration of oxygen, namely 100 per cent oxygen, is indicated. Whether or not pulmonary edema is present, the fact that profound tissue anoxia exists and is one of the important factors resulting in damage to all the organs in the body constitutes sufficient reason for employment of oxygen therapy. In a carefully studied case of peripheral circulatory failure it was shown that the blood flow through the hand showed a marked fall when a patient breathing 50 per cent oxygen in an oxygen tent was subjected to an abrupt lowering of the oxygen concentration to that of atmospheric air. Although peripheral circulatory failure was commonly recognized as the clinical manifestation of surgical shock, occurring frequently after injury, burns, operations, and hemorrhage, the condition is met with frequently in clinical medicine, during pneumonia, in infarction of the coronary or pulmonary arteries, in Addison's disease, in diabetic acidosis, and in other illnesses.

In all these conditions the significance of the increase of the physically dissolved oxygen is important to emphasize. Although the arterial oxygen saturation is normal in the absence of moisture in the lung, a substantial increase of tension of oxygen in the tissue capillaries is provided by breathing 100 per cent oxygen. Although only 0.25 cc. of oxygen is present in the dissolved state in 100 cc. of blood when the patient breathes air, there is an increase to 1.5 cc. due simply to the increased partial pressure of pure oxygen. An additional 1.0 cc. is added by raising the saturation of the hemoglobin from 95 to 100 per cent. Since approximately 5 cc. of oxygen are consumed in 100 cc. of blood passing from artery to vein, an increase of 2.0 to 2.5 cc. in 100 cc. of blood results in a substantial rise in oxygen pressure, manifestly sufficient to relieve in part a profound tissue anoxia, and in that way prevent damage to the cells of the various organs in the body.

The oxygen mask with a flow of 12 and 15 liters of oxygen per minute is the most efficient method of providing 100 per cent oxygen. When concentrations between 50 and 60 per cent oxygen are used, the oxygen tent or the rubber catheter inserted into the nose or oral pharynx may be employed. The duration of treatment is decided by recovery from the state of circulatory failure.

BIBLIOGRAPHY

Aub, J. C., and T. D. Cunningham: Studies on experimental traumatic shock: II. The oxygen content of the blood, Amer. Jour. Physiol., 54:408, 1920.

Barach, A. L.: The contrast between the treatment of heart failure and peripheral circulatory failure, Jour. Michigan Med. Soc., 37:497, 1938.

Blalock, A.: Principles of Surgical Care: Shock and Other Problems, St. Louis, C. V. Mosby Co., 1940.

Boothby, W. M., W. R. Lovelace, and C. W. Mayo: One hundred per cent oxygen: indications for its use and methods of its administration, Jour. Amer. Med. Asso., 113:477, 1939.

Chase, H. C.: Anoxia—its surgical significance, Surg., Gynec., and Obstet., 73: 105, 1941.

Cournand, A., R. L. Riley, S. E. Bradley, E. S. Breed, R. P. Noble, H. D. Lauson, M. I. Gregersen, and D. W. Richards: Studies of the circulation in clinical shock, Surgery, 13:964, 1943.

Davis, H. A.: Physiologic effects of high concentrations of oxygen in experimental shock, Arch. Surg., 43:1, 1941.

Fine, J., B. M. Banks, J. B. Sears, and L. Hermanson: The treatment of gaseous distension of the intestine by the inhalation of 95 per cent oxygen; description of apparatus for the clinical administration of high oxygen mixtures, Ann. Surg., 103:375, 1936.

Freeman, N. E., L. J. Show, and J. C. Snyder: The peripheral blood flow in surgical shock, Jour. Clin. Invest., 15:651, 1936.

Henderson, Y.: Acapnia as a factor in postoperative shock atelectasis and pneumonia, Jour. Amer. Med. Asso., 95:572, 1930.

Meakins, J. C.: Shock, its causes and treatment, Canad. Med. Jour., 43:201, 1940.

Melton, G.: Oxygen therapy in shock, Lancet, 1:481, 1943.

Moon, V. H.: Shock and Related Capillary Phenomena. With a Foreword by Walter B. Cannon, Harvard Medical School, New York, Oxford University Press, 1938.

Schnedorf, J. G., and T. G. Orr: Beneficial effects of oxygen therapy in experimental traumatic shock, Surg., Gynec., and Obstet., 73:79, 1941.

Schnedorf, J. G., and T. G. Orr: Beneficial effects of oxygen therapy in shock, Ann. Surg., 113:1113, 1941.

Schnedorf, J. G., and T. G. Orr: Oxygen therapy in shock due to hemorrhage, Surg., Gynec., and Obstet., 63:495, 1941.

Wiggers, C. J.: Applicability of experimental results to the shock problem in man, Jour. Amer. Med. Asso., 117:1143, 1941.

Wood, G. O., M. F. Mason, and A. Blalock: Studies on the effects of the inhalation of a high concentration of oxygen in experimental shock, Surg., Gynec., and Obstet., 8:247, 1940.

8

Pulmonary Infarction

DEFINITION

Pulmonary infarction is due to an embolus or thrombus occluding a branch of the pulmonary artery, resulting in formation of a pyramidal mass of airless lung tissue infiltrated with blood which has extravasated into the air cells and interstitial pulmonary tissue. In typical cases, the clinical picture includes a sudden pain in the chest, and at times the development of shock or pulmonary edema.

PATHOLOGIC PHYSIOLOGY

If the infarcted area is small, little or no disturbance in respiratory function may be observed. However, in cases in which a large blood vessel is occluded there is interference with the absorption of oxygen by blood passing through the infarcted area. When large emboli obstruct the pulmonary artery there may be sufficient increase in resistance to the flow of blood through the lung to result in failure of the right ventricle. In many cases anoxia and the outstanding symptoms are due to peripheral circulatory failure.

INHALATIONAL THERAPY

Although restoration of the circulating blood volume is indicated in the presence of shock, the existence of right heart failure obviously is a contraindication to the addition of intravenous fluid. The administration of high concentrations of oxygen up to 100 per cent is urgently indicated to overcome the anoxia and to prevent if possible circulatory and respiratory failure. Although morphine is said to be a most valuable drug to relieve the pain and dyspnea from which these patients suffer, it should be borne in mind that anoxia may be increased after this medication and therefore that adequate oxygen therapy should be provided. Any suitable method of administering oxygen may be employed, including the oxygen mask for the administration of pure oxygen, the nasal or oropharyngeal catheter, or the oxygen tent for the inhalation of more moderate concentrations of oxygen.

9

Massive Collapse of the Lung

DEFINITION

Massive collapse of the lung is the term applied to the sudden development of complete atelectasis of one or more lobes of one or both lungs. The main clinical features are severe dyspnea, cyanosis, and prostration.

PATHOLOGIC PHYSIOLOGY

The pathogenesis of massive collapse is not clear in most patients. Although 70 per cent of the cases follow surgical operation and injury, others are associated with the presence of a foreign body or tumor in a primary bronchus, asthma, pneumonia, or various other illnesses. Since the condition frequently occurs after operations in the upper abdomen, with splinting of the bases of the lungs, it has been assumed that tenacious mucus may fail to be expectorated and act as a plug blocking the entrance of air into a lobe of the lung. The gradual absorption of air by the blood passing through the plugged area may thus result in atelectasis. The heart and mediastinum are then pulled toward the affected side. The sudden dyspnea and cyanosis are due only in part to the fact that the collapsed lung is poorly ventilated, with the pulmonary blood continuing to circulate through it, but mainly to the mechanical effect of the shift of the mediastinum. In some cases with an allergic history, muscular spasm of the bronchi with swelling of the mucous membrane may cause complete closure of a good-sized bronchus leading to a lobe of the lung. A reflex etiology of the condition has been described in which a primary atelectasis occurs, followed by retention of secretion in the bronchi leading to the affected area.

INHALATIONAL THERAPY

The inhalation of 5 to 7 per cent carbon dioxide in oxygen has been employed in order to stretch the bronchial walls by maximal expansion of the chest, in the hope that the mucus will be freed and subsequently coughed up. Inhalation of carbon-dioxide–oxygen mixtures for two to four minutes at repeated intervals should be tried in order to accomplish this purpose. Inflation of the lung has at times followed turning the patient from side to side, first on the affected side and then on the sound side. Bronchoscopy has given excellent results in skilled hands in those cases that do not respond to the above measures.

The inhalation of 50 to 70 per cent oxygen is generally indicated to maintain respiratory function until the above measures are tried or in the event that they prove to be unsuccessful. Gradual relief of cyanosis and dyspnea generally takes place in patients who are treated with continuous inhalation of an oxygen-enriched atmosphere. The oxygen tent appears to be the most comfortable method of administering oxygen to these cases, although in many instances the oxygen mask or nasal catheter may be successfully used.

BIBLIOGRAPHY

Barach, A. L.: The therapeutic use of oxygen in acute respiration disturbances, Med. Clin. N. Amer., 9:471, 1925.

Beecher, H. K.: Effects of carbon dioxide hyperventilation on aeration of lungs in patients after operation, Surg., Gynec., and Obstet., 59:734, 1934.

Bergh, G. S.: Prophylaxis of postoperative pulmonary atelectasis, with especial reference to the use of carbon dioxide hyperventilation, Minnesota Med., 16: 105, 1933.

Coryllos, P. N., and G. L. Birnbaum: Alveolar gas exchanges and atelectasis: mechanism of gas absorption in bronchial obstruction, Arch. Surg., 21:1214, 1930.

Henderson, Y., and H. W. Haggard: Hyperventilation of the lungs as a prophylactic measure for pneumonia, Jour. Amer. Med. Asso., 92:434, 1929.

King, D. S.: Postoperative pulmonary complications: II. Carbon dioxide as a preventive in a controlled series, Jour. Amer. Med. Asso., 100:21, 1933.

10

Postoperative Atelectasis

INTRODUCTION

In the majority of instances of atelectasis of the lung following operations, the development of the condition takes place more gradually than that observed in massive pulmonary collapse. The immediate causative factors are: (1) The effect of the anesthetic agent which abolishes the laryngeal and cough reflexes, making it possible for infected secretions from the nasal pharynx to be aspirated into the tracheobronchial tree. If the patient is recumbent and the head lower than the chest, this is less apt to take place. However, in most instances the course of the trachea as it descends leads into the right main bronchus and into the lower lobe, which accounts for the increased frequency of the condition on that side. (2) The abdominal incision reduces the vital capacity and the effectiveness of coughing by weakening the abdominal muscles. The result of both these factors is the tendency for abnormal secretions to stagnate in the tracheobronchial tree and plug a larger or smaller bronchus. After a period of one to three or four days, signs of deficient ventilation may be found in the right lower lobe on physical examination or x-ray. If infection takes place the condition is that of postoperative bronchopneumonia.

TREATMENT

In the prevention of atelectasis in cases in which suppurative disease of the lung is present, repeated bronchoscopy may be indicated. From the standpoint of inhalational therapy, inhalation of the nebulized spray of 2.5 per cent sulfadiazine in ethanolamine solution may accomplish to some degree a disinfection of the involved area. In preventive treatment, as well as when the condition has been discovered after operation, hyperventilation with carbon dioxide or deep-breathing exercises or both are definitely indicated since the walls of the bronchi are separated by these procedures and coughing may be stimulated with the expectoration of large amounts of bronchial exudate. If relief does not follow this procedure, aspiration of the mucus should be attempted either by passing a urethral catheter into the trachea or by bronchoscopy. Previous intubation allows catheter aspiration under more favorable conditions, preventing the larynx from closing in on the catheter.

The recently developed resuscitators that have automatic controls of both negative and positive pressures are safe to use, and may be tried. An important point to emphasize is that few physicians or surgeons are sufficiently experienced in the use of the tracheal catheter to aspirate secretions in the tracheobronchial tree, especially with previous intubation.

BIBLIOGRAPHY

Beecher, H. K.: Effects of carbon dioxide hyperventilation on aeration of lungs in patients after operation, Surg., Gynec., and Obstet., **59**:734, 1934.

Bergh, G. S.: Prophylaxis of postoperative pulmonary atelectasis, with especial reference to the use of carbon dioxide hyperventilation, Minnesota Med., **16**: 105-119, 1933.

Boothby, W. M., W. R. Lovelace, and Charles W. Mayo: The use of oxygen and oxygen-helium, with special reference to surgery, Surg. Clin. N. Amer., **20**: 1107-1168, 1940.

Christie, R. V.: Therapeutic use of carbon dioxide, Canad. Med. Asso. Jour., **27**: 289, 1932.

Coryllos, P. N., and G. L. Birnbaum: Alveolar gas exchanges and atelectasis: mechanism of gas absorption in bronchial obstruction, Arch. Surg., **21**:1214-1281, 1930.

Evans, J. H.: The preoperative and postoperative use of oxygen, Aneth. and Analg., **8**:287, 1929.

Gillespie, N. A.: Endotracheal Anesthesia, Madison, University of Wisconsin Press, 1941.

Henderson, Yandell: Acapnia as a factor in postoperative shock atelectasis and pneumonia, Jour. Amer. Med. Asso., **95**:572-575, 1930.

Henderson, Yandell, and Howard W. Haggard: Hyperventilation of the lungs as a prophylactic measure for pneumonia, Jour. Amer. Med. Asso., **92**:434-436, 1929.

King, Donald S.: Postoperative pulmonary complications: II. Carbondioxide as a preventive in a controlled series, Jour. Amer. Med. Asso., **100**:21-27, 1933.

Schmidt, H. W., L. H. Mousel, and S. W. Harrington: Postoperative atelectasis; clinical aspects and a review of cases, Jour. Amer. Med. Asso., **120**:895, 1942.

Waters, R. M.: Tracheobronchial toilet, Brit. Jour. Anæsth., **18**:1, 1942.

11

Bronchial Asthma

DEFINITION

Bronchial asthma is a disease in which the circular muscles surrounding the smaller bronchi suddenly contract, narrowing their lumen and causing an increased resistance to the flow of air in and out of the lung. Other factors which are involved in the production of this classic example of obstructive dyspnea are swelling of the bronchial mucous membrane and the formation of mucus which also tend to block the passage of air. The disease manifests itself in attacks in which the patient develops a characteristic wheezing type of breathing. In some cases the condition may become chronic and a severe continuous form of difficult breathing takes place, called *status asthmaticus*.

Bronchial asthma is due to the existence of an allergic state, in which the patient becomes hypersensitive to some substance with which he comes into contact, resulting in the most serious manifestation of allergy; namely, spasm of the bronchial muscle and swelling of the mucous membrane. Removal of the offending agent in favorable cases results in a disappearance of the disease. In many instances, however, the cause of the condition is not discovered and more or less recurrent severe dyspnea results. In patients with severe asthma in whom no etiologic agent can be discovered, persisting bronchial spasm may result in prolonged suffering and in pathologic damage to the lung. Although the allergic state of the individual should be investigated carefully, emphasis on this therapeutic approach should not exclude physiologically directed treatment, especially since inhalational therapy may be successful not only in relieving the subjective symptoms but also in preventing the pathologic consequences of obstructive dyspnea, especially a state of chronic overdistention of the lung called pulmonary emphysema.

PATHOLOGIC PHYSIOLOGY

The initial effect of breathing through a constricted orifice is an almost instantaneous sensation of dyspnea which is not due to any decrease in the amount of oxygen in the blood but to an increase in the physical effort necessary to draw air into the lung. Patients with asthma increase their pulmonary ventilation at first as a result of reflex stimulation of proprioceptive reflexes in the lungs and chest wall; later, the consequences of obstructive dyspnea lead to pathologic changes in the lung which are responsible for anoxia, which then becomes a contributory cause of dyspnea and in addition exercises a harmful influence.

Physiologic studies on obstructive dyspnea in animals have contributed to our understanding of the mechanics of respiration in patients with bronchial asthma. When the larynx of a dog is constricted in its lumen to one-eighth of an inch, an immediate increase in the negative intrapleural pressure takes place during the inspiratory cycle, obviously necessary in order to suck air past the point of obstruction. As this pathologically elevated intrapulmonary pressure persists over a long period of time, it exercises a cupping action on the pulmonary capillaries and on the intrathoracic bronchi, which causes an exudation of serum into the alveoli and an outpouring of mucus from the bronchial mucous membrane. Both these factors interfere with absorption of oxygen. As the lung becomes progressively congested and edematous there is a marked increase in the physical effort to breathe, due both to the original obstruction and an increasingly engorged lung. Areas of emphysema appear in the periphery of the lung and pulmonary edema finally takes place, especially at the base of the lung.

This sequence of events occurs during the inhalation of air under a negative pressure of 6 cm. of water, or with resistance interposed to inspiration only. However, no sign of damage to the lung takes place when a comparable resistance to expiration is inserted, or when air is exhaled against a positive pressure of 6 cm. of water, provided inspiration takes place freely. It is as a result of obstruction during the inspiratory cycle that swelling of the bronchial mucous membrane and alveolar ducts produces areas in which the inhaled atmosphere does not come into contact with the pulmonary capillaries, with the production of anoxia, due to the fact that the blood passes through unventilated alveoli. Pathologically elevated negative intrapleural pressure has been demonstrated at the end of inspiration in a patient with severe bronchial asthma.

Although there is no diminution in the oxygen saturation of the arterial blood in the beginning of an attack of asthma, in more severe and long-continued bronchial spasm a decrease in the oxygen saturation of the arterial blood takes place, due to the mechanisms which have been described above. In patients with mild or moderate bronchial asthma the carbon-dioxide content of the arterial blood may be slightly lowered, due to the hyperventilation which a constricted passageway produces. If the obstruction in the bronchial lumen, as a result of spasm or edema, is of long duration, carbon-dioxide elevation in the arterial blood may take place together with a serious arterial anoxia.

When the pathologic consequences of obstructive dyspnea are present in the lung, the inhalation of oxygen-enriched atmospheres decreases the volume of breathing and maintains a higher oxygen saturation in the arterial blood. However, the inhalation of 100 per cent oxygen at the start of an attack of asthma does not diminish the dyspnea since the primary cause of the sensation of difficult breathing is simply the mechanical effort necessary to pull air or oxygen past the point of obstruction. In fact, there is a slight increase in the physical pressure required to breathe oxygen as compared to air in early uncomplicated obstruction, because of the greater specific gravity of oxygen as compared to air. The function of molecular weight of gases in obstructive dyspnea has been clarified by the introduction of helium as a therapeutic agent, used in conjunction with oxygen to lessen the physical effort of breathing.

The velocity of movement of a gas through a constricted orifice is inversely proportional to the square root of the molecular weight of the gas, as shown in the accompanying illustration. Conversely, the heavier the gas the greater will be the pressure required to pass it beyond a point of obstruction. The factor of viscosity is not involved in localized obstruction but if the constriction were continued in a linear direction, Poiseuille's law would then become applicable. To the extent that viscosity itself becomes an influence, there is no advantage in substituting helium for nitrogen, since the latter is slightly less viscous.

Since helium has a specific gravity one-seventh that of nitrogen, a mixture of 20 per cent oxygen and 80 per cent helium, with a density one-third that of air, was employed in the treatment of clinical conditions characterized by obstructive dyspnea. When this mixture was tested by passing it through a narrowed orifice, it was found that the pressure required to move a unit volume of gas was almost one-half that necessary for the passage of a similar volume of air or oxygen through constricted orifices.

When a normal individual was allowed to breathe air through a one-eighth inch orifice the sensation of dyspnea began immediately, but when a mixture of 10 per cent oxygen and 90 per cent helium was substituted the difficulty of breathing was instantly diminished. How-

$$\frac{\text{VELOCITY} \begin{cases} \text{HELIUM 80\%} \\ \text{OXYGEN 20\%} \end{cases}}{\text{VELOCITY AIR}} = \frac{\sqrt{\text{SP. GR. AIR}}}{\sqrt{\text{SP. GR.} \begin{cases} \text{HELIUM 80\%} \\ \text{OXYGEN 20\%} \end{cases}}} =$$

$$\frac{\sqrt{1.0}}{\sqrt{.3315}} = \frac{1.0}{.576} = \frac{1.78}{1.0}$$

Fig. 9. Relative increase in velocity of helium-oxygen mixture as compared to air, due to difference in specific gravity.

ever, if 10 per cent oxygen had been inhaled for more than a short period, dyspnea would have been stimulated by oxygen-want. The effect of inhalation of helium-oxygen mixtures in obstruction of the respiratory passageway was studied in animals. These experiments, carried out under full anesthesia, showed that an 80 per cent helium–20 per cent oxygen mixture could be inhaled with a smaller negative pressure during inspiration than was required when air was inhaled in the presence of a constricted larynx. Furthermore, it was decisively shown that when helium-oxygen mixtures were breathed under a positive pressure of 5 cm. of water, the pathologically elevated negative intrapleural pressure during the inspiratory cycle was even more markedly decreased, and the physical effort of inspiration conspicuously diminished.

The physiologic basis for inhaling helium with oxygen in severe bronchial asthma is, therefore, the reduction in the pathologically elevated negative pressure which occurs during the inspiratory cycle, and the prevention of the consequences of a persistently high negative intrapulmonary pressure on the alveoli and on the mucous membrane in the intrathoracic bronchi. The decrease in the negative intrapulmonary pressure diminishes the suction effect on the mucous membrane and the bronchi, and accomplishes also an alleviation of another result of continued bronchial obstruction; namely, the irregular and unequal ventilation of the alveoli which takes place when some areas of the lung are closed off to air although the blood supply continues to them with the consequence that unoxygenated blood is contributed to the aorta.

Since the introduction of helium as a therapeutic gas in 1934, the physiologic basis for its use in asthma and obstructive lesions of the larynx and trachea has been described by the author (Use of Helium as a New Therapeutic Gas; cf. references at end of chapter).

The physical basis for the use of helium was stated as follows: "According to Graham's law, the rate of diffusion of a gas is inversely proportional to the square root of its density. This law applies also to effusion, i.e., the passage of a gas through small orifices, which is especially applicable to the problem here discussed. Since the viscosity of helium is slightly greater than that of nitrogen, there is no reduction in frictional resistance, and Poiseuille's law does not become involved in an explanation of the results. The point involved is that the obstruction exists for a space so limited in extent as to obey the law of diffusion or effusion rather than Poiseuille's law. Under these circumstances the pressure required for moving a mixture of helium and oxygen would be approximately one-half that required for moving air" (Kernan and Barach: Role of Helium in Cases of Obstructive Lesions in the Trachea and Larynx).

However, Dean and Visscher erroneously reported that Barach ignored viscosity: "It might have been supposed that the greater ease of movement of helium mixtures over nitrogen mixtures would be due to lower viscosity. However, the viscosity of helium is actually about 10% greater than that of nitrogen (see Table 1). Another explanation has been given by Barach who says 'Since work is in general proportional to the density, the pressure required to move helium oxygen mixtures in and out of the lung should be decidedly less than nitrogen mixtures.' This statement is not adequate as a generalization since it ignores viscance" (Dean and Visscher: Kinetics of Lung Ventilation).

Dean and Visscher, admitting that less work is performed in breathing a helium-oxygen mixture under conditions of obstruction in the larger airways, state that they found no significant difference of work done between the two mixtures when the normal airway was preserved.

It has been repeatedly stated by the author that during quiet breathing no change is found in intrapulmonary or intratracheal pressure by the substitution of the helium-oxygen mixture for air, but that when dyspnea is stimulated by markedly increasing the volume of ventilation, the work performed is decreased by the substitution of the lighter-than-air gas mixture, which is manifestly more relevant to clinical disorders of respiration. The mechanics of respiration was described, insofar as the effects of substitution of a helium-oxygen mixture for air is concerned, as follows:

"The physical advantage of helium-oxygen mixture over air was demonstrated by subjecting a spirometer to mechanical movement and having it breathe various gases through a fixed orifice. With an orifice of 0.31 inch the tidal air was 1,070 cc. when the spirometer was connected to a mixture of 21 per cent oxygen and 79 per cent helium, and 705 cc. when it was connected to atmospheric air, representing an increase of 50 per cent in spirometer ventilation. When the orifice was altered to 1.75 inch, the increase in spirometer ventilation was 21 per cent, but this was accomplished with a decrease of 23 per cent in pressure during the period that the spirometer was breathing the helium-oxygen mixture. In summary, an atmosphere containing 21 per cent oxygen can be moved with less pressure or in greater volume when the diluent is helium instead of nitrogen; this experiment applies to clinical dyspnea under circumstances in which the respiratory passageway acts as a constricting force."

We quote again: "When a helium-oxygen mixture is substituted for air in a normal subject breathing against resistance, the pressure required to move the helium-oxygen atmosphere is thus substantially less even when the pulmonary ventilation is maintained the same in both instances. In most cases the normal subject responds by a type of breathing which approaches the normal, in other words by increasing the rate and decreasing the depth of breathing. The swifter entrance of the helium-oxygen mixture makes possible a shorter period of inspiration with the consequence that a more normal flow of respiration is achieved with less effort. The patient with asthma generally responds to the inhalation of helium-oxygen mixture with a decrease in tidal air and in total pulmonary ventilation, the explanation being similar to that just presented concerning the response of normal subjects exposed to respiration against resistance . . .

"Helium may, therefore, be used as a vehicle for oxygen in conditions of respiratory obstruction. Theoretically, the oxygen molecule diffuses faster in an atmosphere of helium than it does in nitrogen, which might raise the tension of oxygen in the alveolar air independent of the increased velocity of movement of the helium-oxygen mixture. The usefulness of helium in the absence of constriction in the respiratory passageway would appear to depend on the volume and velocity of the pulmonary ventilation. In severe dyspnea the normal orifice may act as an obstructing force, and under these circumstances similar physiological advantages might be obtained, reduced somewhat by viscosity which would become a factor in obstruction extended in a linear direction" (Barach: The Therapeutic Uses of Gases).

In our experiments it has been shown that the flow of the helium-oxygen mixture through an oxygen regulator with a fixed orifice is 1.7 times the flow of oxygen through the same fixed orifice in the same regulator. This result is an instance of the gas law of effusion, the formula of which is the same as Graham's law quoted above, and has not been acknowledged as a factor in the relief of obstructive dyspnea by Dean and Visscher. These authors state the physical advantage of helium in decreasing the work performed in obstructive breathing as follows: "When a constricted tube, designed to produce turbulence, is placed in series with the trachea, the pressures accompanying ventilation of the lung are altered and the viscous work is increased. When a helium-mixture is substituted for air this work is markedly decreased. . . . Since helium has a higher streamline resistance but a lower turbulent resistance than nitrogen it is obvious that the lower work in moving the helium mixture is due to its higher critical velocity and lower turbulent viscosity. This effect is very large when constrictions are placed in the upper airways." Graham's law was accepted by Maytum, Prickman and Boothby, Eversole, and Behnke and Yarbrough, the latter reporting experiments in spirometer ventilation in which helium-oxygen mixtures were substituted for air.

When a graphic record is made of the pulmonary ventilation on a high-speed drum in patients with severe asthma, a more complete emptying of the atmosphere in the lung has been shown when a mixture of 20 per cent oxygen and 80 per cent helium is compared to air. In some cases the volume of breathing is reduced about 25 per cent, during inhalation of the lighter-than-air mixture. In a few patients with asthma bronchial relaxation persists for some time afterwards. However, in most cases of severe asthmatic dyspnea the difficulty in breathing returns after the first treatment is concluded but repeated inhalations of helium with oxygen promote progressive and cumulative bronchial relaxation, as the pathologic conditions in the bronchi and in the lungs are themselves improved. Although greater relief of the physical effort of breathing is obtained with a helium concentration of 80 per cent and an oxygen concentration of 20 per cent, the degree of anoxia in many patients with intractable asthma and in all cases of status asthmaticus is such as to indicate a higher oxygen concentration, namely, 30 to 35 per cent oxygen with a corresponding diminution in the helium percentage. When this mixture is administered with positive pressure during inspiration and expiration, the loss in the purely physical relief of dyspnea engineered by lowering of the helium concentration is more than made up by the positive pressure which forces the atmosphere into the lungs during inspiration.

Although the maintenance of a normal saturation of the arterial blood with oxygen and an adequate removal of carbon dioxide are basic requirements that determine the volume of breathing in health and disease, another fundamental respiratory equilibrium consists of the maintenance of an accustomed velocity flow of air in and out of the lung. The sensation of the volume of air delivered to the lung per breath is interpreted through the Hering-Breuer reflex arc which is operative in stimulating and terminating normal respiration. Emphasis has been placed upon the fact that a sensation of dyspnea manifests itself immediately after constriction in the respiratory passageway has been induced, paralleled by an instantaneous increase in effort on the part of the respiratory musculature. It is this increased physical effort in breathing that is diminished by substituting helium for nitrogen in the atmosphere. When a helium-oxygen mixture is inhaled under a continuously positive pressure such as from 3 to 6 cm. of water in a helmet hood, the relief of inspiratory dyspnea is much more marked, since the effect of positive pressure during the inspiratory cycle is to blow the gas mixture into the lung. Even during the inhalation of pure oxygen, without helium, the effect of positive pressure during inspiration is a marked decrease in dyspnea in cases where obstruction in the air passages is present.

An additional physiologic advantage of breathing oxygen under positive pressures of 3 to 6 cm. of water in cases in which obstruction is present is that inspiration is achieved in a far shorter period of time which allows a correspondingly longer period in which expiration may proceed, in that way tending to relieve both inspiratory and expiratory dyspnea.

When positive pressure is applied during both cycles of respiration the effect of the positive pressure during expiration is not uncomfortable for the patient. In fact, it has been shown that patients with bronchial asthma, in whom the intrathoracic bronchi constrict markedly during expiration, accompanying the decrease in the total volume of the chest, are benefited by breathing under positive pressure because the lumen of the bronchi under these circumstances is more patent than when breathing is conducted in the absence of positive

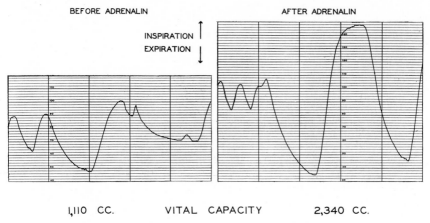

1,110 CC.   VITAL CAPACITY   2,340 CC.

FIG. 10.   Effect of inhalation of 1 cc. of 1:100 adrenalin on the vital capacity of a patient with severe asthma.

pressure. However, when a helium-oxygen mixture or pure oxygen is delivered to the patient through a mask, positive pressure can be provided only during the expiratory cycle. The relief of dyspnea is then due to the mechanical effect of a lighter gas or to the chemical influence of oxygen in lowering the total pulmonary ventilation. When the mask is used, positive pressure in expiration should be kept at a lower range, such as 1 to 2 cm. of water, since a high pressure in expiration alone is not so well tolerated in patients with bronchial asthma as positive pressure during both cycles of respiration. Positive pressure during the *inspiratory cycle* makes for a swift inlet of the helium-oxygen mixture, or pure oxygen, and thus allows a longer period of time for expiration to take place.

The inhalation of the nebulized sprays of 1:100 epinephrine has the advantage over hypodermic administration in that effective relaxation of constricted bronchi may frequently be obtained without systemic effects of the drug. The topical application of bronchodilator substances is preferable for this reason, in addition to its simplicity. In the accompanying illustration, the inhalation of 1 cc. of 1 : 100 adrenalin resulted in an immediate rise in vital capacity from 1,110 cc. to 2,340 cc. The shape of the respiratory tracing reveals the prolonged emptying of the lung during expiration prior to relief of bronchial spasm.

INHALATIONAL THERAPY

Inhalational therapy is indicated in two types of cases: (1) Status asthmaticus, in which continuous bronchial spasm is accompanied by a grave clinical condition in the patient, unrelieved by injection of adrenalin. (2) Intractable asthma, in which frequent seizures of bronchial asthma occur during the day and night with partial or transient relief from epinephrine.

In status asthmaticus the inhalation of an oxygen-enriched atmosphere is indicated to overcome the anoxia from which the patient inevitably suffers. The ideal method of treatment is to place the patient in a helmet-hood apparatus in which a mixture of 30 to 35 per cent oxygen and the remainder helium is administered under a positive pressure of from 3 to 5 cm. of water.

In the early use of helium, patients were kept in the hood for the major part of the time for a period of one to five days. However, subsequent experience showed that breathing the helium-oxygen mixture under positive pressure for two hours, two or three times a day, was also followed by return of sensitiveness to epinephrine and by a disappearance of the asthmatic state when the treatment was continued over a period of three to five days. In 84 cases of status asthmaticus the repeated inhalation of helium-oxygen mixtures was followed by either complete freedom from asthma or very mild asthma in 40 cases; in 36 cases, a return of sensitiveness to epinephrine took place, with a mild or moderate degree of persisting asthma; in 30 patients in this series in whom follow-up observation was satisfactory, 15 maintained either all or a substantial part of their improvement for six months or more. The conclusion was reached that 90 per cent of the 84 patients with status asthmaticus or severe intractable asthma were decisively benefited by a program of helium-oxygen therapy.

Repeated bronchial relaxation, with progressive improvement in the functioning of the respiratory system, as indicated in the preceding section on pathologic physiology, appeared to be responsible for the termination of persistent bronchial spasm. Another mechanism involved in the relief of bronchial asthma by this method of treatment is the consequence of subjective relief of dyspnea in alleviating tension in the central nervous system. The frequency with which spectacular relief of severe asthma at times results from injection of dilaudid is evidence of the rôle which central-nervous-system influences play in maintaining bronchial spasm.

Since the introduction of intravenous injection of aminophyllin in the treatment of status asthmaticus, this drug has been added to a program of helium-oxygen therapy in the therapy of both status asthmaticus and intractable asthma. The difference in the treatment of these two conditions is that the patient with status asthmaticus is generally provided with an oxygen-enriched atmosphere during the periods between helium-oxygen inhalations. Thus, if the patient manifests considerable dyspnea and cyanosis after a two-hour period of helium-oxygen therapy, the oxygen tent or nasal catheter is usually employed until the next helium-oxygen inhalation is due. Aminophyllin was given rectally since it was more convenient for repeated use than intravenous injection, and daily or twice daily administration was combined with repeated inhalations of helium with oxygen in a series of 100 courses of such therapy administered to 71 patients. In the accompanying table, the immediate response to treatment in hospital

TABLE IV

THE EFFECT OF HELIUM-OXYGEN AND AMINOPHYLLIN THERAPY IN HOSPITAL
AND AMBULATORY PATIENTS WITH INTRACTABLE ASTHMA

No. of Cases	Type of Case	No. of Courses of Therapy	Immediate Response to Treatment		
			Disappearance of Asthma or Very Mild Symptoms	Restoration of Epinephrine Sensitivity with Moderated Asthma	Little or No Improvement
26	Hospital	46	34	9	3
45	Ambulatory	54	23	17	14
71		100	57 (57%)	26 (26%)	17 (17%)

Before treatment.

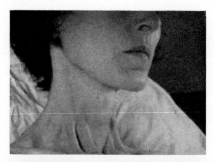

Inspiration.

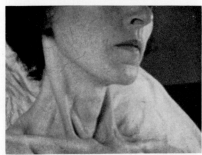

Expiration.

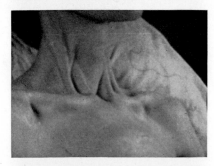

During treatment with helium-oxygen mixtures under positive pressure.

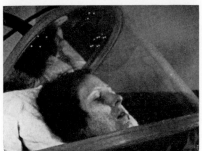

Fig. 11, Part 1

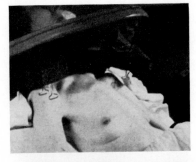

During treatment in
helium-oxygen hood.

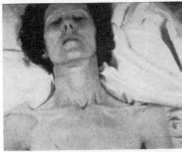

After treatment:
inspiration.

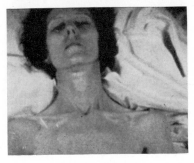

After treatment:
expiration.

Fig. 11, Part 2

and ambulatory patients is presented.[1] It may be seen that in 57 per cent of 100 courses, disappearance of asthma took place or very mild symptoms remained. In 26 per cent of 100 courses of this therapy the response included restoration of sensitivity to epinephrine with the persistence of occasional attacks of asthma of moderate degree. In this group of patients the asthma which persisted after conclusion of treatment generally responded to inhalation of 1 : 100 epinephrine and did not require hypodermic injection of adrenalin. There was little or no improvement in 17 per cent but the larger proportion of cases was contributed by the ambulatory group.

In Table V, the *duration* of improvement after helium-oxygen and aminophyllin therapy is shown in 57 cases who received 91 courses of

TABLE V

DURATION OF IMPROVEMENT AFTER HELIUM-OXYGEN AND AMINOPHYLLIN THERAPY IN HOSPITAL AND AMBULATORY PATIENTS

No. of Cases	Type of Case	No. of Courses of Therapy	Maintenance of All or a Major Pat of Immediate Improvement			
			1 to 4 Weeks	1 to 4 Months	5 to 12 Months	1 Year or More
26	Hospital	44	14	12	10	8
31	Ambulatory	47	22	8	10	7
—		—	—	—	—	—
57	Totals	91	36*	20	20	15

* Many recurrences in this group took place in a relatively small number of cases of severe asthma.

such therapy. In 15 cases there was a maintenance of all or a major part of the immediate improvement for a period of one year or more. It will be seen that in 30 additional cases improvement lasted for one to four months in half and for five to twelve months in the remaining half. In 36 of the 91 courses the improvement lasted less than four weeks, but in this group many recurrences took place in a relatively small number of cases of characteristically recurrent severe asthma.

If the helium-oxygen mixtures are not available, positive pressure

[1] From Barach, A. L.: Jour. Allergy, 14:296, May, 1943.

may be administered with 100 per cent oxygen, under the program outlined below. If it is not possible to employ positive pressure, the continuous inhalation of an oxygen-enriched air atmosphere, such as 50 per cent oxygen for a period of one week, is desirable, to overcome the anoxia and make less likely the chance of respiratory failure. The inhalation of the nebulized solutions of adrenalin and neosynephrin either by the hand bulb or preferably by a stream of oxygen from a high-pressure tank are at times helpful when hypodermic injection of adrenalin is ineffective.

An oxygen-enriched air atmosphere may be provided by an oxygen tent, the catheter in the nasal or oral pharynx, or a mask oxygen apparatus. If the latter is used it is of great importance that a high flow of oxygen from the tank be employed to prevent any negative pressure from developing in the mask. If the injector Meter mask is used a liter flow from the tank of 6 to 8 liters per minute will generally prevent collapse of the collecting bag if the meter is set at 50 per cent oxygen. If the B.L.B. mask is employed it is safer to give 8 to 10 liters per minute in order to prevent collapse of the rebreathing bag and the drawing of air through the sponge-rubber disks at the expense of the patient's own effort. If 100 per cent oxygen is used in severe cases of status asthmaticus a flow of 15 liters of oxygen per minute should be employed in either the Meter or the B.L.B. mask.

The program of inhalational therapy at Presbyterian Hospital has recently been described as follows:[2]

"The patient in severe status asthmaticus was placed continuously in a helium-oxygen hood under a positive pressure of 3 to 5 cm. of water. The majority of the patients who were treated in the hospital were placed in the hood. In ambulatory patients, including clinic and private patients, helium oxygen mixtures were administered with the Meter injector mask.

"The program of treatment for a patient with intractable asthma admitted to the hospital was as follows:

"A rectal injection of 0.5 to 0.6 Gm. of aminophyllin in 20 cc. of water was given immediately. The patient then inhaled the spray of 0.5 cc. of 1 : 100 epinephrine, vaporized by a stream of 5 liters per minute of oxygen from a high-pressure tank to a nebulizer.[3] In some

2 Barach, A. L.: Jour. Allergy, 14:296, May, 1943.

3 The nebulizer generally used was that made by the Vaponefrin Company (see section on methods). The form of epinephrine employed was in most instances that contained in Vaponefrin solution.

instances the inhalation of the epinephrine spray was followed by inhalation of the spray from 1 cc. of 1 per cent neosynephrin. Hypodermic injection of adrenalin was not used because a refractory state had already taken place. In patients who were very excitable or nervous a hypodermic injection of 1 or 2 mg. of dilaudid was then given. In some cases 2 mg. of dilaudid were placed in the aminophyllin solution administered by rectum. Following the epinephrine spray and administration of aminophyllin the patient was put in the helium-oxygen hood for two hours. The nebulizer was used more frequently when it was necessary. In most cases no more helium-oxygen therapy was given that day. In a few very severe patients an additional two hours was given in the evening. The oxygen concentration was generally set at 25 per cent but in patients with pulmonary emphysema this was increased to 35 per cent, the remainder helium. A positive pressure of 3 to 4 cm. of water was employed in most cases. In a few patients with severe inspiratory dyspnea the positive pressure was raised to 5 or 6 cm. In the evening before bedtime a rectal instillation of 0.5 or 0.6 Gm. of aminophyllin was repeated. In a number of patients to whom dilaudid was not given on admission, it was added to the evening aminophyllin mixture. In cases who had persisting severe asthma, dilaudid was added to the evening dose of rectal aminophyllin for two or three or sometimes four nights.

"The combined use of aminophyllin by rectum and helium-oxygen inhalations in the hood twice a day was kept up for a five-day period and then abruptly stopped in most instances. In a number of patients the rectal injection of aminophyllin was continued at home for a period of one to three weeks after discharge from the hospital.

"During the period of residence in the hospital potassium iodide in a saturated solution was given, 1 cc. three times a day, and after discharge 1 cc. twice a day for a period of two or three weeks and then a maintenance dose of 1 cc. every evening before retiring.

"Hypodermic injection of adrenalin was dispensed with in the majority of patients. The result of treatment was not considered satisfactory if it was necessary to employ hypodermic injection of adrenalin. The patient was given a nebulizer with 1 : 100 epinephrine and instructed to use it if wheezing or a paroxysm of asthma took place. If the asthmatic seizure was so severe as not to be controlled by inhalation of the spray of epinephrine, hypodermic injection of adrenalin was allowed.

"In office practice these patients were given a spray of nebulized

1 : 100 epinephrine and a rectal injection of 0.5 to 0.6 Gm. of aminophyllin, followed by inhalation of a helium-oxygen mixture through the Meter mask, the flow of the mixture being set between 7 and 9 liters per minute, for a one-hour period. This was continued for a five-day period, during which time the patient was instructed in the administration of aminophyllin by rectum, in order that it might be continued for a period of one to four weeks after the course of office treatment. A tank of 20 per cent oxygen and 80 per cent helium was used, but an addition of 1 to 2 liters a minute of oxygen was added through a Y-tube to the helium-oxygen mixture, thus increasing the percentage of oxygen in the inspired air to 22 to 25 per cent oxygen. In patients who had pulmonary emphysema the oxygen proportion was increased to 3 or 4 liters a minute with 7 liters of the helium-oxygen mixture."

BIBLIOGRAPHY

Barach, A. L.: Use of helium as a new therapeutic gas, Proc. Soc. Exper. Biol. and Med., 32:462, 1934.

Barach, A. L.: The use of helium as a therapeutic gas, Anesth. and Analg., 14:210, 1935.

Barach, A. L.: The use of helium in the treatment of asthma and obstructive lesions in the larynx and trachea, Ann. Int. Med., 9:739, 1935.

Barach, A. L.: Effects of the inhalation of helium mixed with oxygen on the mechanics of respiration, Jour. Clin. Invest., 15:47, 1936.

Barach, A. L.: The therapeutic use of helium, Jour. Amer. Med. Asso., 105:1273, 1936.

Barach, A. L.: Physiological methods in the diagnosis and treatment of asthma and emphysema, Ann. Int. Med., 12:454, 1938.

Barach, A. L.: The Therapeutic Uses of Gases: Modern Medical Therapy in General Practice. Edited by D. P. Barr. Baltimore, Williams & Wilkins Co., 1940.

Barach, A. L.: Repeated bronchial relaxation in the treatment of intractable asthma, Jour. Allergy, 14:296, 1943.

Barach, A. L., and H. A. Cromwell: Recent advances in oxygen and helium therapy with special reference to the treatment of bronchial asthma, M. Clin. N. Amer., 24:621, 1940.

Barach, A. L., and Paul Swenson: Effect of breathing gases under positive pressure on lumens of small and medium-sized bronchi, Arch. Int. Med., 63:946-948, 1939.

Behnke, A. R., and O. D. Yarbrough: Respiratory resistance, oil-water solubility and mental effects of argon, compared with helium and nitrogen, Amer. Jour. Physiol., 126:409, 1939.

Dean, R. B., and M. B. Visscher: Kinetics of lung ventilation, Amer. Jour. Physiol., 134:450, 1941.

Eversole, U. H.: The use of helium in anesthesia, Jour. Amer. Med. Asso., 110:878, 1938.

Kernan, J. D., and A. L. Barach: Role of helium in cases of obstructive lesions in the trachea and larynx, Arch. Otolaryngol., 26:419-447, 1937.

Kerr, W. J.: Discussion of paper by Barach, A. L., on The Therapeutic Use of Helium, Jour. Amer. Med. Asso., 107:1273, 1936.

Maytum, C. K.: Helium and oxygen mixture in status asthmaticus, Jour. Allergy, 10:266, 1939.

Maytum, C. K.: Helium and oxygen treatment of intractable asthma, Proc. Staff Meet., Mayo Clin., 13:788, 1938; Modern Med., 7:32, 1939.

Maytum, C. K., L. E. Prickman, and W. M. Boothby: Use of helium and oxygen in the treatment of severe intractable asthma, Proc. Staff Meet., Mayo Clin., 10:785, 1935.

Meakins, J. C., and H. W. Davies: Respiratory Function in Disease, London, Oliver & Boyd, 1925.

Metz, C. W., A. A. Wearner, and A. E. Evans: Therapeutic use of helium, South. Med. Jour., 33:34, 1939.

Oertel, M. J.: In Von Ziemssen's Handbook of Therapeutics, Translated from the German by J. B. Yeo, William Wood & Co., 1885.

Poulton, E. P.: Left-sided heart failure with pulmonary edema treated with the pulmonary plus pressure machine, Lancet, 231:983, 1936.

Richards, D. W., Jr., A. L. Barach, and H. A. Cromwell: Use of vaporized bronchodilator solutions in asthma and emphysema; a continuous inhalation method for severe asthmatic states, Amer. Jour. Med. Sci., 199:225, 1940.

Rowe, A. H.: Bronchial asthma, its diagnosis and treatment, Jour. Amer. Med. Asso., 111:1827, 1938.

Schwartz, A. L.: The relief of status asthmaticus by helium, Cincinnati Jour. Med., 19:122, 1938.

Segal, M. S.: Inhalation therapy in the treatment of serious respiratory disease, New England Jour. Med., 229:235, 1943.

12

Obstructive Lesions in the Larynx, Trachea, and Bronchi

INTRODUCTION

Obstructive dyspnea may be caused by lesions in the upper air passages, such as: (1) Swelling of the mucous membrane due to infection or irritation, (2) tumors, (3) enlarged glands or aneurysms, (4) foreign bodies. In adults, due to the relatively larger lumen of the respiratory tubal passage, obstructive dyspnea is less common as a result of infection than it is in children. In the latter, however, difficult breathing frequently progresses to the point of requiring tracheotomy, as in acute laryngitis or croup. Infection with *H. influenzae* bacillus may result in acute swelling of the glottis with severe obstructive dyspnea. In other cases, a descending infection may be present with varying degrees of inflammation of the smaller bronchi, called capillary bronchitis or tracheobronchitis. In adults metastatic cancer with external pressure on the bronchi, primary cancer of the bronchus, tumors in the larynx, and aneurysm are the more common causes of obstructive dyspnea.

PATHOLOGIC PHYSIOLOGY

The pathologic physiology of obstructive dyspnea was described in part in Chapter 11, Bronchial Asthma. It may be pointed out here that when obstruction is present within the thorax, respiration modifies the degree of obstruction, since the lumen of the bronchi enlarge on inspiration and contract during expiration. In asthmatic dyspnea inspiration is generally short and forcible, whereas expiration is prolonged. The long-drawn-out character of expiration may be explained by the constriction of the bronchi during the expiratory cycle. A slow exhalation appears to be more efficient than a more powerful and abrupt expiratory effort which might produce an even greater narrowing of the smaller bronchi and trap air in the alveoli. In fact, a prolonged expiration in which the patient maintains an arbitrary back pressure by exhaling through partially closed lips will in many instances clear wheezing râles during mild asthma. In severe bronchial asthma forcible inspiration results in a distention of the alveoli, and in the succeeding expiration incomplete emptying of the alveolar cells takes place.

When the respiratory passageway is not exposed to varying intrathoracic pressures and consequently does not enlarge during inspiration and constrict during expiration, its lumen remains relatively constant; it is also protected from alteration in size by strong cartilaginous rings. In obstructive dyspnea due to lesions in the extrathoracic larynx and trachea, inspiration and expiration are both prolonged. As a result of the lengthened period of the inspiratory cycle carbon dioxide gradually accumulates in the blood during this period and is responsible for further increase in depth of breathing until respiratory fatigue takes place. The increased percentage of carbon dioxide found in the alveolar air, however, allows a greater elimination of carbon dioxide per breath and is not necessarily an indication that the acid-base equilibrium has shifted to the acid side. Retention of carbon dioxide and increased blood acidity may take place as a result of prolonged and severe obstructive dyspnea in which pathologic changes in the lung have been produced.

The sequence of events in the production of pulmonary congestion and edema due to tracheal stenosis may be briefly reviewed. There is an immediate increase in the negative intrapleural pressure during the inspiratory cycle. The resistance of the pulmonary bed is lessened, and there is first an increase in pulmonary blood flow. Blood continues to enter the lungs through the right ventricle but the passage of blood through the lungs into the left auricle and from the left ventricle into the extrathoracic aorta is hindered by a high negative pressure within the chest during the inspiratory cycle. During expiration, as powerful expiratory movements are made, the intrapleural pressure approaches that of the atmosphere. The progressive accumulation of blood in the lung results in an increase in pressure in the pulmonary capillaries with a greater hydrostatic pressure directed outward. The high negative pressure within the lung during inspiration exerts a direct suction on the pulmonary capillaries, tending to cause exudation of serum. The progressive increase in engorgement of the lungs necessitates increased effort which results in a vicious circle of progressive elevation in the intrapulmonary negative pressure that encourages further development of pulmonary edema. Anoxia becomes more and more severe as diffusion of oxygen through the edematous pulmonary membrane is retarded, with additional factors of rapid shallow breathing and inadequate ventilation of alveoli that are closed off by swollen alveolar ducts and bronchioles. Increased permeability of the pulmonary capillaries results from the progressively severe anoxia which is the final cause of respiratory failure.

INHALATIONAL THERAPY

Although the treatment of respiratory obstruction depends in a large measure on the pathogenesis of the condition, inhalational therapy is primarily directed to measures which will lower the pathologically elevated negative intrapulmonary pressure. The provision of positive pressure continuously during both phases of the respiratory cycle in a helmet-hood apparatus is the method of choice. Although mixtures of 25 to 30 per cent oxygen in helium are more effective in relieving dyspnea, pure oxygen may also be employed with expectation of very considerable benefit when positive pressures between 3 and 6 cm. of water are provided.

In children with acute inflammatory swelling of the larynx, helium-oxygen inhalation, preferably with positive pressure, may avert tracheotomy. However, the swift increase in the pathology that sometimes takes place makes it necessary for cases of this type to be under close supervision in order to make possible an immediate tracheotomy should complete or almost complete closure of the larynx or glottis take place. Since apprehension and subjective distress will increase the pulmonary ventilation and therefore further elevate the pathologically elevated negative pressure present in the lungs, adequate sedation is indicated to diminish unnecessary respiratory effort due to excitement.

If helium is not available 50 to 100 per cent oxygen may be administered under a pressure of 2 to 4 cm. of water with very considerable relief. The atmosphere should contain a relatively high humidity and therefore Baralime instead of shell natron is employed in order not to absorb moisture. The patient is kept in the helmet-hood apparatus until the obstruction is relieved by subsidence of the infection. By gradually lowering the pressure from 4 to 1 cm., and then to that of the atmosphere, the return of a patent lumen can be easily verified. In these cases the attempt to provide nourishment by mouth is unwise. It generally promotes dyspnea and coughing and in that way actually aggravates the obstruction by increasing the swelling of the mucous membrane. Subcutaneous administration of 5 per cent glucose in normal saline is adequate to take care of the needs of these patients for periods of one to two days.

The problem is made difficult in children and infants by the constant necessity of giving the child confidence and reassurance sufficient to free him from struggling against the therapy. This can be obtained only when expert technical supervision and sympathetic nursing care are provided. Under these circumstances a severe degree of obstruction in the larynx may frequently be compensated for by administration of positive pressure, either with a helium-oxygen atmosphere or 100 per cent oxygen. In small infants positive pressure may be difficult to apply with the helmet-hood apparatus. Helium-oxygen mixtures may then be used with the patient entirely enclosed in a leak-tight tent, or one with closure at neck. In the latter case, a higher flow of helium with oxygen may be necessary.

In milder cases of narrowing of the larynx which are seen in croup, periodic inhalations of steam in a so-called croup tent at times give relief, probably due to a loosening of tenacious mucus by contact of the warm moist air with the laryngeal mucous membrane. However, when the obstruction becomes more severe reliance should not be placed on steam alone. Anoxia is a serious influence when the breathing becomes rapid and shallow, and constitutes an urgent indication for the inhalation of 50 to 70 per cent oxygen. An open-top tent may frequently be employed under these circumstances, since it will provide a high oxygen concentration at a flow of 6 to 8 liters per minute, and at the same time a relatively high humidity. By decreasing the volume of breathing as a result of inhalation of a 50 per cent oxygen atmosphere, the child is not only saved the effort of continued dyspnea and therefore the consequences of increased negative intrapulmonary pressures but he also avoids the consequences of severe anoxia, which ultimately leads to respiratory failure.

An apparatus which vaporizes a considerable quantity of water is being perfected at this time by Walton, and may prove useful in conjunction with oxygen-tent therapy in patients with tracheobronchitis. In this method a cool oxygen-enriched atmosphere may be provided with a relative humidity as high as 80 per cent. The hot air so often obtained in a croup tent is not desirable, since it is the moisture which is probably the therapeutically effective agent in steam inhalation. The nasal catheter is generally not well tolerated by children, either in the nasal or oral pharynx, although it may be used with good supervision. Mask oxygen therapy is also not apt to be comfortable to little children as it requires more cooperation than they are able to give. Furthermore, the special precaution of avoiding negative pressures in the mask must be observed at all times in obstructive dyspnea.

Although a relative humidity of 60 to 90 per cent may be helpful in tracheobronchitis, the temperature should not be above room temperature except in very young infants. In order to obtain a relatively high humidity with temperatures that are not excessively elevated, half of the ice may be removed and the air circulation set at the low or mid-position of the rheostat in the motor-blower closed oxygen tents. This provides air movement of the oxygen-enriched atmosphere surrounding the child, without undue precipitation of water vapor on ice.

Although the application of helium-oxygen therapy in infants and young children with severe obstructive dyspnea is a difficult clinical and technical problem, it has been clearly shown to have averted tracheotomy in 5 of 16 cases in which dyspnea was present which was sufficiently severe to constitute an indication for this procedure. A conservative attitude toward tracheotomy is therefore warranted in those patients in whom it is possible to supply expert technical supervision. However, anxiety unrelieved by sedation and by effective treatment of dyspnea results in restlessness and struggling, which undoubtedly promotes progressive swelling of the mucous membrane of the larynx, and in those cases in which psychic and physiologic distress cannot be controlled, early tracheotomy is the method of choice.

Unfortunately, complications arise from tracheotomy itself, not the least of which is oozing of mucus from the bronchi and serum from the alveoli after sudden termination of the backward pressure which the patient had engineered to accomplish adequate ventilation during expiration. When tracheotomy has been performed after obstructive dyspnea, a tracheotomy tube should be inserted which projects beyond the neck margins in order that expiration may be conducted under positive pressure of 2 to 5 cm. of water and in that way avert the necessity for continued aspiration of fluid from the trachea and bronchi. This may be done by breathing through an inspiratory valve and

Before treatment: expiration.

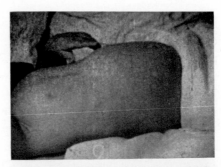

Before treatment: inspiration.

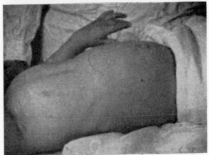

During treatment with helium-oxygen mixtures under positive pressure.

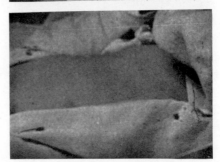

FIG. 12, Part 1

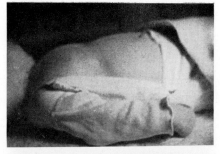

Before treatment: inspiration.

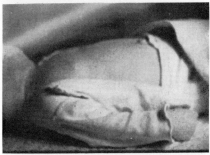

Before treatment: expiration.

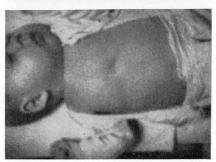

During treatment with helium-oxygen mixtures under positive-pressure inspiration.

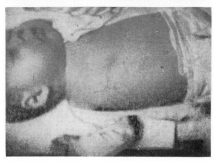

Expiration.

FIG. 12, Part 2

exhaling into a water bottle with a glass tube inserted 2, 3, or 5 cm., as is found desirable.[1]

If the decision has been made to employ inhalational therapy, either with a simple oxygen-enriched atmosphere, with positive pressure in a hood, or with a helium-oxygen atmosphere, a far better opportunity to avoid tracheotomy is obtained if the child is disturbed as little as possible. This requires a willingness to employ codeine and pheno-barbital in doses sufficient to accomplish either sleep or a relaxed state. If a high oxygen atmosphere is provided there is no justification in being concerned with the development of anoxia as a result of depression of the respiratory center. Another frequent cause of apparent failure of inhalational therapy is the attempt to introduce nourishment through the mouth as well as the performance of physical examinations that are not urgently indicated.

Obstructive dyspnea in adults is handled with far greater effectiveness due to willingness on the part of the patients to cooperate and through their understanding of the aim of treatment. Even in severe constriction of the trachea or larger bronchi which may take place as a result of intrathoracic metastatic tumors or aneurysm, the dyspnea can be controlled by the continuous application of positive pressures of 4 to 6 cm. of water, preferably in a helium-oxygen atmosphere containing 20 to 30 per cent oxygen and 70 to 80 per cent helium, but also with considerable effectiveness in an atmosphere of 100 per cent oxygen. Many cases have been observed in which marked supra- and infrasternal retraction was present with pronounced sucking-in of the soft parts of the intercostal spaces during inspiration, in which either complete or very marked relief was provided by a positive-pressure hood. If tumors exerting compression are radiosensitive, patients treated in this way may be tided over a period of difficult breathing until recession of the growth makes such therapy no longer necessary.

If a therapeutic procedure such as the introduction of wire into an aneurysm is contemplated, the helium-oxygen hood may be employed both before and after the operation to tide the patient over a period of severe obstructive breathing. In some cases of swelling of the larynx and bronchi after either laryngoscopy or bronchoscopy, the use of the helium-oxygen hood with positive pressure will maintain a patent airway until the inflammation has receded. When the technical supervision of this type of positive-pressure hood therapy is adequate,

---

[1] A special apparatus has been made by Pilling and Sons, Philadelphia, to combat the post-tracheotomy oozing from the tracheobronchial tree and lungs.

it should be possible to compensate for narrowing of the larynx or bronchi of one-fourth the normal diameter.

The use of the nebulized solutions of 1: 100 epinephrine and of 1 per cent neosynephrin is indicated in many cases of obstructive dyspnea in order to overcome bronchial spasm, and also by vasoconstriction to increase the patency of the bronchial lumen. Although these substances may be inhaled, after being vaporized by the pressure of a hand-bulb nebulizer, it is more effective, as described in the section on asthma, to create a nebulized vapor by running a stream of 4 to 5 liters per minute of oxygen through the end of the nebulizer. In the absence of definite bronchial spasm, inhalation of epinephrine solutions should not be continued but the nebulin of neosynephrin is frequently found helpful and may be repeated at intervals of two to three hours in doses of 0.5 to 1.0 cc. of the 1 per cent solution.

BIBLIOGRAPHY

Barach, A. L.: The use of helium as a new therapeutic gas, Anesth. and Analg., **14**:210, 1935.

Barach, A. L.: The use of helium in the treatment of asthma and obstructive lesions in the larynx and trachea, Ann. Int. Med., **9**:739-765, 1935.

Barach, A. L.: Obstructive lesions in the trachea and bronchi, Modern Medical Therapy in General Practice, Baltimore, Williams & Wilkins Co., 1940.

Boothby, W. M., W. R. Lovelace, and Charles W. Mayo: The use of oxygen and oxygen-helium, with special reference to surgery, Surg. Clin. N. Amer., **20**: 1107-1168, 1940.

Boothby, W. M., and H. L. Moersch: The value of oxygen following bronchoscopy in children, Arch. Otolaryngol., **6**:542, 1927.

Davies, H. W., J. S. Haldane, and J. G. Priestley: The response to respiratory resistance, Jour. Physiol., **53**:60, 1919.

Davison, F. W.: Some observations on the control of temperature and humidity in oxygen tents, Ann. Otol., Rhinol., and Laryngol., **49**:1083, 1940.

Delfs, G.: Helium-oxygen inhalation—recent advances in treatment of laryngitis and tracheitis, Arch. Dis. Childhood, **16**:52, 1941.

Eversole, Urban H.: The use of helium in anesthesia, Jour. Amer. Med. Asso., **110**:878, 1938.

Haines, S. F., and W. M. Boothby: Value of oxygen treatment after thyroidectomy, Amer. Jour. Surg., **6**:1, 1929.

Kernan, J. D., and A. L. Barach: Role of helium in cases of obstructive lesions in trachea and larynx, Arch. Otolaryngol., **26**:419, 1937.

Moore, R. L., and C. A. L. Binger: (a) Observations on resistance to the flow of blood to and from the lungs, Jour. Exper. Med., **45**:655, 1927. (b) Response to respiratory resistance: a comparison of the effects produced by partial obstruction in the inspiratory and expiratory phases of respiration, Jour. Exper. Med., **45**:1065, 1927

Woodman, M.: On the control of air pressure in the lungs after tracheotomy, Jour. Laryng. and Otol., **50**:214, 1935.

13

Pulmonary Emphysema

DEFINITION

Pulmonary emphysema is a disease in which progressive distention of the alveoli takes place with rupture of the pulmonary membrane and the formation of enlarged air sacs of greater or less degree. A so-called functional form of pulmonary emphysema takes place after any form of obstructive dyspnea, especially severe asthma. Under these circumstances the constriction of the smaller bronchi during expiration creates a valvelike obstruction that admits air without allowing it an exit at the same rate. Overdistention of the lung temporarily takes place, but with the subsidence of the cause of the respiratory obstruction the alveoli may resume their normal state. However, pulmonary emphysema as a primary disease is due to a degenerative change in the alveolar epithelium. Narrowing of the bronchioles appears to be consistently present, either due to muscle spasm, swelling of the bronchial mucous membrane, or torsion of the alveolar ducts. As a result of the atrophic change in the alveolar membrane stretching of the lungs during inspiration results ultimately in tearing of their walls and consequent merging of air cells. The outstanding symptoms are dyspnea, cough, and cyanosis.

PATHOLOGIC PHYSIOLOGY

In the normal individual the elastic recoil of the pulmonary membrane results in an effortless decrease in the volume of the lungs. The chief factor in the disturbance in respiratory function in pulmonary emphysema is the loss of the elastic element in the pulmonary epithelium as a result of either local infection or atrophy. During expiration the lungs do not empty passively because of the absence of this mechanism of elastic recoil of the lungs, and active muscular effort is required. At the end of expiration the pressure in the intrapleural space

114

approaches that of the atmosphere and this consequently retards the expiratory ascent of the diaphragm. In addition, the overdistended lung tends gradually to flatten the diaphragm, with the result that inspiration does not produce the enlargement of the volume of the chest that occurs in normal individuals. For this reason the chest is elevated by the muscles in the neck and the intercostal muscles in order to effect an increase in lung volume. The stretching of the pulmonary membrane during inspiration results in a further interference with nutrition and increases the likelihood of weakening the wall with subsequent rupture.

As air cells are joined by tearing of their walls, and as many of the pulmonary capillaries have been destroyed, there are large areas of lung in which there is diminished circulation of blood through them, with resultant anoxia. Since the elastic element in the lung tissue has been lost, the expansion of the chest affects the periphery of the lung directly and the region at the hilus to a lesser extent. Areas at the surface of the lung are therefore overdistended, and the pulmonary capillaries that course through them are often collapsed. Although hyperventilation takes place the result is inefficient in providing oxygen to the arterial blood. An important factor in the production of arterial anoxia is the presence of some degree of obstruction in the smaller bronchioles and the alveolar ducts. If there is partial or complete closure of some of the alveoli, unoxygenated blood will pass into the aorta. The shallow type of breathing and the decreased vital capacity add to the lowering of the arterial oxygen saturation which in many cases falls to levels between 60 and 80 per cent. The carbon-dioxide content in both arterial and venous blood is also elevated under these circumstances. It is characteristic of this disease that the patient does not respond to inhalation of 5 to 7 per cent carbon dioxide with as striking an increase in volume of breathing as takes place in normal subjects.

However, in some patients with pulmonary emphysema and pulmonary fibrosis the arterial oxygen saturation may be normal and nearly normal even in the presence of severe dyspnea. The interpretation of this finding is comparable in some respects to the situation in cardiac dyspnea due to congestive heart failure. In these patients it may generally be shown that an augmented volume of breathing is maintained with the result that arterial anoxemia is thereby avoided; a lack of understanding of this mechanism has prompted some observers to assume that anoxia was not significantly involved in the production of the dyspnea of pulmonary emphysema and pulmonary fibrosis. It has been shown in a number of patients that continuous inhalation of an oxygen-enriched atmosphere, such as 50 per cent oxygen, is regularly followed by progressive and in many instances almost complete relief of dyspnea as long as the patient lives in the oxygen-enriched atmosphere.

An illustration of the response of a patient with advanced pulmonary emphysema to inhalation of oxygen will serve to explain the mechanism of this type of dyspnea as well as the procedure of oxygen therapy itself. An arterial oxygen puncture at rest revealed a saturation of the arterial blood of 92.9 per cent oxygen, a small decrease from the 95 per cent normal level. At that time the pulmonary ventilation was 10.7 liters per minute. The immediate effect of inhalation of 100 per cent oxygen was a rise in the arterial oxygen saturation to 100 per cent, with an additional increase in physically dissolved oxygen of approximately 1 cc. per 100 cc. of blood. The pulmonary ventilation dropped to 7.6 liters per minute, with complete relief of the sensation of dyspnea.

The pathophysiologic disturbances in breathing referred to above and the impairment of the mechanism for diffusing oxygen into the lungs are responsible for increased pulmonary ventilation in most of these patients, and the maintenance of an adequate respiratory exchange is the fundamental physiologic problem. Expressed differently, it may be said that although mechanical difficulties in breathing initiate proprioceptive reflexes from the lungs, it is noteworthy that a 35 per cent decrease in the volume of breathing was followed by a disappearance of dyspnea. It is characteristic of patients with severe pulmonary emphysema that a heightened volume of breathing exists at rest and although this degree of hyperventilation, namely between 10 and 12 liters per minute, does not promote the sensation of difficult breathing in the normal individual, it is consistently productive of dyspnea in the presence of an impaired respiratory apparatus.

Since the dyspnea in this case of pulmonary emphysema was relieved when the pulmonary ventilation dropped toward a normal level, conclusive evidence was presented of the importance of impaired respiratory function in respect to diffusion of oxygen as the fundamental cause of his difficulty. In many other cases of pulmonary emphysema, the relief of dyspnea and cough takes place more gradually, during a period of two days to a week of continuous oxygen administration. The difficulty in diffusion of oxygen is the primary cause of the dyspnea and not an actual impairment of carbon-dioxide elimination. The response of the case just mentioned to three weeks' oxygen therapy illustrates the functional significance of carbon-dioxide excretion in pulmonary emphysema. In a course of oxygen treatment of two weeks' duration, in which the patient breathed 50 per cent oxygen continuously in an oxygen room, the carbon-dioxide content of the arterial blood rose from 51.9 to 78.6 volumes per cent. At this time the patient was free from the sensation of dyspnea. As pointed out in the discussion on oxygen therapy in congestive heart failure, the decrease in volume of breathing is associated with an increased concentration of carbon dioxide in the blood. With an increased content of carbon dioxide in the blood and, therefore, an increased percentage of carbon dioxide in the expired air, carbon dioxide is eliminated with a smaller volume of breathing. The increased carbon-dioxide tension in the blood does not represent a shift in acid-base equilibrium to the acid side, since the measurement of the hydrogen-ion concentration shows only a very transient shift toward acidity at the start of therapy, and regularly an unaltered pH after continuous oxygen therapy.

The increased tension of carbon dioxide in the blood thus represents not simply a difficulty in eliminating carbon dioxide in the presence of an impaired respiratory apparatus and a lowered pulmonary ventilation initiated by oxygen inhalation, but an adaptive mechanism which makes possible a larger elimination of carbon dioxide per unit of air exhaled, since the expired air contained an increased percentage of carbon dioxide, paralleling the increased carbon-dioxide content of the blood. Surprising as it may at first seem, the high tension of carbon dioxide in the blood actually makes possible a progressive *lowering* of the pulmonary ventilation initiated by inhaling oxygen; this remarkable homeostatic mechanism is peculiarly efficient in getting rid of carbon dioxide.

In a patient with progressive pulmonary fibrosis who was treated for six months in an oxygen chamber with 60 per cent oxygen, the arterial carbon-dioxide content was 132 volumes per cent in the presence of a normal acid-base equilibrium. In this case inhalation of a 60 per cent oxygen atmosphere was finally required to prevent dyspnea, since her vital capacity became equal to her tidal air; namely, 250 cc. It is evident that her pulmonary ventilation could not have been lowered to the extent which relieved dyspnea had it not been for an unusually high concentration of carbon dioxide in the expired air, which allowed the full elimination of carbon dioxide produced by the patient. In the presence, therefore, of very severely damaged lungs, there was completely adequate elimination of carbon dioxide by homeostatic employment of a mechanism in which a high tension of carbon dioxide existed in the blood and made necessary an extraordinarily swift diffusion of carbon dioxide into the alveolar air and hence into the outer atmosphere. It must be emphasized, therefore, that retention of carbon dioxide is not the *primary* cause of the dyspnea of emphysema (or congestive heart failure) since it is possible for either the congested and edematous or the emphysematous and fibrotic lung to diffuse carbon dioxide through it by means of a high blood carbon-dioxide concentration, provided an adequate tension of oxygen is obtained in the arterial blood.

In patients in whom no recovery of lung function takes place, such as in a progressive fibrosis due to cancer or some other cause, the elevated blood carbon dioxide continues to remain high, since carbon dioxide cannot be eliminated at a normal concentration through damaged lungs as long as the pulmonary ventilation is kept lowered by oxygen inhalation. From a homeostatic point of view, a high blood carbon dioxide is necessary to permit a lower pulmonary ventilation to take place as a result of oxygen therapy. However, in patients with pulmonary emphysema in whom a decrease in the distention of the lung takes place as a result of the lower pulmonary ventilation and some recovery in the elastic quality of the alveolar epithelium occurs, the arterial carbon-dioxide content declines even in the presence of continuous oxygen administration. Thus, in the first case cited above, the carbon-dioxide content in the arterial blood fell from 78.6 volumes to 65.8 volumes per cent even during the continuous inhalation of oxygen. However, the arterial carbon-dioxide content did not return to the original level of 51.9 volumes per cent.

The interpretation of this residual increase in carbon-dioxide content is that the patient did not improve to the extent that would allow a normal pulmonary ventilation in the absence of oxygen treatment. In other words, the inhalation of 50 per cent oxygen made possible a lowered pulmonary ventilation consistent with subjective relief of dyspnea, but only with the retention of carbon dioxide in the blood and therefore the provision of a higher percentage excretion of carbon dioxide in the expired air per unit of volume of breathing. In this patient it was possible to breathe an air atmosphere for a period of four hours at a time, twice daily, without recurrence of severe dyspnea. Nevertheless, residence in 50 per cent oxygen was always accompanied by a definite decrease in the volume of breathing and consequently in the sensation of dyspnea. A few remarks concerning his clinical history may illustrate the method of oxygen treatment in patients who can afford prolonged therapy.

The patient was a man 74 years of age who had developed progressively severe dyspnea three years before admission to the hospital. During the previous year severe shortness of breath was created by the slightest exertion, such as eating or talking. The dyspnea was characteristic of that of pulmonary emphysema. The lower costal infrasternal margins were drawn inward during inspiration. The lungs were hyperresonant, breath sounds were prolonged, and there were a number of wheezing râles scattered throughout both lungs. The heart was not enlarged but the rate was elevated to 110, the blood pressure 145 systolic and 100 diastolic. Hemoglobin, 98 per cent; red blood cells, 4.5 million. Venous pressure, 85 mm. with a rise of 4 mm. on expiration. X-ray of the chest revealed a moderately flattened diaphragm with an essentially normal cardiac shadow. He did not appear cyanotic.

Analysis of the arterial blood showed an oxygen saturation of 92.9 per cent and a carbon-dioxide content of 51.9 volumes per cent. As observed above, the pulmonary ventilation was 10.7 liters per minute at rest, and fell to 7.6 liters per minute after the inhalation of 100 per cent oxygen. Oxygen treatment was begun by residence in the oxygen room for a period of two weeks at a concentration of 50 per cent oxygen. He was allowed out of the oxygen room for periods of four hours each day. Night and morning he was given an inhalation of the nebulized spray of 0.5 cc. of neosynephrin. During his stay in the hospital the reaction of the patient to inhalation of 100 per cent oxygen was tested many times. At the start of treatment the pulmonary ventilation in the morning was 11.5 liters per minute breathing air and 6.5 liters per minute during the inhalation of pure oxygen, a reduction of 43 per cent.

When the patient returned home he resided in a portable oxygen room for approximately 17 hours during the 24, including the night, early morning and a two-hour rest period from 4 to 6 in the afternoon. He went out for lunch and frequently for dinner in the early evening. The effect of oxygen therapy was a striking relief of dyspnea, a disappearance of the paroxysmal attacks of morning coughing, and a progressive gain in strength as well as subjective feelings of well-being. At the beginning of treatment the vital capacity was 1,430 cc., and 6 months later 2,100 cc., which was further increased by the inhalation of 1 per cent neosynephrin to 2,300 cc. The patient was now able to walk 60 steps to and from the dining room without undue distress. It was possible for him to go to a hotel for lunch and dinner, and entertain his friends without the severe dyspnea which had formerly made this impossible.

His pulse rate had decreased from an average of 110 to 90 beats per minute. The pulmonary ventilation in air had decreased to a range between 7.5 to 8.0 liters per minute, if he were not exposed to atmospheric oxygen longer than one hour. There was also a very conspicuous decrease in infrasternal and intercostal retraction during residence in the oxygen chamber. The following year and a half the patient continued to live comfortably without the dyspnea from which he formerly suffered. The patient was not allowed to go longer than four hours without return to the oxygen room. However, the patient himself showed no resentment at this restriction of activity out of doors but was continuously grateful for the relief of severe shortness of breath

Air   Oxygen

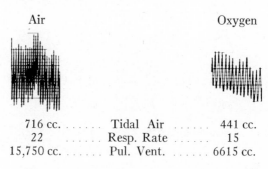

716 cc. . . . . . . Tidal Air . . . . . . 441 cc.
22   . . . . . . Resp. Rate   15
15,750 cc. . . . . . . Pul. Vent. . . . . . . 6615 cc.

Fig. 13. Decrease in pulmonary ventilation in a patient with emphysema, bronchiectasis, and pulmonary fibrosis after eight days of inhalation of 50 per cent oxygen.

which had affected him for the previous three years. The development of cancer of the prostate with complete urethral obstruction necessitated insertion of a tube into the bladder from which the patient developed a pyelonephritis and died.

It should be pointed out that improvement in this patient was made possible by the provision of exceptional facilities for oxygen treatment at home. In patients in whom this type of extensive oxygen therapy is not possible it is unwise to provide continuous oxygen therapy except during acute infections, such as acute bronchitis which may temporarily impair respiratory function but which on subsidence of the infection leaves them in a state comparable to that previously present. In advancing pulmonary fibrosis the improvement which consistently takes place during continuous inhalation of 50 per cent oxygen does not continue when oxygen therapy is dispensed with. The patient may then be worse than he was prior to treatment, since he has the knowledge that he could be more comfortable if he had a life-long supply of oxygen. The return of cough and expectoration appears to be due

Before oxygen treat-
ment: inspiration.

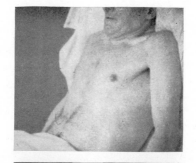

Before oxygen treat-
ment: expiration.

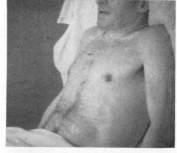

After oxygen treat-
ment: inspiration.

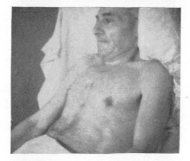

After oxygen treat-
ment: expiration.

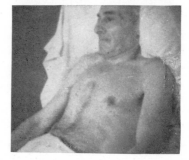

Fig. 14.   Emphysema.

to the increased volume of breathing in atmospheric oxygen, and the consequent heightened negative intrapulmonary pressure in certain areas of the lung that are partially obstructed.

In the accompanying illustration (Fig. 13), the decrease in pulmonary ventilation due to inhalation of 50 per cent oxygen for eight days is illustrated in a patient with pulmonary emphysema, fibrosis,

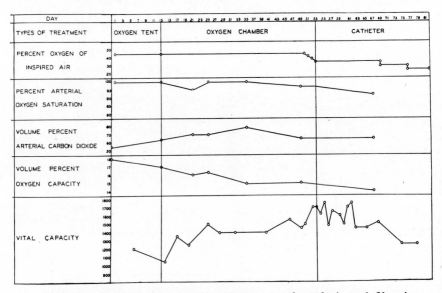

FIG. 15. Patient with chronic pulmonary tuberculosis and fibrosis. Prolonged treatment with oxygen resulted in increased arterial oxygen saturation, increased blood carbon dioxide, decreased hemoglobin, and marked rise in vital capacity.

and bronchiectasis. It will be seen that the patient had a volume of ventilation of 15.7 liters per minute before treatment and 6.6 liters per minute at the end of eight days' therapy. In this patient there was also a marked diminution in expectoration as well as a feeling of increased well-being. However, the advanced state of pulmonary fibrosis did not make it possible to discontinue oxygen therapy in this case except with the return of dyspnea, from which he had suffered prior to treatment.

The sequence of physiologic events during prolonged oxygen treatment in a patient with severe pulmonary fibrosis due to progressive tuberculosis is shown in the accompanying illustration.

For the first 13 days he was in an oxygen tent at a concentration of 45 per cent oxygen. The arterial oxygen saturation was promptly elevated to 98 per cent. The arterial carbon dioxide rose from 55 to 63 volumes per cent. The oxygen capacity fell from 18 volumes per cent to 17.4 volumes per cent. The fall in hemoglobin concentration is a consistent finding in patients of this type who are treated with oxygen. In those cases in which there is subsequent removal to air, a gradual rise in oxygen capacity takes place. It is of interest that the vital capacity of 1,200 cc. at first fell to 1,080 cc. This is a not infrequent finding and may accompany relief of dyspnea; it may be related to the decrease of respiratory movement and lessened blood flow. The patient was transferred to the oxygen room and there revealed a disappearance of most of the symptoms of dyspnea, cough, and expectoration, with progressive rise in the vital capacity to 1,800 cc. The oxygen capacity fell to 15.3 volumes per cent. The oxygen saturation of his arterial blood continued high until, between the fifty-first and fifty-third day, there was a gradual lowering of the oxygen concentration to 35 to 30 per cent.

The carbon-dioxide content of the arterial blood rose progressively from 55 volumes per cent to 78 volumes per cent on the thirty-fifth day of oxygen treatment, and then fell moderately to 68 volumes per cent, the fall indicating a functional capacity for a better diffusion of both oxygen and carbon dioxide.

After administration of a low oxygen percentage by nasal catheter, the improvement in his clinical condition began to recede. This was especially manifested as the inspired air was lowered to 25 per cent oxygen on the eighty-first day of oxygen treatment, at which time the vital capacity had fallen to 1,200 cc.

Several conclusions were reached as a result of these studies. In the first place the clinical symptoms were strikingly relieved during the period of residence in 45 per cent oxygen. Secondly, an attempt to substitute a lower oxygen concentration by nasal catheter and at the same time maintain improvement was unsuccessful, as shown by recurrence of the symptoms of cough, dyspnea, and expectoration and also the progressive fall in the vital capacity. In this patient with pulmonary fibrosis and pulmonary tuberculosis, the impaired respiratory function was improved by continuous oxygen treatment but required for the maintenance of this improvement the provision of adequate oxygen therapy at home.

The mechanism of the changes in respiratory function produced by oxygen treatment in cases of pulmonary emphysema and fibrosis will be reviewed since similar tendencies exist in other examples of anoxemic dyspnea. The fundamental response to inhalation of a high oxygen atmosphere in a patient with pulmonary emphysema is an immediate or a gradual reduction in the volume of breathing. When the pulmonary ventilation approaches that of the normal, subjective relief of dyspnea, diminution or absence of cough, and decrease or disappearance of expectoration may take place. A gradual elevation in vital capacity of the lung and a diminution in the degree of pulmonary distention occur in cases that respond favorably. When a patient of this type is replaced in an air atmosphere the pathologic physiology shows a change for the worse, characterized first of all by an increase in the quantity of air moved in and out of the lung. As the volume of breathing continues to be elevated, a progressive distention of the alveoli takes place, due to a ball-valve mechanism which traps air within the air cells. This may be generally demonstrated in a patient with pulmonary emphysema or pulmonary fibrosis by taking a graphic record of the breathing on a basal metabolism spirometer. If the individual is made to increase his ventilation, either artificially or as a result of exercise, it will be observed that a forcible inspiration will cause a sharp downward movement of the pen on the graphic chart but that the expiration which follows will not return to the level of the previous inspiration. As forcible breathing continues, the level of the respiratory curve will be markedly elevated, indicating that air has been held within the lung and fails to obtain its customary exit. The reason for this has been referred to elsewhere in the section on asthma, but it must be remembered that patients with pulmonary emphysema consistently manifest constriction either in the smaller bronchi or in the alveolar ducts of such a degree as to result in impaired emptying of the lung.

During expiration the bronchi normally constrict, but in the presence of bronchial spasm or bronchiolar edema the constriction of the bronchi is relatively augmented so that air has a smaller lumen to pass outward than it had to pass inward during inspiration, when an enlargement of the chest and the diameter of the bronchi take place. This progressive trapping of air within the alveoli results in distention, atrophy, and finally rupture of the weakened alveolar walls, in a large increase in residual air, and in a progressive fall in vital capacity.

The mechanism of improvement may now be more clearly visualized. When the inhalation of a high oxygen atmosphere is begun the lungs of the patient are distended. As a result of the higher oxygen tension in the arterial blood and as a consequence of the subsequent retention of carbon dioxide in the blood, which actually makes possible a more efficient elimination of carbon dioxide, the volume of breathing decreases. Because of the lowered pulmonary ventilation, when an oxygen-enriched atmosphere is inhaled, more time is available in which a unit volume of air may be exhaled. Thus, trapping of air within the air cells is less apt to take place because a more efficient emptying of the lung is provided. When dyspnea and an augmented pulmonary ventilation occur, an incomplete emptying of the air cells results, because of the narrowing of the lumen of the alveolar ducts and the smaller bronchioles. However, with a lower volume of breathing, more complete emptying of the alveolar spaces ensues, pulmonary distention is progressively diminished, the alveolar ducts and bronchi are relatively more patent, aeration of the alveoli is better, anoxia and dyspnea are relieved, and improvement in the elastic tissue in the lungs may result.

In most cases of pulmonary emphysema the heart is not enlarged; in some instances it is smaller in its transverse diameter than normal, as the vertical diameter of the chest is increased. However, strain on the right side of the heart is present in most patients and right heart failure may be seen in advanced cases of emphysema, associated with disease in the pulmonary arteries. In one such patient in whom previous bed rest and digitalis had not been effective in terminating dyspnea, oxygen treatment for one month restored cardiac compensation and made possible ambulatory activity with very little dyspnea. The decrease in heart size and in pulmonary congestion is shown in the accompanying x-ray pictures. Whenever cardiac insufficiency is present in association with either pulmonary emphysema or pulmonary fibrosis, continuous oxygen inhalation is justified, for it may achieve a more lasting improvement than when emphysema is present with normal heart function.

It is noteworthy that the intrapulmonary pressure during expiration generally approaches that of the atmosphere. The elevation in pulse rate is in part due to the associated anoxia and in part to the effort made in connection with the maintenance of an adequate ventilation, for in most instances the pulse rate returns to normal after residence in a high oxygen atmosphere.

INHALATIONAL THERAPY

In patients who suffer from severe dyspnea on slight exertion, the inhalation of 50 to 100 per cent oxygen for one-half hour in the morning and before going to bed is in most cases a palliative remedy of some value. As explained in the above section, the inhalation of an oxygen-enriched atmosphere is accompanied by a progressive decrease

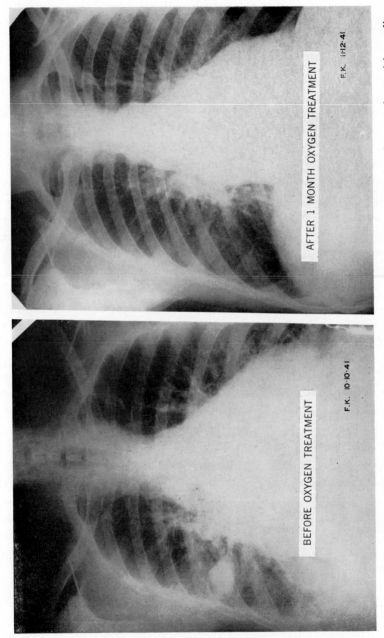

FIG. 16. Decrease in heart size after continuous inhalation of 50 per cent oxygen in a patient with cardiac insufficiency and pulmonary fibrosis.

in the distention of the lungs and is apt to promote sleep at night. In addition, the oxygen debt from which these patients frequently suffer is temporarily paid off. The inhalation of the nebulized solution of 1 per cent neosynephrin night and morning is also a helpful procedure. This may be used with the ordinary hand-bulb nebulizer, or a more effective method is to inhale the nebulized suspension of the drug during the passage of 4 liters of oxygen per minute from a high-pressure tank through the nebulizer. A dose of 0.5 cc., 7 to 8 drops, of the solution is adequate to cause some increase in vital capacity and to decrease dyspnea. Neosynephrin in milder cases is preferred to epinephrine since the former does not result in the development of a refractory state. However, in patients with more severe bronchospasm the inhalation of 1:100 epinephrine is frequently more efficient. It is generally adequate to use the hand-bulb nebulizer and four to ten forceful squeezes of the bulb during the inspiratory cycle will provide considerable relief. If the oxygen tank is at hand, however, a better result will then be obtained if 6 drops of the 1:100 epinephrine solution is placed in the nebulizer and the end held within the open mouth during the passage of a stream of 4 liters per minute of oxygen through the nebulizer. These three procedures performed night and morning will result in a temporary decrease in pulmonary distention.

In patients who are unable to afford a more ambitious type of oxygen therapy, the inhalation of 50 per cent oxygen should not be encouraged for periods oftener than three times a day. As discussed in the preceding section, the improvement that takes place under *continuous* oxygen therapy is not maintained on cessation of treatment unless a liberal provision of oxygen such as 16 hours of the 24 can be maintained, or a *gradual adaptation* to air is provided.

In well-to-do patients with either pulmonary fibrosis or pulmonary emphysema, continuous oxygen treatment for a period of four weeks or more may be undertaken if expert supervision is available. The decision to embark on a course of oxygen therapy in patients of this type should be made after full discussion with the patient and the family of the possible benefits and disadvantages. It may be said that in all likelihood the patient will be much improved, with relief of dyspnea and cough, and a marked diminution of expectoration during the period of oxygen treatment. A substantial part of this improvement can be maintained if sufficient oxygen therapy is provided at home, for approximately 16 hours of the 24. Acknowledgment should be made that pulmonary emphysema and pulmonary fibrosis are progressive diseases. Although adequate oxygen therapy retards the progress of the condition by preventing distention of the lung and consequent damage to the pulmonary epithelium, inhalational therapy does not do away with the underlying pathology.

When a course of continuous oxygen therapy is decided upon, the patient is in most instances placed in an environment of 50 per cent oxygen, either in an oxygen room or an oxygen tent for a period of four weeks. The nasal catheter or an oxygen mask may also be used. If the latter is employed care must be observed that no negative pressure whatsoever develops in the inspiratory cycle as a result of resistance within the mask. There is little or no advantage in oxygen therapy if the patient is forced to employ more effort to inspire than he does breathing atmospheric oxygen. The total flow of an oxygen-enriched atmosphere delivered through a mask should therefore exceed his pulmonary ventilation, i.e., above 12 liters per minute. In the Meter mask this can be obtained by admitting 5 to 7 liters of oxygen from the regulator, with the meter set at 40 to 50 per cent oxygen. In the B.L.B. mask the patient should be prevented from inhaling air through the sponge-rubber disk because this would entail increased effort during the inspiratory cycle, and a flow of approximately 10 liters per minute should come from the tank itself. However, since patients are to embark on a plan of oxygen treatment for the rest of their lives, the oxygen tent is generally used rather than the mask because it is in all respects more comfortable and suitable for this purpose. Either the motor-blower, the thermal-circulation or the open-top tent may be employed.

During the first four days of treatment a conspicuous decrease in the symptoms of the disease will take place. But another influence of oxygen therapy in patients who have had previous severe chronic anoxia must be looked for. In those patients who have shown a cyanotic hue of the nail beds or the lips prior to oxygen treatment, a temporary period of either deep sleep, coma, or irrationality may take place as a result of the sudden change in oxygen tension of the brain. Headache is an additional symptom in some cases. This reaction has been frequently misinterpreted and not understood as a transient response to oxygen therapy. In one instance the patient was in deep sleep for a period of six days and awoke on the seventh day bright and cheerful. No matter what degree of mental disorientation may take place during the early days of oxygen therapy, the condition has always been found by the author to be temporary and clears on continuance of oxygen treatment. It is in no sense a contraindication to further therapy and may be avoided if a gradual increase in oxygen concentration is provided. It is noteworthy also that the patient is apt to recover from the preliminary period of either depression, sleep, or disorientation with a state of cheerfulness which he had not had previously for many years. The first reaction to oxygen treatment is a shift in arterial pH to the acid side, with increase in carbon-dioxide tension, which may be linked to the symptoms mentioned above. However, a normal acid-base equilibrium is soon established.

If facilities are not available for determining the carbon-dioxide content of arterial blood the venous plasma bicarbonate may be done at intervals of four to seven days. There will be at first a gradual rise in arterial carbon-dioxide content or in the plasma bicarbonate, for a period of two to three weeks. If and when improvement in lung function takes place, the plasma bicarbonate begins to fall, and although it will not return to the level before oxygen treatment, it may show a decrease perhaps of 5 to 10 volumes per cent below the maximal level. When such a diminution in plasma bicarbonate is found while the patient is continuously receiving 50 per cent oxygen, the prognosis may be understood to be far better than if no such lowering takes place. If the plasma bicarbonate becomes elevated to 80 volumes per cent and does not decrease, it is an indication that the patient will be unable to do without oxygen except at the expense of considerable dyspnea and loss of the improvement obtained.[1]

In patients with pulmonary emphysema who do not at the same time have advancing fibrosis, the arterial carbon dioxide or the plasma bicarbonate will generally be found to have dropped somewhat by the end of the fourth week. By this time the patient is prepared to come out of the oxygen environment at first for a period of one hour, followed by an hour in the morning and in the afternoon, and then by one hour three times a day. It is helpful at the start to give the patient a spray of either 1 per cent neosynephrin or 1:100 epinephrine with the hand-bulb nebulizer or with the solution vaporized by an oxygen stream before going into the outside atmosphere. Depend-

---

[1] Recent observation of a patient whose plasma bicarbonate rose to 106 vol. per cent during oxygen therapy revealed that gradual reduction of nasal catheter oxygen, i.e., 0.5 liters per min. every 2 days, was followed by a remarkable adaptation to an air atmosphere in a three-week period. This patient became acclimatized to air without severe dyspnea, although with residual dyspnea increased by slight effort.

ing upon individual circumstances the length of time in which the patient is in the outer atmosphere may be varied from two hours three times a day to four hours twice a day. When patients breathe air for longer than four hours at one time there is apt to be a return of definite dyspnea. In most instances 50 per cent oxygen is provided, but there are patients in whom inhalation of 40 per cent oxygen is adequate to lower the pulmonary ventilation sufficiently to achieve a therapeutic result. The decrease in the pulmonary ventilation to such an extent as to relieve the feeling of difficulty of breathing is rarely obtained by concentrations of oxygen under 40 per cent.

A portable or a permanent oxygen room is unquestionably the most comfortable way in which patients of this type may be relieved of anoxia and the progressive pulmonary distention which hyperventilation causes. However, an oxygen tent may be used with considerable comfort. If the patient is to sleep without nursing care at night, a thermal-circulation tent which would not require a motor-blower unit and is therefore not dependent upon electricity may be found more practical, although it is generally less comfortable than the larger motor-ventilated tents. Care should be taken, however, that carbon dioxide does not accumulate within thermal-circulation tents as a result of oxygen flows below 9 liters per minute. A method of overcoming this is to use an injector such as is employed on the Meter mask and deliver 60 per cent oxygen into the tent from the meter attached to the oxygen regulator. If a flow of 7 to 8 liters per minute from the regulator is maintained with the meter set at 60 per cent, this will result in an adequate washing out of carbon dioxide given off by the patient and the maintenance of approximately 50 per cent oxygen. During the day a simpler form of oxygen therapy may be employed, depending upon the personal preference of the patient. The choice of apparatus under these circumstances is properly made by the patient and not by the physician. In some instances the catheter in the nasal or oral pharynx will provide a comfortable and efficient method of obtaining 40 to 50 per cent oxygen. In other cases the nasal mask is found more agreeable. For this type of patient the Meter mask is to be preferred since 40 to 50 per cent oxygen in the inspired air may be provided with a flow from the regulator of approximately 5 to 7 liters per minute, in the absence of any effort on the part of the patient and without accumulation of carbon dioxide.

In cases in which a program of this kind, which is actually a regimen of a liberal provision of oxygen for life, is impractical, the use of intermittent oxygen treatment for half an hour before going to bed or twice a day may be employed as a palliative measure, as indicated above, in conjunction with inhalation of the nebulized spray of 1 per cent neosynephrin or 1 : 100 epinephrine. However, if an ambulatory patient develops acute bronchitis and is then faced with a state of severe and possibly fatal dyspnea, continuous inhalation of 50 per cent oxygen is justified until the bronchitis has subsided. During this period of acute inflammatory swelling of the bronchi, repeated inhalation of neosynephrin and epinephrine solutions, at two-, three-, or four-hour intervals is of value in maintaining a partially patent airway through the smaller bronchi. With the subsidence of the acute infection oxygen therapy should be progressively curtailed, the patient being taken out of the tent for one hour the first day, two hours the second day, three hours the third day, and so on until he is entirely free from oxygen therapy or it is offered to him for half an hour once or twice a day.

There is little evidence that climate has any effect on the course of pulmonary emphysema. Particular care must be exercised under all circumstances to prevent the recurrence of acute upper-respiratory infection. There are patients who are aided by wearing an abdominal belt that increases the intra-abdominal pressure and facilitates an elevation of the diaphragm during expiration. When the condition is accompanied by congestive failure, digitalis may be tried, but it is generally found ineffectual. However, oxygen treatment in combination with strict elimination of sodium chloride and sodium bicarbonate often results in dramatic improvement in the state of the circulation. In one patient with advanced pulmonary fibrosis treated in this way there was a weight loss of 30 pounds in a period of approximately three weeks. Limitation of fluids is seldom necessary or advisable, but in the presence of pretibial edema the omission of sodium in any form from the diet is a procedure of unquestionable value. However, when the edema has cleared caution must be exercised in the maintenance of a too strict salt-elimination diet. This is especially true during the summer months when excessive perspiration may be followed by weakness and prostration due to the absence of sufficient salt in tissue fluids.

In extremely severe dyspnea in patients with pulmonary emphysema in whom either acute infection has taken place or severe bronchial spasm has been added to the picture, inhalation of 100 per cent oxygen may not be sufficient to relieve the dyspnea. In these instances, a positive pressure of 3 to 4 cm. of water may accomplish the desired result. If considerable difficulty in breathing is still present during inhalation of 100 per cent oxygen under a positive pressure of 4 cm. of water, a mixture of 40 per cent oxygen and 60 per cent helium may be tried. In some cases in which the element of bronchial spasm is a significant factor, the inhalation of either pure oxygen, or oxygen and helium, under positive pressure is the only effective method of relieving the dyspnea. It must be borne in mind that positive pressure in this situation should be continuously provided during inspiration, and that positive pressure in expiration alone is inadequate. Therefore, the helmet hood should be employed if it is available. Otherwise, an oxygen mask should be used with 100 per cent oxygen but under these circumstances the pressure on expiration generally should be sufficient only to maintain a slightly more patent bronchial lumen; namely, 1 to 2 cm. of water.

BIBLIOGRAPHY

Alexander, H. L., and W. B. Kountz: Symptomatic relief of emphysema by an abdominal belt, Amer. Jour. Med. Sci., **187**:687, 1934.

Barach, A. L.: Physiological methods in the diagnosis and treatment of asthma and emphysema, Ann. Int. Med., **12**:4, 1938.

Barach, A. L.: The therapeutic use of gases: the therapeutics of internal diseases. Edited by George Blumer. Vol. I, New York, D. Appleton-Century Co., 1940-1941.

Barach, A. L., and D. W. Richards, Jr.: Effects of oxygen treatment over long periods of time in patients with pulmonary tuberculosis, Amer. Rev. Tuberc., **26**:241, 1932.

Campbell, J. M. H., G. H. Hunt, and E. P. Poulton: An examination of the blood gases and respiration in disease, with reference to cause of breathlessness and cyanosis, Jour. Pathol. and Bacteriol., **26**:234, 1923.

Christie, R. V.: Elastic properties of emphysematous lung and their clinical significance, Jour. Clin. Invest., **13**:295, 1934.

Darling, R. C., A. Courand, J. S. Mansfield, and D. W. Richards, Jr.: Studies on intrapulmonary mixture of gases: I. Nitrogen elimination from blood and body tissues during high oxygen breathing. II. Analysis of rebreathing method (closed circuit) for measuring residual air. III. Open circuit method for measuring residual air, Jour. Clin. Invest., **19**:591, 1940.

Eckman, M., and A. L. Barach: Horizontal graphs by automatic intake of oxygen into basal metabolism machine, Proc. Soc. Exper. Biol. and Med., **36**:138, 1937.

Knipping, H. W., and G. Zimmerman: Oxygen therapy in patients with cardiac and pulmonary disease, Ztschr. f. klin. Med., **124**:435, 1933.

Kountz, W. B., H. L. Alexander, and M. Prinzmetal: The heart in emphysema, Amer. Heart Jour., **11**:163, 1936.

Meakins, J., and Christie, R. V.: Treatment of emphysema, Jour. Amer. Med. Asso., **103**:384, 1934.

Richards, D. W., Jr., and A. L. Barach: Oxygen therapy in pulmonary fibrosis, Am. Rev. Tuberc., 26:253, 1932.

Richards, D. W., Jr., and A. L. Barach: Prolonged residence in high oxygen atmosphere: effects on normal individuals and on patients with chronic cardiac and pulmonary insufficiency, Quart. Jour. Med., 3:437, 1934.

14

Accidental Asphyxia

INTRODUCTION

Under this heading will be included the treatment of carbon-monoxide poisoning, drowning, electric shock, and poisoning due to morphine, the barbiturates, or alcohol. In these conditions the respiration is generally depressed. Although an increased content of carbon dioxide is found in the blood as well as a state of tissue anoxia, there is good physiologic reason for administering 5, 7 or 10 per cent carbon dioxide in oxygen, especially in carbon-monoxide poisoning. The respiratory center is stimulated, resulting in an increased pulmonary ventilation and a swifter relief of anoxia.

PATHOLOGIC PHYSIOLOGY

Carbon-monoxide poisoning is the most important entity in this group. Carbon monoxide is formed as a result of the incomplete oxidation of gasoline, coal, and other substances. Since the affinity of hemoglobin for carbon monoxide is 300 times stronger than it is for oxygen, a relatively low concentration of this poisonous gas in the atmosphere will displace oxygen from the hemoglobin and produce varying degrees of asphyxia. The inhalation of 5, 7, and 10 per cent carbon dioxide in oxygen for 15 to 30 minutes not only augments the volume of breathing of gassed subjects, producing a swifter elimination of carbon monoxide from the blood, but also the affinity of carbon monoxide for hemoglobin is diminished by the presence of a high carbon-dioxide pressure in the blood; the oxygen dissociation curve is shifted to the right under these circumstances and oxygen is given up to the tissues more readily. Since the introduction of carbon-dioxide–oxygen treatment for carbon-monoxide poisoning, deaths from this cause have decreased, but the critical factor involved is the speed of administration of oxygen rather than the oxygen–carbon-dioxide mixture.

Although there is a somewhat faster elimination of carbon monoxide when carbon dioxide is added to the oxygen mixture, recovery takes place almost as fast if the patient is promptly provided with pure oxygen. The important factor is the speed with which 100 per cent oxygen or oxygen with carbon dioxide is administered to the patient. If the breathing has completely stopped, artificial respiration with the Sharpey-Schaefer prone-pressure method should be instituted while the mask is held to the patient's face. The carbon-dioxide–oxygen mixture should be administered for approximately 15 to 30 minutes, or until the patient is breathing normally.

A very efficient agent for resuscitation in accidental asphyxia is the positive and negative pressure resuscitator, either the E. and J. or Emerson type. Mechanical resuscitation is accomplished by inflating the lung to a pressure of 14 mm. Hg and aspirating air from the lung to a pressure of 9 mm. Hg. Although considerable prejudice exists against this kind of resuscitation, largely derived from knowledge of the old pulmotor, the new resuscitators have been used in adults and newborn infants without any evidence of harm to the lungs. Indications for its employment include electric shock, carbon-monoxide poisoning, drowning, accidents in industry, war injuries, and postoperative shock.

Positive and negative pressure by the resuscitator has been shown to have advantages over other methods in experimental investigations. In studies by Thompson and Birnbaum, the effects of rhythmic suction (negative pressure), rhythmic inflation (positive pressure), and manual artificial respiration were compared to the results achieved by the positive-negative pressure resuscitator. When advanced asphyxia was produced, with failure of respiration and circulation, the recovery rate with the resuscitator was the rule, whereas with the other methods recovery of the circulation and the respiration was the exception. Furthermore, when inhalation asphyxia was produced by an inert gas, such as nitrogen, the employment of the resuscitator, even with persisting inhalation of the inert gas, resulted in recovery in 85 per cent of the dogs treated, whereas the recovery rate in dogs treated with rhythmic suction was 20 per cent, with rhythmic positive-pressure inflation 17 per cent, and manual artificial respiration 15 per cent. These results indicate that the use of both positive and negative resuscitation gives the most effective ventilatory excursion independent of the state of tonus of the chest. Inflating the lungs with positive pressure, with subsequent fall to atmospheric pressure, is not adequate to achieve recovery in severely asphyxiated dogs. The employment of intermittent application of negative and positive pressure restores the circulation first and the respiration later. In all probability the negative pressure produced within the lungs facilitates the entrance of blood into the chest, and the application of positive pressure aids in the delivery of blood from the lungs into the left heart. The resuscitator thus acts as a circulatory pump. In peripheral circulatory failure, use of positive pressure alone does not appear on theoretical grounds to be of as much value as the employment of both negative and positive pressure, since the flow of blood into the right heart would tend to be retarded.

For clinical purposes either oxygen or carbon-dioxide–oxygen mixtures may be used to promote recovery of cardiorespiratory function. However, it should be emphasized that the respirator may be used with air when oxygen is not available. A compressor may be motivated by either the hand or the foot. This may be of value in military situations in which an oxygen cylinder may not be immediately available or when the oxygen supply has been used up. An aspirator is attached to the respirator which is convenient for the removal of mucus or secretions in the air passages of the patient.

The evidence available at present indicates that mechanical positive and negative pressure resuscitation will be more apt to give a favorable result in accidental asphyxia than either an H-H inhalator, the Drinker respirator, or resuscitators which employ either negative or positive pressure only. It is exceedingly unlikely that either the positive or negative pressure *in the degree employed* in this type of apparatus will result in damage to the pulmonary epithelium. This is especially true if aspiration of mucus is performed when present in sufficient amount to cause obstruction in the air passages.

The inhalation of 7 to 10 per cent carbon dioxide in individuals in coma from excessive intake of alcohol results in symptomatic improvement and in some cases in a state of mental clarity. Alcohol is said to produce a histotoxic anoxia, a form of tissue oxygen-want in which the catalyst required for tissue oxidation is impaired. There is some evidence that loss of control of certain postural reflexes due to alcohol is slightly improved by inhaling pure oxygen. In human subjects the acute symptoms of intoxication can be counteracted by inhalation of

100 per cent oxygen only in those patients in whom intoxication has been produced as a result of a relatively small intake of alcohol. Patients with delirium tremens have been said to be somewhat improved during the inhalation of an oxygen-enriched atmosphere.

In the treatment of patients poisoned by drugs such as morphine and the barbiturates it may be of crucial importance to maintain respiratory function by the inhalation of 50 per cent oxygen for a long period. If respiratory depression is severe, as evidenced by a respiratory rate of four to eight per minute, low concentrations of carbon dioxide such as 3 per cent may be administered in a 50 per cent oxygen concentration for stimulation of the respiratory center. Patients poisoned by excessive doses of sedative drug may be comatose for days and yet survive if inhalation of high oxygen mixtures is provided, together with the administration of suitable quantities of normal saline and 5 per cent glucose solutions by hypodermoclysis.

The method of treatment in carbon-monoxide poisoning may make use of a mask, either that devised by Henderson and Haggard that is part of the carbon-dioxide–oxygen equipment, or any other type of oxygen mask may be employed. In barbiturate poisoning, in which the respiratory depression may last over a period of days, the oxygen tent or nasal catheter may also be employed.[1]

---

[1] Yandell Henderson has recently (Science, December 24, 1943) made a vigorous denunciation of resuscitators, despite the fact that they have been accepted by the Council on Physical Therapy of the American Medical Association. Since the introduction in 1921 by Henderson and Haggard of the method of resuscitation by inhalation of oxygen with enough carbon dioxide to induce a maximum minute volume of respiration, many lives have been saved with the employment of the H-H inhalator. The many studies of these authors on asphyxia and its prevention by inhalation of oxygen–carbon-dioxide mixtures represent a noteworthy contribution in medicine. Their emphasis on the sensitiveness of the brain to anoxia has been responsible not only for the saving of life but also for the recovery of patients without the neurologic effects of improperly treated asphyxia.

Henderson's recent condemnation of resuscitators indicates that this apparatus should be carefully investigated. However, I have been sufficiently impressed by the experimental studies of Thompson and Birnbaum to include use of the resuscitator as an effective agent in the treatment of advanced asphyxia. Furthermore, I have not seen evidence that the modern resuscitator has produced mechanical injuries to the lung, dangerous degrees of acapnia, and failure of the circulation. The resuscitator can be used with oxygen and carbon-dioxide mixtures. The use of mechanical artificial respiration in accidental asphyxia will be and should be studied in both animal and clinical investigation. The improvements in the design of the modern resuscitator and its effectiveness in relieving experimental asphyxia in dogs warrant an impartial trial in human cases of asphyxia resulting from partial drowning, electric shock, anesthesia, and carbon-monoxide poisoning. In maintain-

BIBLIOGRAPHY

Barach, A. L.: Action of oxygen in counteracting alcoholic intoxication, Amer. Jour. Physiol., **107**:610, 1934.

Beck, H. G., and G. M. Suter: Role of carbon monoxide in the causation of myocardial disease, Jour. Amer. Med. Asso., **110**:1982, 1938.

Douglas, C. G., J. S. Haldane, and J. B. S. Haldane: The laws of combination of hemoglobin with carbon monoxide and oxygen, Jour. Physiol., **44**:275, 1912.

Drinker, C. K.: The efficiency of the oxygen carbon dioxide treatment of carbon monoxide poisoning, Jour. Indust. Hyg., **7**:1, 1925.

Haggard, H. W.: The elimination of carbon monoxide and a method of acceleration, Proc. Soc. Exper. Biol. and Med., **17**:205, 1920.

Haldane, J. B. S.: The dissociation of oxyhemoglobin in human blood during partial CO poisoning, Jour. Physiol., **45**:22, 1912.

Henderson, Y.: Treatment of acute alcoholism, Jour. Amer. Med. Asso., **64**:106, 1936.

Henderson, Y.: The return of the pulmotor as a "resuscitator": a back-step toward the death of thousands, Science, **98**:547, 1943.

Henderson, Y., and H. W. Haggard: The treatment of carbon monoxide poisoning, Jour. Amer. Med. Asso., **77**:1065, 1921.

McFarland, R. A., and A. L. Barach: The relationship between alcoholic intoxication and anoxemia, Amer. Jour. Med. Sci., **192**:186, 1936.

Palthe, P. M. Van W.: Über Alkoholvergiftung, Deutsche Ztschr. f. Nervenh., **92**: 79, 1926.

Review of carbon monoxide poisoning, Public Health Bulletin No. 195, 1936.

Sayers, R. R., and Yant, W. P.: The elimination of carbon monoxide from the blood by treatment with air, with oxygen and with a mixture of carbon dioxide and oxygen. Pub. Health Rep., **38**:2053, 1923.

Stadie, W. C., and K. A. Martin: The elimination of carbon monoxide from the blood: a theoretical and experimental study, Jour. Clin. Invest., **2**:77, 1925.

Thompson, S. A., G. L. Birnbaum, and E. Ostrow: Resuscitation in advanced asphyxia, Surgery, **12**:284, 1942.

---

ing this opinion I wish to acknowledge to the full the importance and value of the significant studies in the treatment of accidental asphyxia carried out by Henderson and Haggard in the past two decades.

15

Asphyxia of the Newborn: Antenatal Fetal Anoxia and Atelectasis of the Lungs of the Newborn

INTRODUCTION

The question of adequate treatment of asphyxia of the newborn is of great importance and deserves continued study. In a recent analysis Yandell Henderson stated that 150,000 deaths per year in this country alone resulted from combined stillbirth and neonatal deaths due to respiratory complications, approximately 7 in 100 births.

PATHOLOGIC PHYSIOLOGY

Fetal anoxia in the period before delivery is the cause of many stillbirths, and also of death in infants who die shortly after delivery, due to cerebral pathology inflicted by severe anoxia during delivery. Fetal anoxia may be caused by interference with the maternal supply of oxygen and also by factors which prevent the fetus from receiving oxygen. In the first category is included the low oxygen concentration present in certain anesthetic mixtures of nitrous oxide. Although nitrous oxide is of inestimable value in preventing labor pain, it may be administered with a low concentration of oxygen so continuously that the mother experiences anoxia for a prolonged period. The failure to interrupt administration of anesthetic mixtures with inhalations of high concentrations of oxygen, preferably with 100 per cent oxygen, accounts for the mother and, therefore, the fetus undergoing relatively severe oxygen-want in many instances.

When excessive doses of analgesic drugs have produced relaxation of the lingual and pharyngeal musculature, respiratory obstruction may be produced with accumulation of mucus and at times gastric contents from emesis. In addition, drugs which slow the respiratory rate result in a lowered volume of ventilation with resultant arterial anoxia.

The fetus may fail to receive oxygen even when the maternal blood stream is well saturated with it, due to disturbances in the placental circulation, such as in placenta previa or cord entanglement. Long-sustained contraction of the uterus due to the use of oxytocics may interfere with placental circulation to such an extent as to produce fetal anoxia.

Recognition of intra-uterine anoxia is of great importance and should be attempted routinely by auscultation of the fetal heart rate. Although an increase in the pulse rate is the usual sign of anoxia in adults, a slowing of the fetal heart rate, either in the form of a rather sudden drop of 25 or more beats per minute or a persistent slowing below 100 or 110 beats per minute, points to the development of severe fetal anoxia. The diagnosis may be confirmed by the thera-peutic response to oxygen. It appears that the majority of cases of fetal anoxia respond to maternal oxygen therapy. As a result of the inhalation of 100 per cent oxygen for 5 to 10 minutes the quality of the fetal pulse generally returns to normal. Since the time of prepa-ration of a patient for operative delivery is usually more than 5 or 10 minutes, inhalation of 100 per cent oxygen to the mother may be carried out while the preparations are being made. Under these cir-cumstances no hazard is created for the infant and in many instances the improvement in the fetal heart rate may be so marked as to obviate the necessity for exigent operative delivery with its attendant danger to both mother and infant.

In the newborn infant the lung is airless until the first breath is inhaled. Gradually the collapsed alveoli expand as repeated inspira-tory enlargement of the chest increases the negative pressure within the lung and air is admitted to more and more alveoli. The dilatation of the alveoli is followed by opening up of the capillaries and of the pulmonary arteries. The blood of the pulmonary arteries now flows through the lungs as the foramen ovale closes. However, in many cases there is a prolongation of the time in which the major part of the lung expands which results in marked impairment of respiratory function, specifically, severe anoxia. When small areas of the lung remain atelectatic, the infant first suffers from oxygen-want and then frequently from a superimposed infection resulting in bronchopneu-monia or lobar pneumonia. In some instances obstruction in the respiratory passageway is caused by mucous exudate or by aspiration of amniotic fluid.

PREVENTIVE INHALATIONAL THERAPY IN FETAL ANOXIA

Prophylaxis of fetal anoxia should be carried out by the obstetrician in all ways that are available for the prevention of both maternal anoxia and failure of the fetal supply of oxygen. When fetal anoxia has made itself apparent by changes in the rate and rhythm of the fetal heart, especially slowing of the heart rate as indicated above, inhalation by the mother of 100 per cent oxygen is urgently indicated. When the fetal heart rate persists below 100 after 10 minutes' inhalation of pure oxygen, it is a sign that the response to oxygen will probably not be seen and that the delivery should not be further delayed. However, if delivery is impossible, deep anesthesia may be continued with simultaneous continuation of as high an oxygen concentration to the mother as possible.

INHALATIONAL THERAPY

When breathing does not begin soon after birth, inflation of the lung of the newborn baby by mouth-to-mouth insufflation is the best of all empiric methods, provided it is done gently. Although it has been shown that the infant who fails to breathe adequately at birth has a high carbon-dioxide content in his blood, inhalation of 5 per cent carbon dioxide in oxygen has been advocated for short periods of two to three minutes to overcome the possible cohesion of collapsed alveolar walls. However, inhalations of carbon dioxide should not be relied upon for treatment of atelectasis of the lungs since this may require one to six weeks for sufficient expansion to take place. Residence in a 50 per cent oxygen atmosphere in a tent or, if the infant is premature, in an oxygen incubator, is the safest method to pursue. Under continuous oxygen treatment the infant is protected against the damaging effects of anoxia and the possibility of respiratory failure, until the lungs gradually expand. When the infant no longer becomes cyanotic on removal from the oxygen environment inhalational therapy may be discontinued. It should be remembered that the capacity of the lungs during the first hour rarely exceeds 50 cc., and that expansion of the lungs is a slow process probably accomplished through forcible expiratory movements with the glottis partially closed as when the baby cries. There is, therefore, no urgent indication to completely expand the lung by carbon-dioxide administration during the first day or two.

Although sudden respiratory failure and severe cyanosis may take place as a result of hemorrhage in the brain, infants who are cyanotic at birth should invariably be treated with continuous inhalation of 50 to 60 per cent oxygen in recognition of the fact that failure of complete expansion of the lungs may be the cause of the condition and that completely normal opening up of the alveoli may ultimately take place if sufficient time is afforded by maintenance of respiratory function through oxygen inhalation.

In cases in which it is suspected that mucus or amniotic fluid is in the tracheobronchial tree, the method of intratracheal suction with preliminary intubation or catheter aspiration may be of crucial value. In a method of suction in which there is a control of the pressure used, it may be employed to clear the larynx, trachea, and the larger bronchi of obstructing secretions. In premature infants oxygen incubators are of special value in maintaining the temperature of the infant and preventing severe anoxia at the same time.

An improved type of pulmotor called the resuscitator has been used in a series of 500 infants without any apparent harmful influence. This is a mechanical device that provides positive and negative pressures which result in alternate inflation and deflation of the lungs. No injury to the lung after the use of this resuscitator has been reported in cases which came to autopsy due to cerebral hemorrhage. The procedure employed was to aspirate the mucus that might be present from any baby who did not cry immediately and to apply the resuscitator with pure oxygen.

Although Henderson has advocated carbon-dioxide inhalation, Kane, Eastman, and Kreiselman believe that oxygen without carbon dioxide is preferable in the treatment of atelectasis of the lungs of the newborn. In cases treated by the author, continuous inhalation of 50 per cent oxygen has been responsible for ultimate recovery when carbon-dioxide inhalations did not seem of value. In one instance, disappearance of atelectasis did not take place until six weeks of treatment had elapsed. In another patient who had a markedly increased respiratory rate from birth, dyspnea was accompanied by recurrent infections in the lungs until, at the age of five months, emphysema of both lower lobes was seen on x-ray examination. Residence in an oxygen tent at 50 per cent oxygen was accompanied by gradual disappearance of dyspnea and the signs of infection. In this patient oxygen therapy was continued for one and a half years, 16 to 20 hours of the day, before full expansion of the lungs took place. No signs of emphysema are now evident, two years after cessation of oxygen-tent therapy.

The inhalation of helium and oxygen in atelectasis of the lungs seems logical since this mixture might enter the lung cells through alveolar ducts that might not be patent to the oxygen-nitrogen mixture, and in fact this procedure has apparently been successfully used in this condition. Helium-oxygen inhalations have also been reported to be of value in unresolved pneumonic consolidation.

The oxygen tent is more suitable as a method of administration of oxygen than either the catheter or mask. Although the motor-blower or thermal-circulation tent may be employed, the open-top tent is the most convenient, simplest, and most effective method for infants, since they do not require a cool dry atmosphere. A relatively high concentration of oxygen such as 60 per cent may be obtained with a flow of 6 to 7 liters of oxygen per minute.

BIBLIOGRAPHY

Amberg, S.: Oxygen incubator, Proc. Staff Meet., Mayo Clin., **9**:132, 1934.

Amberg, S.: Oxygen in the treatment of pertussis, Proc. Staff Meet., Mayo Clin., **9**:133, 1934.

Benedict, F. G., P. White, and R. C. Lee: An infant incubator; employing controlled mixtures of helium and oxygen to combat respiratory failure, Amer. Jour. Obstet. and Gynecol., **39**:63, 1940.

Buffum, W. P., and G. F. Conde: Use of oxygen in the care of feeble premature babies, Jour. Pediat., **4**:35, 1934.

Clifford, S. H.: Asphyxia of the fetus and the newborn infant: a study of the clinical and pathologic changes produced by intrauterine asphyxia due to placenta previa and a consideration of methods to prevent or minimize fetal anoxemia, Amer. Jour. Obstet. and Gynecol., **39**:388, 1940.

Eastman, N. J., R. B. Dunn, and J. Kreiselman: Relative value of pure oxygen and carbon dioxide in experimental resuscitation, Amer. Jour. Obstet. and Gynecol., **36**:571, 1938.

Flagg, P. J.: Treatment of asphyxia neonatorum, Maine Med. Jour., **31**:1, 1940.

Henderson, Y.: Incomplete dilatation of the lungs as a factor in neonatal mortality Jour. Amer. Med. Asso., **96**:495, 1931.

Kane, H. F.: Use of helium and oxygen in treatment of asphyxia neonatorum: preliminary communication, Amer. Jour. Obstet. and Gynecol., **40**:140, 1940; Jour. Amer. Med. Asso., **115**:963, 1940.

Kane, H. F., and J. Kreiselman: The carbon dioxide content of the blood in the newborn, Amer. Jour. Obstet. and Gynecol., **20**:826, 1930.

Lund, C. J.: The recognition and treatment of fetal heart arrhythmias due to Anoxia, Amer. Jour. Obstet. and Gynecol., **40**:946, 1940.

Martinez, D. B.: The mechanical resuscitation of the new-born, Jour. Amer. Med. Asso., **109**:489, 1937.

Nicodemus, R. E.: Oxygen tent therapy in the treatment of eclampsia, Jour. Amer. Med. Asso., **117**:1238, 1941.

Schreiber, F.: Apnea of the newborn and associated cerebral injury, Jour. Amer. Med. Asso., **111**:1263, 1938.

Waters, R. M.: Tracheobronchial toilet, Brit. Jour. Anæsth., **18**:1, 1942.

16

Hemorrhage

INTRODUCTION

Although severe hemorrhage is frequently followed by shock, in which the function of inhalational therapy has been discussed under that section, it is not sufficiently realized that profuse loss of blood is accompanied by serious anoxia even in the absence of peripheral circulatory failure. Marked loss of blood may occur in the course of clinical illness, such as duodenal ulcer, pulmonary tuberculosis, hemorrhagic diseases, and as a result of wounds and injuries.

PATHOLOGIC PHYSIOLOGY

The effect of marked loss of blood is that of acute oxygen-want in all the tissues of the body, so-called anemic anoxia. When shock takes place the syndrome is that of peripheral circulatory failure, with clinical evidence of deficient return of venous blood to the right heart. In the absence of shock a rapid pulse rate, pallor, apprehension, or loss of consciousness may be present. The normal content of oxygen carried in 100 cc. of arterial blood is 19.5 cc. When the blood loss has been sufficient to decrease this by one-half or one-third, the patient may expire from a combination of shock and acute anoxia. During the passage of 100 cc. of blood from arteries to the veins, 6 cc. are ordinarily removed by the intervening tissues, resulting in a venous oxygen content of 13.5 cc. When a severe hemorrhage has been responsible for lowering the content of oxygen in 100 cc. of arterial blood to 9 cc. per 100 cc. of blood, only 3 cc. of oxygen would theoretically remain in 100 cc. of venous blood unless compensation was made by an increase in cardiac output. The pressure of oxygen in the tissues would fall rapidly and be insufficient to maintain consciousness and even life itself. However, elevation in pulse rate and an increased blood flow raise the tissue oxygen pressure, decreasing the difference between the arterial and venous oxygen content. Nevertheless, the deficiency in available oxygen may lead to severe anoxia and a lowering of the total oxygen consumption.

INHALATIONAL THERAPY

Since patients with serious blood loss are not cyanotic, the swift employment of inhalation of 100 per cent oxygen has not been generally recommended as a routine emergency measure until transfusions restore adequate blood. The need for an increased oxygen pressure in the tissues is nonetheless urgent and breathing 100 per cent oxygen through a mask will increase the physically dissolved oxygen from 0.25 cc. to 1.5 cc. per 100 cc. of blood. If the patient has sufficient hemoglobin to carry 8 cc. of oxygen in 100 cc. of blood, inhalation of 100 per cent oxygen will increase its saturation from 95 to 100 per cent. This would mean an additional 5 per cent of 8 cc. or 0.4 cc. of oxygen. which would then be added to the 1.5 cc. present in physical solution or a total of 1.9 cc. of oxygen in 100 cc. of circulating blood. This increased content of oxygen may raise the tissue-oxygen pressure sufficiently to prevent impairment in the functioning of the brain, heart. and other organs and also pathologic changes in the brain. Inhalation of pure oxygen is best provided by the Meter or B.L.B. oxygen mask. Oxygen therapy should be continued until it is evident that the clinical condition of the patient has improved to such an extent that anoxia is no longer present.

The decision to operate on a patient who has internal bleeding, such as from an ulcer in the intestine, is at times difficult to make, but the immediate institution of oxygen therapy is desirable either in order to prepare the patient for operation, in which case oxygen treatment should be continued during and after it, or, if the condition of the patient is such as to forbid the attempt to get rid of the cause of hemorrhage, inhalation of pure oxygen should be made continuous in order to give the patient an additional opportunity for spontaneous clotting of the bleeding vessel, or for subsequent improvement in his condition through transfusion so as to make operation possible. Omission of oxygen therapy in severe blood loss allows the maintenance of a state of anemic anoxia with inevitable deterioration in the functioning of all the organs.

17

Peripheral Arteriosclerosis

INTRODUCTION

Arteriosclerotic disease manifests itself frequently in the lower extremity, resulting in symptoms of pain, numbness, tingling, and cramps of the muscles. Local ulcer and gangrene may develop. Ischemia may also be caused by allied conditions such as thromboangiitis obliterans, embolism, and thrombosis of peripheral arteries.

PATHOLOGIC PHYSIOLOGY

As a result of either gradual or abrupt occlusion of an artery, the tissues supplied by it undergo a varying degree of anoxia and necrosis. Pain is a common symptom and, as described in the section on coronary occlusion, is due to the local tissue anoxia and the substances produced as a result of deficient oxygenation. Depending upon the nature and character of the lesions and the individual patient, collateral circulation may develop adjacent to the obstructed artery.

INHALATIONAL THERAPY

In respect to inhalational therapy in conditions of local occlusion of peripheral arteries, the inhalation of a high oxygen mixture is at times followed by relief of pain, especially when 100 per cent oxygen is used. In some cases the more continuous employment of 50 to 70 per cent oxygen has been followed by healing of gangrenous ulcers due to an ischemic circulation. The use of oxygen therapy in conditions of this type has been much neglected. Although the physiologic basis for its employment is a valid one in certain individuals, a careful study of its clinical value has not yet been made. The fact that permanent restoration of an intact blood supply is not to be expected in most instances does not diminish the importance of oxygen therapy in those

147

cases in which there is a borderline possibility of spontaneous healing. This applies especially to patients with peripheral arteriosclerosis, embolism, and thrombosis of peripheral arteries, and also in patients in whom the existence of diabetes mellitus is a predisposing and complicating influence. Any of the current methods may be employed for inhaling high concentrations of oxygen. More continuous use of moderate concentrations of oxygen may be had with the employment of the catheter inserted in the oropharynx. The Meter mask makes possible a long-continued inhalation of 70 per cent oxygen, without fluctuation of the prescribed percentage. More investigation in this field seems indicated.

BIBLIOGRAPHY

Hill, L.: A simple oxygen bed tent and its use in a case of edema and chronic ulcer of the leg, Jour. Physiol., Proc. Physiol. Soc., 55:20, 1921.

Poulton, E. P.: Local tissue anoxia and its treatment, Lancet, 2:305, 1939.

Starr, I., Jr., and A. Stengel: Conservative treatment of gangrene of the feet by a selected temperature, oxygen and desiccation, Jour. Amer. Med. Asso., 99: 253, 1932.

18

Migraine, Seasickness, Gas Gangrene, and Tetanus

Brief mention of the administration of oxygen in these conditions is warranted although clinical experience is very limited.

Patients with migraine who have prodromal symptoms warning them of an attack of headache and nausea are at times apparently benefited by inhalation of 100 per cent oxygen for one hour. If the attack is not aborted, it is likely that further administration of oxygen will be useless. In a few cases of alcoholic headache and nausea which occur the morning after, the administration of oxygen has been said to be helpful.

In severe seasickness headache, nausea, vomiting, and prostration may be present, with in some cases a varying degree of peripheral circulatory failure. The inhalation of 100 per cent oxygen may be beneficial under these circumstances. In a few cases the nausea and vomiting of seasickness have been relieved.

Since the organisms of gas gangrene and tetanus are known to be anaerobic, there is justification for the inhalation of 100 per cent oxygen in these conditions. By producing a sharp increase in tissue oxygen tension the growth of these organisms may be retarded. In cases of gangrene in which subcutaneous emphysema has occurred, the inhalation of pure oxygen will permit the elimination of nitrogen and hydrogen via the blood stream. In experimental infection of guinea pigs with tetanus spores, inhalation of 60 per cent oxygen has prevented infection although control animals acquired tetanus (Chapter 33).

BIBLIOGRAPHY

Alvarez, W. C.: A new treatment for migraine, Proc. Staff Meet., Mayo Clin., 14: 173, 1939.
Boothby, W. M.: Oxygen administration—the value of high concentrations of oxygen for therapy, Proc. Staff Meet., Mayo Clin., 13:641, 1938.

Campbell, J. A., and Paul Fildes: Tetanus X: the effect of the oxygen tension of the tissue fluids in controlling infection of *B. tetani*, Brit. Jour. Exper. Pathol., **12**:77, 1931.

Starr, I., Jr., and A. Stengel: Conservative treatment of gangrene of the feet by a selected temperature, oxygen and desiccation, Jour. Amer. Med. Asso., **99**: 253, 1932.

19

Anesthesia and Anoxia

INTRODUCTION

During the administration of anesthetic agents, anoxia may be produced by respiratory depression and by exclusion of oxygen from the inhaled atmosphere. Physiologically minded anesthetists have delivered many warnings in recent years against allowing anoxia to take place during the course of anesthesia. The finding of degeneration of brain tissue in infants and adults who have been exposed to nitrous-oxide anesthesia has been explained as due to anoxia and not to nitrous oxide. Many cases of disturbed cerebral functioning have been reported as a result of an asphyxial episode associated with the administration of an anesthetic agent. In all these instances it is clear that the anesthetic agent is itself not responsible for damage to the cortical cells but the continued existence of a state of severe oxygen-want is the sole etiologic factor. In experiments on animals and in severe accidental asphyxia in man, such as carbon-monoxide poisoning, pathologic changes in the brain of a specific kind have been described repeatedly. As pointed out in previous chapters, the brain is the organ most sensitive to oxygen deprivation in terms of impairment of mental functioning. The heart is also regarded as an oxygen-sensitive organ, but the muscles and joints may endure severe anoxia for a prolonged period without evidence of disturbance in subsequent function.

PATHOLOGIC PHYSIOLOGY

Anoxia may be produced in the course of anesthesia by excessive preliminary sedative medication and by the inhalation of anesthetic agents which replace an excessive percentage of oxygen. In the former category both morphine and the barbiturates lower the minute volume of ventilation and when large doses of these drugs are prescribed, an arterial anoxia may be produced simply because the air in the alveoli is renewed at an insufficiently frequent rate. Administration of avertin by rectum is also not free from danger since respiratory depression may take place as a result of large doses. In addition to the effect of drugs in lowering the pulmonary ventilation, their effect in depressing pharyngeal and lingual reflexes may result in obstruction in the upper respiratory passageway due to the failure to expectorate mucus and consequent plugging of bronchi.

In considering the agent which may produce anoxia by displacement of oxygen, nitrous oxide may be emphasized as dangerous if unskillfully used. Valuable as this anesthetic agent admittedly is, a mixture of 14 per cent oxygen and 86 per cent nitrous oxide will not provide anesthesia to pain, in the absence of other anesthetic drugs. Although this degree of oxygen-want produces no pathologic damage to the normal young adult, it is possible that patients with coronary disease may develop anoxia of the heart muscle of sufficient extent as to be followed by coronary and cardiac insufficiency. Lower oxygen concentrations, however, are less free from this danger. If reliance is to be placed upon nitrous-oxide anesthesia alone, sufficient relaxation of the patient cannot be obtained in many operations unless severe asphyxia is also produced. This state of affairs is remedied to some extent by preliminary medication, which consists of morphine, barbiturates, or avertin. However, when sufficient relaxation has been obtained in this way, respiratory depression must be guarded against.

A combination of preliminary sedation may be used with nitrous-oxide anesthesia provided that a low oxygen concentration—i.e., below 21 per cent—is not permitted during the course of the operation. It is possible to compensate for preoperative sedation, which may produce a lowered volume of ventilation and arterial anoxemia, by the administration of approximately 30 per cent oxygen with the remainder nitrous oxide. In many cases, however, the attempt to maintain anesthesia with nitrous oxide, even with the preliminary drug medication, is less desirable than the introduction into the anesthetic mixture of ether, chloroform, cyclopropane, or some other agent which will effect anesthesia in the presence of a high oxygen atmosphere. It may become desirable to test the oxygen concentration of anesthetic mixtures in closed-circuit methods of administration. In inhalational therapy this is considered essential for the safety of the patient by all students of the subject. Precautions would have to be taken to prevent absorption of anesthetic gases by the solution which absorbs oxygen.

The inhalation of oxygen has been highly recommended in spinal anesthesia from the beginning to end of anesthesia and for eight hours afterwards. Since the nausea and vomiting are quickly relieved by administration of oxygen, the hypothesis that anoxia is the cause of the symptoms appears to be confirmed. The administration of oxygen from 24 to 36 hours after spinal anesthesia will almost always prevent the postoperative headache.

Special precautions should be observed in operations on patients with heart disease since those with coronary sclerosis are especially sensitive to oxygen deprivation. In a series of patients with advanced heart disease in whom the operation of total thyroidectomy was employed, a program of oxygen treatment before, during, and after operation was accompanied by an exceedingly smooth postoperative course and by the absence of any mortality in a series of 11 cases. This exceptionally good response to an operation of this sort in patients as severely ill as were included in the group referred to is evidence of the importance of maintaining a high oxygen concentration in patients with heart disease.

In the presence of anemia, the employment of both preoperative and operative anesthetic agents should be undertaken with the recognition that these patients are handicapped by a disturbance in oxygen carrying power. The inhalation of a 14 per cent oxygen and 86 per cent nitrous oxide mixture to patients whose hemoglobin is between 50 and 70 per cent is apt to be accompanied by severe tissue anoxia.

When the patient is in shock, a situation of extreme difficulty presents itself, since the patient already is suffering from the most severe form of tissue anoxia. The administration of an anesthetic agent which in any way decreases the oxygen tension in the tissues is unquestionably harmful. Under these circumstances, the employment of as high an oxygen concentration as is possible, with the selection of an anesthetic agent that would make this feasible, is indicated.

Fortunately, the field of anesthesia today includes physiologists who recognize that anoxia is a specific problem of the anesthetist. Since the brain is admittedly the organ most sensitive to anoxia both in terms of mental functioning and of susceptibility to pathologic and therefore permanent damage, the employment of an agent which renders the patient unconscious is fraught with unquestionable hazard. Because the results of anoxic anesthesia include not only unnecessary risk but also neurologic and psychiatric effects that may be more or less lasting, it is evident that a sound physiologic and technical experience is desirable in those who administer anesthesia.

The methods of giving oxygen include the catheter or mask, during local or spinal anesthesia. When preoperative sedation is employed in patients with cardiac or anemic conditions, or older patients in whom anoxia may be a special hazard, the preoperative and operative use of nasal-catheter administration of oxygen will prevent the harmful influence of continuous respiratory depression.

Respiratory depression after operations is overcome by suitable administration of oxygen either by routine placement in an oxygen tent after surgery on the chest and upper abdomen, or by insertion of a catheter in the nasal or oral pharynx. Postoperative depression and the prevention of atelectasis may be treated by periodic inhalations of 5 per cent carbon dioxide with oxygen in order to expand the bronchi and promote coughing with expectoration of retained secretion. Deep breathing and turning the patient from side to side are also employed for this purpose.

BIBLIOGRAPHY

Barach, A. L., D. W. Richards, Jr., and W. B. Parsons: Oxygen treatment and thyroid ablation in the treatment of heart disease, Ann. Int. Med., 9:1513, 1936.

Behnke, A. R., Jr.: Some physiological considerations of inhalation anesthesia and helium, Anesth. and Analg., 19:35, 1940.

Behrend, A., and H. E. Riggs: II. Factors which predispose to cerebral anoxia, Arch. Surg., 41:772, 1940.

Burford, G. E., and H. Leigh: Routine oxygen inhalation during spinal anesthesia: a factor for increased safety, Anesth. and Analg., 18:312, 1939.

Carraway, C. N.: Pentothal sodium with nasal oxygen: a report of 3810 consecutive cases, Anesth. and Analg., 18:259, 1939.

Chornyak, J.: Structural changes produced in the human brain by oxygen deprivation (anoxemia) and their pathogenesis, Ann Arbor, Mich., Edwards Brothers, 1938.

Courville, C. B.: Asphyxia as a consequence of nitrous oxide anesthesia, Medicine, 15:129, 1936.

Eversole, U. H.: The use of helium in anesthesia, Jour. Amer. Med. Asso., 110:878, 1938.

Flagg, P. J.: The Art of Anesthesia, Philadelphia, J. B. Lippincott Co., 6th Ed., 1939.

Gillespie, N. A.: Endotracheal Anesthesia, Madison, University of Wisconsin Press, 1941.

Jones, G. W., and G. J. Thomas: Prevention of cyclopropane-oxygen explosions by dilution with helium. Anesth., 2:138, 1941.

Kreiselman, J.: A new resuscitation apparatus, Anesthesiology, 4:608, 1943.

McClure, R. D., F. W. Hartman, J. G. Schnedorf, and V. Schelling: Anoxia: a source of possible complications in surgical anesthesia, Ann. Surg., 110:835, 1939; Jour. Amer. Med. Asso., 114:189, 1940.

Murphy, F. J.: Anoxemia in relation to use of nitrous oxide anesthesia, Surg., Gynec., and Obstet., **70**:741, 1940.

O'Brien, J. D., and A. T. Steegmann: Severe degeneration of the brain following nitrous oxide-oxygen anesthesia, Ann. Surg., **107**:486, 1938.

Schnedorf, J. G., P. H. Lohran, and T. G. Orr: Problem of anoxia in surgery and anesthesia, Arch. Surg., **43**:169, 1941.

Schreiber, F.: Cerebral anoxia and anesthesia, Trans. Am. Soc. Anesth., **5**:1, 1939.

Schreiber, F.: Cerebral anoxia and craniocerebral injuries, Mich. State Med. Soc. Jour., **40**:603, 1941.

Schreiber, R., and Gates, N.: Jour. Michigan State Med. Soc., **37**:145, 1938.

Shaw, J. L., B. F. Steele, and C. A. Lamb: Effect of anesthesia on blood oxygen: II. Study of effect of spinal anesthesia on oxygen in arterial and venous blood, Arch. Surg., **35**:503, 1937.

Smart, E. P.: Helium in anesthesia and therapeutics particularly in thoracic surgery, Jour. Thoracic Surg., **10**:709, 1941.

Waters, R. M.: Toxic properties of carbon dioxide, West Virginia Med. Jour., **34**: 289, 1938.

Waters, R. M.: Anoxia, the anesthetist's point of view, Jour. Amer. Med. Asso., **115**:1687, 1940.

Waters, R. M.: Tracheobronchial toilet, Brit. Jour. Anæsth., **18**:1, 1942.

Waters, R. M., A. J. Wineland, and M. H. Seevers: Carbon dioxide and oxygen problems in anesthesia, Anesth. and Analg., **10**:10, 1931.

20

Aero-embolism

DEFINITION

Aero-embolism refers to the production in the blood and tissues of the body of nitrogen bubbles caused by ascent to high altitudes. This is not a new concept in medicine since the same phenomenon long has been encountered in caisson workers and divers who have been allowed to come up from increased pressures under water to that of sea-level atmosphere at too rapid a rate. The condition has been often called bends among divers since the pain is sometimes so severe as to cause them to bend over; it is also called caisson sickness. The nitrogen bubbles frequently lodge in the joints, causing local pain, in other instances in the lungs, in which case edema may take place locally, called the chokes; bubbles may end in the central nervous system, causing paralysis. Symptoms of aero-embolism in the skin are those of itching and urticaria.

PATHOLOGIC PHYSIOLOGY

The possibility that aero-embolism may take place in aviators was mentioned by Boycott and Haldane in 1908; Armstrong carefully studied the condition as it occurred in lowering of the barometric pressure in chambers. The condition is now met with in high-altitude flying, particularly when the altitude reached is above 25,000 feet. The condition does not occur until altitudes above 18,000 feet are encountered; namely, above one-half an atmosphere.

In combat military aviation the pilot may bring his plane to 35,000 feet in seven to ten minutes. After this swift rate of ascent brings him to a barometric pressure of 190 mm. Hg or one-quarter of the sea-level barometric pressure of 760 mm. Hg, the relative decompression is similar to that experienced by a diver ascending from 100 feet under water, which is equivalent to four atmospheres, to the surface level. Nitrogen bubbles may be produced in the tissues and blood stream in each instance although a smaller number of bubbles may be formed in the air because of the relatively decreased amount of nitrogen dissolved in the blood at sea level as compared to a pressure of four atmospheres.

The bubble is originally composed of nitrogen, and subsequently carbon dioxide, oxygen, and water vapor may diffuse into it. This is because at sea level nitrogen has a pressure of 573 mm., carbon dioxide 47 mm., water vapor 47 mm., and oxygen 35 mm., in the tissues and venous blood. At the altitudes reached by aviators, the pressure of carbon dioxide and oxygen is insufficient to cause formation of bubbles but nitrogen is obviously present at a pressure sufficiently high so that it goes out of solution in the blood or in the tissue fluid. The symptoms produced apparently depend upon the localization of the nitrogen bubble. Recent investigations have been made on the complex nature of aero-embolism, but they cannot be fully discussed at this time.

It has long been known that inhalation of pure oxygen results in the diffusion of nitrogen from the blood into the alveolar air and thence into the outer atmosphere. If this is continued for a period of five hours, 95 per cent of the dissolved nitrogen is eliminated from the body. Inhalations of helium and oxygen may also be employed to rid the body of dissolved nitrogen. Ascent to high altitudes may then be undertaken with better results than if nitrogen desaturation had not been performed. This is because there is a swifter elimination of helium since its diffusion rate is twice that of nitrogen and also because helium is one-half as soluble in blood as nitrogen. However, inhalation of 100 per cent oxygen is the method of choice since it has been shown that pure oxygen is not irritating to the human lung in periods of inhalation which would be required for this purpose.

Newborn rats exposed to explosive decompression at a simulated altitude of 50,000 feet die of severe abdominal distention and related circulatory failure, both of which are largely prevented by breathing pure oxygen for five hours prior to this test.

Tissues with a high fat content give up their nitrogen more slowly, which accounts for the fact that one-half the total nitrogen may be eliminated by breathing 100 per cent oxygen for 40 minutes, but it requires at least 80 minutes for half the nitrogen dissolved in fatty tissues to be eliminated.

It may be pointed out that helium is only one-third as soluble in fat as nitrogen and therefore the quantity of this gas available for bubble formation, especially in bone marrow, which may be 90 per cent fat, is greatly reduced.

INHALATIONAL THERAPY

Although certain individuals are more sensitive to aero-embolism than others, and a method of preselection of pilots has been employed in order to weed out the subjects more apt to get aero-embolism, at the very high altitudes almost everyone will sooner or later develop symptoms that indicate formation of nitrogen bubbles. Inhalation of 100 per cent oxygen is the only sure method of preventing this syndrome. Although in military operations the time required to accomplish full nitrogen desaturation is longer than is frequently feasible, an attempt to rid the body of as much nitrogen as is consistent with the combat mission should be pursued. Relatively short periods of inhalation of 100 per cent oxygen, such as one hour, protect a good many individuals from altitudes between 25,000 and 30,000 feet. In exposure to altitudes between 30,000 and 40,000 feet inhalation of oxygen must be pursued for periods of two to three hours to insure the probability that none of the members of the airplane crew will get symptoms of aero-embolism. For altitudes above 40,000 feet more prolonged inhalation of oxygen must be carried out, especially if the airplane is to be at this altitude for a long period of time.

Any leak-tight mask may be employed for inhalation of 100 per cent oxygen. The use of the pressure suit or pressure cabin has been advocated in order to produce a pressure at high altitudes equivalent to that of sea level or to that comparable to a level of 8,000 feet (or higher), since in this way the dangers of anoxia and aero-embolism both would be removed. The disadvantage of pressurized cabins or suits is that a sudden leak would result in explosive decompression, the consequences of which would depend upon the pressure differential. The sudden anoxia might be compensated for by immediate use of a mask containing 100 per cent oxygen. The symptoms of aero-embolism might then have to be countered by swift descent to an altitude of 18,000 feet. In probably all instances in which aero-embolism may take place, the symptoms will disappear if there is opportunity for the individual to return promptly to a barometric pressure of less than one-half an atmosphere.

BIBLIOGRAPHY

Armstrong, H. G.: Principles and Practice of Aviation Medicine, Baltimore, Williams & Wilkins Co., 1940.

Barach, A. L., N. Molomut, and S. Landy: The effect of pre-oxygenation on newborn rats exposed to a simulated altitude of 55,000 feet (barometric pressure 67.8 mm. Hg), Jour. Aviation Med., 13:190, 1942.

Bauer, L. H.: Aviation Medicine, Baltimore, Williams & Wilkins Co., 1926.

Bauer, L. H.: Aviation Medicine, New York, Oxford University Press, 1943.

Behnke, A. R., Jr.: High atmospheric pressures; physiological effects of increased and decreased pressure; application of these findings to clinical medicine, Ann. Int. Med., 13:2217, 1940.

Behnke, A. R., Jr., L. A. Shaw, E. C. Messer, R. M. Thomson, and E. P. Motley: Acute circulatory and respiratory disturbances of compressed air illness and administration of oxygen as a therapeutic measure, Amer. Jour. Physiol., 114: 526, 1936.

Fulton, J. F.: Physiology and high altitude flying: with particular reference to air embolism and the effects of acceleration, Science, 95:207-212, 1942.

Gemmill, C. L.: Physiology in Aviation, Springfield, Ill., Charles C. Thomas, 1943.

Lovelace, W. R., Jr., W. M. Boothby, and O. O. Benson: Aeroembolism: a medical problem in aviation at high altitude, Scient. Monthly, 53:30, 1941.

21

War Gas Poisoning and Lung Irritants

INTRODUCTION

The chemical agents employed in the last war which produced edema of the lung will be referred to in the following section. Irritant gases also cause pulmonary edema in civil life since substances such as chlorine and nitric acid are also produced in commercial plants for industrial use. Whether lung irritants initiate edema of the lungs in war or industrial gas poisoning, the treatment is the same. Mixtures of one or more substances frequently take place, which makes identification of the individual gas more difficult. The chemicals used in war include liquids and solids as well as gases. Since the gases are heavier than air they tend to collect in low-lying areas, which should be remembered in the event that gas poisoning is attempted. The liquid may persist for days in enclosed places in which gas is relatively quickly dissipated. Chemical agents may be disseminated by bombs, shells filled with liquid, including gases liquefied by pressure, by discharging gases from cylinders, by spraying liquids from aircraft, and by detonating mixtures of solid substances.

The signs of lung irritation are cough, tightness, and pain in the chest, followed by shortness of breath and expectoration of frothy mucus. In severe cases cyanosis, nausea, vomiting, and prostration take place.

Poison gases which affect only the skin, eyes, and ears will not be discussed in this section since there is no specific inhalational therapy indicated.

LUNG IRRITANTS

Gas masks give adequate protection against the known lung irritants and would of course be used if an attack were recognized in time. When exposure has taken place the symptoms depend upon the nature of the individual gas.

Phosgene ($COCl_2$). Phosgene is a colorless gas at temperatures above 8° C. with an odor like that of musty hay. Soluble in water, it hydrolyzes to hydrochloric acid and carbon dioxide. It has caused pulmonary edema in peacetime when carbon-tetrachloride (Pyrene) fire extinguishers have been used in enclosed places since this compound when in contact with hot metal liberates phosgene. In military operations it is employed in shells and bombs, or liberated from cylinders.

Although it causes damage to the lining of all the respiratory passages, the pulmonary alveoli are more seriously affected. Since there is little immediate irritation in the larynx and trachae, the gas may reach the lung in high concentrations. Pulmonary edema, tearing of the alveoli, thrombosis, and concentration of blood in the pulmonary blood vessels constitute the main pathology. Bronchopneumonia frequently follows after several days if the patient survives pulmonary edema.

The symptoms may not manifest themselves for two to eight hours, although exposure to moderate concentrations of the gas results in watering of the eyes, catching of the breath, and a feeling of tightness in the chest. Deep breathing may cause painful coughing. After a period of several hours the characteristic symptoms of edema of the lungs manifest themselves, with moist râles in the lungs and the patient coughing up bloody or frothy sputum.

INHALATIONAL THERAPY. Complete rest and warmth are universally prescribed with inhalation of oxygen-enriched atmospheres to prevent anoxia, but this therapy is deemed insufficient.

Oxygen can be administered by a rubber catheter in the nasal or oral pharynx, by a mask apparatus of the B.L.B. or Meter type, or by an oxygen tent. If a mask is employed for oxygen therapy, without positive pressure, caution should be exercised to prevent negative pressure from developing in it as a result of collapsing of the rubber bag at end of inspiration, since this would in all probability increase pulmonary edema. Use of the Meter mask with the injector set at 40 per cent oxygen makes possible a high flow of oxygen-enriched air, with an economical oxygen flow and without negative pressure in the mask. This is especially important in the metered positive-pressure mask; positive pressure cannot be obtained in the B.L.B. apparatus.

The most valuable and at times apparently specific procedure is the administration of positive pressure from 2 to 6 cm. of water. The physiology and clinical application of positive-pressure respiration, discussed fully in the section on pulmonary edema, need not be reviewed here. Carlisle has used the Meter mask with the resistance provided on expiration in a large series of cases of pulmonary edema occurring in the course of industrial gas poisoning, and has reported clearing of edema and ultimate recovery in each instance, even after heavy fumes of chlorine and nitric acid. In the mask referred to, positive pressure may be obtained by exhaling through constricted orifices which gives positive pressure during expiration from 1 to 4 cm. of water. The patient is first exposed to 4 cm. of water until the signs of edema clear. It seems likely that the full development of pulmonary edema and subsequent bronchopneumonia would be less apt to take place if treatment were begun early, before serious symptoms manifest themselves. As the edema clears, the pressure against which the patient breathes may be gradually lowered.

The physiologic advantages of positive-pressure respiration have been described in the section on pulmonary edema, including (1) a direct opposing pressure on the external surface of the pulmonary capillaries, (2) a more patent lumen of the intrathoracic bronchi during expiration, and (3) a diminished flow of blood into the right heart.

When a patient has been exposed to a high concentration of phosgene or other irritant gases, a swift exitus may follow or the damage done to the lung may be too extensive for any therapy. However, in the group in which the permeability of the pulmonary capillaries has been increased without irreversible damage, the use of positive pressure may be of decisive value, with oxygen if feasible or with air if cylinders of oxygen are not available.

If oxygen is not available, the Meter mask may be employed with inhalation of air by removing the collecting bag. The closure of the inspiratory valve allows the exhalation to proceed outward through the expiratory flutter valve and then through the varying-sized disks that represent the positive pressure required. During inspiration the inspiratory flutter valve allows air instead of oxygen to come into the mask. When no mask is available, the patient should be instructed to breathe outward through a hand-made device such as a cigarette holder. Even in the absence of any appliance, it is possible for the patient to take a natural inhalation and then purse the lips together so that the expiration may proceed against the positive pressure of the patient's own arbitrarily created orifice.

An alternate method is to close the glottis during expiration, as the patient with lobar pneumonia does in producing the expiratory grunt.

It appears likely, on the basis of evidence previously presented, that grunting in lobar pneumonia has a physiologically advantageous purpose. In the absence then of any device for the creation of positive pressure in expiration, the gassed individual may be told to employ grunting and groaning respiration, the purpose being explained to him.

Although 5 to 10 per cent carbon dioxide with oxygen has been advocated in phosgene poisoning, its use seems to be contraindicated because of the fact that the deep breathing engineered by inhaling carbon dioxide will increase the negative intrapulmonary pressure and in that way accelerate the formation of the edema fluid from the pulmonary capillaries.

In certain types of gas poisoning in which the bronchi are affected, inhalation of helium-oxygen mixtures may be an advantage since a swifter effusion of a helium-oxygen mixture may take place in the presence of obstruction. Under these circumstances the administration of positive pressure during inspiration and expiration, such as provided by the helmet-hood apparatus, would be the procedure of choice. If helium were available a mixture of 40 per cent oxygen and 60 per cent helium could be provided by admitting an oxygen stream from one cylinder and a helium-oxygen mixture from the usual 80 per cent helium–20 per cent oxygen cylinders and joining them with a Y-tube before entrance into the hood.

Artificial respiration by a pulmotor or a resuscitator should not be used since damage to the lungs may take place because of the relatively high positive and negative pressures; positive pressure may cause rupture of the alveolar membrane and negative pressure increased edema.

Certain gases are more apt to produce spasm of the bronchioles, in which event the inhalation of the nebulized spray of 1 per cent epinephrine may be used as described in the section on asthma. It may also be helpful similarly to inhale the spray of 1 per cent neosynephrin. Although these may be nebulized by hand bulbs, larger quantities are provided by running a stream of 4 liters a minute of oxygen through the nebulizer. Venesection has been employed in the stage of blue cyanosis where there is distention of the superficial veins. When peripheral circulatory collapse has taken place with a gray hue to the face and a weak pulse, it is contraindicated. The usual measures for combating shock are employed when this condition is present. In the treatment of pulmonary edema the employment of digitalis and hypodermic adrenalin are not of value. However, injection of caffeine sodium benzoate, metrazol, or neosynephrin hydrochloride may be of temporary help in the presence of peripheral circulatory failure. The employment of adrenal cortical solution may be helpful. Intravenous injections of 50 cc. of 50 per cent glucose may be of value as a palliative procedure, provided the heart is not showing signs of failure.

A brief description of other gases follows:

Diphosgene ($ClCOOCCl_3$). This is an oily liquid which smells like phosgene; it is used in bombs and shells. It affects the eyes more than phosgene but otherwise is similar.

Chlorine. Chlorine is a greenish-yellowish gas with a characteristic familiar odor similar to that of bleaching powders. Used in shells and bombs, and liberated from metal cylinders during the First World War, it is not considered likely that it will be used in this war, although the possibility of its employment must be guarded against. It produces a marked irritation in the upper respiratory tract, at times necrosis of the tracheal mucous membrane and bronchi, and also alveolar damage with severe pulmonary edema.

The symptoms are more acute than those of phosgene poisoning, consisting of violent paroxysms of coughing, a burning painful sensation in the respiratory passageway, and the onset of edema of the lungs within a period of 10 to 20 minutes.

Chloropicrin (CCl_3NO_2). This is a colorless oily liquid of high vapor pressure, relatively nonpersistent, with a smell like licorice. It is employed in shells and bombs.

The fumes of this agent produce extremely irritating effects throughout the entire respiratory tract, with plugging of the bronchi, obstructive emphysema, and, less frequently, pulmonary edema. The absorption of the poison may result in nephritis. The symptoms are similar to phosgene poisoning but the tearing and burning in the eyes is marked and the coughing is more severe.

Nitrous Fumes. They arise mostly from nitric oxide (NO), nitrogen dioxide (NO_2), or nitrogen tetroxide (N_2O_4). These gases are reddish-brown with a pungent odor, and form nitrous and nitric acid when dissolved in water.

The fumes are formed in industrial accidents by the action of nitric acid on organic matter and are incidentally produced in military operations in which explosives are incompletely burned in a confined state. Ulceration of the bronchiolar mucous membrane and edema of the lungs may take place, with symptoms similar to those of phosgene poisoning. In addition, the toxic effect of the nitrite may cause collapse or the production of methemoglobin.

Irritation of the eyes takes place immediately, as well as in the nose and pharynx, followed by a latent period of four to eight hours after which edema of the lungs develops.

Ammonia (NH_3) has a characteristic pungent odor and is a colorless gas lighter than air and very soluble in water. Although not employed in warfare it may be liberated by refrigerating apparatus. The ordinary gas mask does not give protection against it. The symptoms produced include severe irritation of the eye and upper respiratory tract, and edema of the glottis with a pseudomembranous laryngitis. The reflex cessation of respiration may produce asphyxia with spasm and edema of the glottis, larynx, and trachea.

Discussion. The significant factor in pulmonary edema caused by industrial or war gases is the increased permeability of the pulmonary epithelium. In addition to this effect the already existing hydrostatic pressure in the capillaries is also responsible for the outpouring of serum from them. Since it has been decisively shown that inhalation of air under negative pressures as small as 5 cm. of water produces congestion in the lungs of animals, and ultimately edema, the first requirement for inhalational therapy is to prevent the patient from being compelled to inhale a therapeutic gas at the expense of physical effort on the part of the respiratory musculature. In other words, the gas provided to him should be presented without any additional negative pressure. Furthermore, the weight of physiologic and clinical evidence in the treatment of pulmonary edema in the course of respiratory and cardiac disease is such as to offer legitimate support for its employment in irritant lung edema. Although further evidence concerning its value in the treatment of gas poisoning is desired, there is already sufficient testimony to make a trial of its use amply justified.

Although oxygen therapy without pressure will be of value in maintaining respiratory function until the cessation of serous oozing from the capillary takes place, and although a lessened volume of ventilation and consequently a lessened intrapulmonary negative pressure would take place as a result of its use, a large amount of serous fluid in the smaller bronchi forms an obstruction, with impaired drainage, infection of the retained secretions, and bronchopneumonia as a frequent result. Many years ago the author observed a patient who developed edema of the lungs from chlorine-gas poisoning. He was treated in an oxygen tent for seven days and although he was more comfortable and less anoxic, death ultimately took place as a result of bronchopneumonia. At this time it is likely that the administration of the sulfonamide drugs may prevent in small part the consequences of infection in the lungs. However, the employment of positive pressure, if it is effective in preventing or retarding the outpouring of serous fluid, would be valuable from the standpoint of both prevention of infection as well as ultimate recovery.

An additional source of evidence that positive pressure may be of help in irritant gas poisoning is obtained from the behavior of patients who have had tracheotomy for previously existing obstruction in the larynx. As pointed out in that section, a very frequent occurrence is the outpouring of mucus and serum into the tracheobronchial passage within a short time after tracheotomy has relieved the obstruction. This is a clear example of alteration of permeability, both in the pulmonary capillaries and in the mucous glands in the bronchi, due to a sudden withdrawal of a previously existing positive pressure. Since the clinical use of positive pressure has been shown to be effective in clearing this type of pulmonary edema also, an example is available to support the argument of the probable effectiveness of inhalation of air or oxygen under positive pressure in cases in which the permeability of the pulmonary capillary has been diminished by direct irritation.

Since it is generally admitted that there is no intention on the part of our military forces to employ war gases until this practice has been previously employed by the enemy, it seems legitimate and desirable that the probable effectiveness of positive pressure breathing in the treatment of this type of pulmonary edema be given a wide hearing among medical as well as lay audiences, and that the facts now available be given to organizations responsible for civilian defense.

Inhalational Therapy. Oxygen under positive pressure during inspiration and expiration would overcome to a considerable extent the narrowing of the upper respiratory passageway. If helium is available a mixture of 30 per cent oxygen and 70 per cent helium under pressure of 4 to 6 cm. of water in the helmet-hood apparatus would compensate for a marked degree of constriction in the respiratory passageway. If helium is not available, oxygen under pressure provides considerable relief. When the obstruction is confined to the glottis and larynx, tracheotomy may give complete relief.

Mustard gas and Lewisite both irritate and destroy the skin. The inhalation of these gases may be followed by ulceration and infection in the bronchi and finally by bronchopneumonia. In most instances edema of the lungs is not produced except as a complication.

The administration of positive pressure is indicated whenever pulmonary edema occurs. Inhalation of oxygen-enriched atmospheres is indicated if anoxia is present. The methods and results of positive-pressure respiration were discussed in the treatment of phosgene poisoning.[1]

BIBLIOGRAPHY

Barach, A. L.: The treatment of pulmonary edema due to gas poisoning in war and in civilian life, with special reference to the use of positive pressure respiration, New England Jour. Med., March, 1944.

Barach, A. L., J. Martin, and M. Eckman: Positive pressure respiration and its application to the treatment of acute pulmonary edema, Ann. Int. Med., 12: 754, 1938.

Barach, A. L., and P. Swenson: Effect of breathing gases under positive pressure on lumens of small and medium-sized bronchi, Arch. Int. Med., 63:946, 1939.

Barcroft, J. H., G. H. Hunt, and D. Dufton: The treatment of chronic cases of gas poisoning by continuous oxygen administration in chambers, Quart. Jour. Med., 13:179, 1920.

Carlisle, J. M.: Personal communications.

Carlisle, J. M.: Pulmonary edema, Jour. Amer. Med. Asso., 123:947, 1943.

Haldane, J. S.: The administration of oxygen, Brit. Med. Jour., 2:517, 1918.

Segal, M. S., and M. Aisner: The management of certain aspects of gas poisoning with particular reference to shock and pulmonary complications, Ann. Int. Med., 20:219, No. 2, 1944.

Treatment of War Injuries, Merck & Co., 1942.

Welch, W. H.: Zur Pathologie des Lungenödems, Virchows Arch. f. path. Anat., 72:375, 1878.

Winternitz, M. C.: Collected Studies on the Pathology of War Gas Poisoning, New Haven, Yale University Press, 1920.

[1] A case of advanced pulmonary edema due to irritant gas poisoning has recently been described in which the application of positive pressure with the Meter mask appeared to be responsible for a swift clearing of edema and ultimate recovery of the patient. (This patient was treated by E. A. Rovenstine and the details of the case history are given in the paper by Barach, New England Jour. Med., March, 1944.)

22

Postencephalographic Headache

DEFINITION

Following encephalography, headache, nausea, and other disagreeable symptoms take place due to the slowness with which the introduced air escapes from the subarachnoid space and the ventricles.

PATHOLOGIC PHYSIOLOGY

The rate of escape of a gas from the ventricles is dependent upon certain physical factors. Since it is impractical to aspirate gas from the subarachnoid space, the only method of eliminating the introduced air is for this material to be picked up by the blood stream, delivered to the lung, and diffused to the outer atmosphere. The introduction of oxygen into the ventricles is followed by the diffusion of nitrogen and carbon dioxide from capillary blood into the oxygen atmosphere. However, when the patient *breathes* 100 per cent oxygen following encephalography with pure oxygen, most of the physically dissolved blood nitrogen is eliminated swiftly through the lungs, which prevents introduction of nitrogen into the subarachnoid space. This procedure has unquestionably lessened the duration of headache.

A recent improvement is the introduction of helium into the subarachnoid space and the inhalation of 100 per cent oxygen after the roentgenograms have been taken. The value of this procedure may be explained as follows: The diffusion of a gas depends upon the difference in pressure between the gas in the subarachnoid space and the same gas in the blood stream, and on the inherent diffusibility of the gas itself. Helium will diffuse from the subarachnoid space into the capillary blood since the latter contains only an infinitesimal quantity of physically dissolved helium. In addition, the diffusibility of helium according to Graham's law is far swifter than that of nitrogen or oxygen. Since the diffusion rate of a gas is inversely proportional to the square root of its molecular weight, helium with a molecular weight of 4, nitrogen with a molecular weight of 28, and oxygen with a molecular weight of 32 have diffusion rates inversely proportional to 2, 5.3, and 5.7, respectively. In other words the diffusion rate of helium is almost three times that of either oxygen or nitrogen. There is, therefore, from this theoretical consideration an anticipated advantage in the employment of helium. However, since the solubility of helium is one-half that of nitrogen, the circulating blood carries only one-half as much helium as it can nitrogen, which would tend to delay the removal of helium from the subarachnoid space. Nevertheless the procedure is effective when oxygen is breathed. Nitrogen is then eliminated largely through the lung without diffusing into the subarachnoid space. A small amount of carbon dioxide and oxygen does enter the helium area.

The symptoms which follow encephalography with air last 58.5 hours if no oxygen inhalation is permitted and 15 hours if pure oxygen is inhaled. When oxygen is introduced into the subarachnoid space and followed by inhalation of pure oxygen, the symptoms last nine hours. When helium encephalography is performed without inhalation of oxygen the headache and other disturbances persist for 18 hours or longer but this period is said to be strikingly reduced to three to four hours if pure oxygen is inhaled after the introduction of helium.

Pure oxygen may be given either with the B.L.B. or the Meter-mask apparatus.

BIBLIOGRAPHY

Cleveland, D., and E. End: Helium in encephalography, Surg., Gynec., and Obstet., **74**:760, 1942.

Schwab, R. S., J. Fine, and W. J. Mixter: Reduction of postencephalographic symptoms by inhalation of 95 per cent oxygen, Arch. Neurol. and Psychiat., **37**:1271, 1937.

23

Anoxia and Brain Lesions Following Fever Therapy

INTRODUCTION

Pathologic studies in patients and animals autopsied after exposure to heat therapy have revealed hemorrhage, edema, and degeneration of cells throughout the cerebrum and cerebellum. In addition, degeneration and hemorrhage of the adrenal glands, and edema and congestion in the lungs have been reported.

PATHOLOGIC PHYSIOLOGY

When animals were exposed to fever therapy, such as temperatures induced to a range of 104° to 108° F. for 4 to 14 hours, the measurement of the arterial blood revealed a marked decrease in oxygen saturation, in many instances as low as 60 per cent oxygen. Due to the increased blood flow the arterial venous-oxygen difference is reduced. In patients exposed to fever therapy alkalosis is severe, since a pH of the blood averaging 7.6 is found, as a result of the rapid breathing and blowing off of carbon dioxide. This is in itself conducive to anoxia, both by its effect on the hemoglobin which holds on to oxygen more tightly and by producing capillary constriction and ischemia of tissues. The shallow breathing is in part the cause of the marked lowering of the oxygen saturation of the arterial blood. An additional factor is the increased temperature of the blood which has been shown to decrease the oxygen saturation at a time when the oxygen consumption is notably increased as a result of the fever; a 40 per cent rise in basal metabolic rate accompanies a temperature of 106° F. It should be remembered, however, that the increased temperature of the blood facilitates unloading of oxygen to the tissues, similar to the action of an acid shift in pH.

The hypothesis has been advanced that the pathologic changes in the brain and other organs found in autopsied cases of fever therapy that ended in mortality are in large measure due to severe anoxia, since the changes are very comparable to those produced by asphyxia.

INHALATIONAL THERAPY

On the basis of the demonstration of serious anoxia during fever therapy, inhalation of oxygen during the course of heat therapy has been employed with clinically beneficial results. Considering the evidence presented it seems likely that pathologic changes resulting from fever therapy which are typical of anoxia produced in other ways are prevented by adequate oxygen administration. The most practicable method is the administration of oxygen by the nasal catheter, preferably in the oral pharynx.

One of the striking evidences of benefit from oxygen therapy during fever treatment is the slowing of the pulse rate which takes place after oxygen administration as compared to the rapid mounting of the pulse rate in non-oxygen-treated cases. In addition to the increase in the tension of oxygen in the blood, the undue loss of carbon dioxide and the alkaline blood pH are largely prevented when effective oxygen therapy is given continuously.

Although the arterial oxygen tension falls 25 per cent with the development of the desired level of fever, and *continues* to fall as the treatment progresses in routinely treated cases, the patients in whom oxygen was administered during the whole treatment showed no drop in arterial oxygen tension, but rather a continuous rise.

BIBLIOGRAPHY

Cullen, S. C., E. F. Weir, and E. Cook: The rationale of oxygen therapy during fever therapy, Anesthesiol., **3**:123, 1942.

Hartman. F. W.: Lesions of the brain following fever therapy: etiology and pathogenesis, Jour. Amer. Med. Asso., **109**:2116, 1937.

24

Head Injuries

INTRODUCTION

Head injuries may take place with or without skull fracture and at times accompanied by concussion of the brain.

PATHOLOGIC PHYSIOLOGY

Anoxia follows severe head injury when shock is present or when a neurogenic hyperthermia takes place due to disturbance of the temperature-regulating center. A decreased circulation in the brain may take place as a result of increased intracranial pressure, vasodilatation, edema, and hemorrhage. In experimental studies in dogs it has been shown that concussion is accompanied by arterial anoxia, and that this type of oxygen-want may be markedly relieved by inhalation of oxygen-enriched atmospheres. In 12 patients with recent concussion of the brain in whom six had a fracture of the skull, the oxygen saturation was lowered in 10 cases; in two of them the lowering was 34 and 44 per cent. Since brain concussion with or without fracture of the skull results in a lowering of the arterial oxygen saturation of from 5 to 44 per cent below the normal, in both dogs and human beings, there is indication for recommending inhalation of high oxygen concentrations in order to overcome the anoxia. This appears to be all the more legitimate since the brain is sensitive to anoxia.

INHALATIONAL THERAPY

In patients with mild or moderate anoxia inhalation of 50 per cent oxygen with nasal catheter or tent may be employed. In cases in which severe injury has been followed by anoxia and shock, inhalation of concentrations approaching 100 per cent oxygen is suggested in order to increase as much as possible the oxygen physically dissolved in the plasma. Under these circumstances the B.L.B. or Meter mask may be employed with a flow of oxygen of 12 to 15 liters per minute. The length of oxygen therapy should include the period in which the patient is unconscious and in which concussion may be presumed to be present.

BIBLIOGRAPHY

Fulton, J. F.: Blast and concussion in the present war, New England Jour. Med., **226**:1, 1942.

Schnedorf, J. G., R. A. Munslow, A. S. Crawford, and R. D. McClure: Anoxia and oxygen therapy in head injury, Surg., Gynecol., and Obstet., **70**:628, 1940.

25

Paralysis of the Respiratory Musculature

INTRODUCTION

The most frequent cause of paralysis of the respiratory musculature is poliomyelitis. Syringomyelia, lethargic encephalitis, and other nerve diseases may occasionally result in impairment or paralysis of the intercostal muscles due to involvement of the cervical and dorsal spinal cords. Although objective dyspnea may not be apparent because the chest fails to move, the patient is nevertheless aware of extreme distress and generally reveals marked anxiety or fear of death.

PATHOLOGIC PHYSIOLOGY

In an adult complete paralysis of the intercostal muscles may not be followed by respiratory distress if he lies quietly in bed. The rate of respiration is increased and the excursion of the diaphragm is larger than under normal conditions. The rigidity of the adult thorax is sufficient to protect the upper thorax against retraction in the transverse diameter when the diaphragm descends, which allows the patient full respiratory value of the fall of the diaphragm. The costal margins are drawn toward the midline during inspiration and there is an exaggeration of normal abdominal breathing.

In a child paralysis of the upper intercostal muscles is, however, more apt to result in grave impairment of respiratory function. The flexible ribs do not prevent the upper thorax from retracting, and the sternum and the first two ribs are apt to be pulled downward by the powerful contraction of the diaphragm. Consequently, the volume of the upper lungs is decreased during inspiration and air may pass from them into the stream of air inhaled in the lower portion of the lung. During expiration the upper parts of both lungs are then increased in volume and air from the lower lung may be in part expelled into the upper lung, with the production of a variable amount of rebreathing, resulting in severe anoxia, cyanosis, and dyspnea on very slight exertion. In paralysis of the lower five intercostal muscles in a child the upper lung is enlarged during inspiration and the lower lung also, as a result of descent of the diaphragm. Although the volume capacity of the lower lungs is diminished, there would be no rebreathing between upper and lower lungs, and consequently the patient would have no dyspnea as long as he did not undergo moderate exertion.

Paralysis of all the intercostal muscles in a child will unquestionably result in a certain amount of rebreathing between the upper and lower parts of the lungs. In an adult the chest wall is immobilized after paralysis of all the intercostals and the only movement discerned is in the costal margins which move toward the midline during inspiration, the inspiratory descent of the diaphragm resulting in more marked abdominal protrusion. When any part of the lung is unventilated or filled with air that has been previously employed in another part of the lung, the area contributes unrespired blood to the arterial circulation. The arterial oxygen saturation is inevitably lowered, but in most cases the increased ventilation of the remainder of the lung results in an adequate elimination of carbon dioxide.

In two cases of paralysis of the intercostal muscles in lethargic encephalitis the control arterial oxygen saturation was 64 and 60 per cent, and 84 and 82 per cent respectively after inhalation of 80 per cent oxygen. The arterial carbon-dioxide content rose after treatment with oxygen, in one case from 64 to 88 volumes per cent and in the other from 51 to 62 volumes per cent. In these two cases extreme shallow breathing was an additional cause of the severe anoxia. The mechanism of the increase in carbon-dioxide content as a result of the inhalation of high oxygen concentrations in patients with anoxia has already been discussed in the sections on congestive heart failure and in pulmonary emphysema. It may merely be mentioned here that the retention of carbon dioxide in the blood due to decreased volume of breathing also made possible an increased elimination of carbon dioxide per unit of pulmonary ventilation.

INHALATIONAL THERAPY

In the treatment of acute anterior poliomyelitis the Drinker respirator has been of inestimable value. It has accomplished the aim of maintaining artificial respiration in a manner which provides the patient with as much comfort as possible and at the same time achieves an efficient form of ventilation. In one series of 23 children who had paralysis of the intercostal muscles or the diaphragm of sufficient extent to bring about serious impairment of respiratory function, three died of pneumonia. Although it cannot be proven that all of the others would have died, life was preserved in a number of them who otherwise apparently would have succumbed. Certainly the relief given to children with paralysis of the intercostal muscles or the diaphragm is sufficiently great to justify its use. In patients who are under 12 years of age the respirator is run at a rate between 20 and 30 times per minute. In the presence of obstruction to the passage of air due to secretions in the air passages, the patient cannot accommodate himself readily to changes in rate. In some cases the maintenance of a rate of 48 times per minute has been used. The negative pressure in the respirator is usually between 15 and 20 cm. of water. Passive expiration is almost always adequate, even in patients with the most extensive paralysis. Positive pressure very rarely may be helpful in bringing about a more forceful expiration in patients with paralysis of the abdominal muscles who cannot cough effectively.

In patients with respiratory paralysis of the spinal type (i.e., paralysis of the intercostal muscles and the diaphragm), the machine should be used early, before the appearance of cyanosis, in order to prevent the adverse effect of anoxia on the course of the disease. Since destruction of the nerve cells is considered due to a local tissue anoxia produced in the anterior horns due to edema and lymphocytic infiltration, it is entirely reasonable to prevent generalized anoxemia and inadequate ventilation of the lung. Furthermore, the relief obtained by the patient as shown by relaxation and sleep is itself an indication for the early use of the machine. The patient should be kept in the apparatus for a long time since early removal may result in recurrence in difficulty in breathing and fatigue of the muscles of respiration.

Respiratory failure may also be brought about by involvement of the medulla with the production of pharyngeal paralysis. The diagnosis of this condition is made by hearing audible gurgling in the throat during breathing. Frequent severe choking attacks threaten the patient with asphyxia. A deep inspiration tends to aspirate fluid into the larynx and is frequently interrupted by a forced expiration. Three dangers occur from this form of paralysis: (1) Choking attacks with severe anoxia, (2) aspiration of mucus, and (3) excessive fatigue. Treatment consists in the maintenance of an adequate ventilation in the respirator and measures which will keep the pharynx free from food, vomitus, and secretions. Fluids are administered by rectum or parenterally.

Respiratory failure may also take place as a result of involvement of the respiratory center. Thirteen of a series of 20 patients treated in a Drinker respirator survived. In the patients who survived it was believed that the respirator was an important factor in their ultimate recovery.

In paralysis of the respiratory musculature due to marked bulbar involvement, the condition may be too far advanced and hopeless to try a therapeutic procedure. In other more favorable cases the maintenance of respiratory function may be followed by relatively normal activity of the muscles of respiration and the patient may ultimately be restored to complete health. Unfortunately, patients with poliomyelitis may live for weeks and months in a respirator and finally succumb to pulmonary infection. There are also other patients who are unable to do without the respirator for years.

The respirator designed by Drinker and his collaborators is generally employed to maintain continuous artificial respiration. A negative pressure of 15 cm. of water is sufficient to produce inspiratory enlargement of the chest in most instances. Restoration of pressure to that of the atmosphere causes expiration. The speed and depth of respiration may be varied depending upon individual indications. Patients may take nourishment without interruption of the treatment and at the present time most nursing care may be given through appropriate portholes in the chamber.

A modification of this method has been employed in which a metal plate is fitted to the anterior chest wall by an appropriate rubber leak-tight gasket. A negative pressure is produced between the chest wall and the inner surface of the metal dome which results in inspiratory descent of the diaphragm. Another apparatus employed abroad is the Bragg-Hall pulsator which consists of a flat rubber bag that encircles the chest, being fastened in position by an inextensible outer covering. Air is forced into the bag by contraction of a bellows which is in turn activated by an electric motor. This method of alternated compression of the ribs by air pressure has been used for long periods in a case of progressive muscular atrophy.

When paralysis of the respiratory musculature takes place before mechanical methods of maintaining respiratory function are available, the Sharpey-Schaefer prone method of manual artificial respiration should be employed. The ribs are compressed so that expiration is forced and inspiration follows due to the natural resilience of the bony thorax. A small pad is placed underneath the abdomen with the patient in the prone position. The physician kneels astride the subject and, placing his hands on the lower part of the chest on each side, he employs his body weight to press firmly on the back of the chest, producing expiration in this way. Withdrawal of his weight is followed by inspiration. This method of manual inflation and deflation of the lung is generally carried out from 12 to 15 times a minute.

The modern resuscitator, which uses positive pressure to inflate the lung and negative pressure to cause it to collapse, is an effective remedy for maintaining artificial respiration, and with the blow-off valves now in use should not be considered in the same dangerous category as the old pulmotor. The duration of treatment depends upon the rate at which recovery of the function of the muscles of respiration takes place. In some patients with impairment of activity of the respiratory musculature, especially in the absence of involvement of the diaphragm, inhalation of oxygen in 50 to 60 per cent concentrations may relieve the dyspnea. The diminution in the volume of respiration may also provide the patient with rest to the muscles of breathing. Inhalations of helium with oxygen have also been described in paralysis of the respiratory musculature with subjective relief. The problem in the treatment of these cases is the difficulty in being able to tell in advance whether or not return of function of the respiratory musculature will take place.

BIBLIOGRAPHY

Barach, A. L., and M. N. Woodwell: Studies in oxygen therapy with determination of the blood gases, etc.: I. In cardiac insufficiency and related conditions. Arch. Int. Med., 28:367, 1921. II. In pneumonia and its complications, Arch. Int. Med., 28:394, 1921. III. In an extreme type of shallow breathing occurring in encephalitis, Arch. Int. Med., 28:421, 1921.

Birnbaum, G. L., and S. A. Thompson: Resuscitation in advanced asphyxia, Jour. Amer. Med. Asso., 118:1364, 1942.

Drinker, P., and C. F. McKhann: The use of a new apparatus for the prolonged administration of artificial respiration: I. A fatal case of poliomyelitis, Jour. Amer. Med. Asso., 92:1658, 1929.

Eversole, U. H.: The use of helium in anesthesia, Jour. Amer. Med. Asso., 110:878, 1938.

Wilson, J. L.: Acute anterior poliomyelitis: treatment of bulbar and high spinal types, New England Jour. Med., 206:887, 1932.

26

Cerebral Embolism and Thrombosis

INTRODUCTION

Occlusion of one of the cerebral blood vessels may take place as a result of an embolus or thrombus, the latter usually incident to arteriosclerosis. Degeneration and necrosis of the brain tissue supplied by the artery take place to a varying degree as a result of tissue ischemia and anoxia. Symptoms depend upon the localization of the lesion but paralysis of one side, speech defects, and mental disturbances are frequent. Death occurs in 30 per cent of patients with cerebral hemorrhage, in 15 per cent of those with thrombosis, and in 7.5 per cent of those with embolism. The disturbance which remains in patients that recover is subject to wide variation, depending upon the character and extent of the lesion.

PATHOLOGIC PHYSIOLOGY

Occlusion of a cerebral artery results in acute local anoxia of the area supplied by the blood vessel. Thrombosis may obliterate the entire lumen but occasionally there is absorption and recanalization of the thrombus. In the cortex of the brain collateral circulation is more readily established than in the brain stem.

Since brain tissue is more sensitive to oxygen-want than any other body organ, the attempt to remedy local anoxia by increasing the physically dissolved oxygen in conditions of total or partial occlusion of a cerebral blood vessel is amply justified. It has been shown that the cortex is most sensitive to anoxia. The newer phyletic and higher anatomic portions of the central nervous system possess a higher metabolic rate and are therefore the first parts to be overcome by lack of oxygen. The function of the cerebral cortex shows impairment before that of the midbrain and the medulla. From a pathologic point of view hemorrhage in the brain appears as a result of anoxia before it occurs in other organs.

Therefore, since the brain is the organ most readily damaged by anoxia and since the damage of brain tissue results in a most disturbing form of invalidism, there is a definite indication to prescribe the inhalation of 70 to 100 per cent oxygen in these cases. In the treatment of coronary thrombosis and of shock, the increase in the physically dissolved oxygen in the blood has been shown to be followed by clinical improvement, even in the absence of arterial anoxemia, an argument which applies to the treatment of cerebral hemorrhage, thrombosis, and embolism. In the small series reported by Poulton, oxygen therapy appeared to be clinically valuable and it is conceivable that more severe brain damage was prevented. It may be remembered that in the early development of oxygen therapy, inhalation of oxygen-enriched atmosphere in patients with obliterative endarteritis was helpful in promoting healing of ulcers due to ischemia.

INHALATIONAL THERAPY

Although oxygen therapy is not conventionally employed in the treatment of occlusion of cerebral blood vessels, the inhalation of 70 to 100 per cent oxygen is recommended in every case where it is feasible to do so. Recognizing that 2.5 cc. of oxygen may thus be added to 100 cc. of circulating blood, and that the average quantity of oxygen removed from this amount of blood circulating from artery to vein is 5 to 6 cc., the provision of this additional amount of oxygen should be helpful. In experiments in dogs in shock 1.5 to 2 cc. of additional oxygen have actually been found in right-heart blood during inhalation of 100 per cent oxygen. Every precaution, therefore, should be taken to prevent not only impairment of brain functioning but pathologic permanent damage in brain structure.

The oxygen-mask apparatus should be employed with a sufficiently high flow to provide 70 to 100 per cent oxygen until the patient has recovered from the effect of the cerebral embolus, thrombosis, or hemorrhage. This might require as long as five to eight days. The rationale of adding this significantly increased quantity of physically dissolved oxygen is that a substantial increase in oxygen pressure in the capillaries of the collaterals bordering on the occluded blood vessel may prevent additional edema and hemorrhage. If oxygen therapy is conducted longer than 48 hours, the inhalation of 70 per cent oxygen is to be preferred to 100 per cent.

BIBLIOGRAPHY

Poulton, E. P.: Local tissue anoxia and its treatment, Lancet, 2:305, 1939.

27

Chronic Pulmonary Tuberculosis

INTRODUCTION

The purpose of this section is to describe a method of achieving local lung rest through a new type of inhalational therapy in which the force applied to the outer and inner surfaces of the chest wall is made equal by air pressure.

The ultimate objective of therapy in active pulmonary tuberculosis is clearing of the inflammatory tuberculous process. Pneumothorax and other collapse measures are employed for this purpose, as well as to close cavity. Our intention is to present a practical procedure which accomplishes an immobilization of the lungs, decreasing the functional activity of the diseased organs by providing an adequate pulmonary ventilation without lung movement, and in this way initiating or accelerating the healing process. The equalizing pressure chamber has been employed in the treatment of seven patients of advanced bilateral pulmonary tuberculosis with cavities of greater or lesser extent, with complete arrest or clearing of the disease in five cases.

PATHOLOGIC PHYSIOLOGY

Rest of the diseased lung is still regarded as the most effective principle in the treatment of active tuberculosis. Although lying in bed is of considerable therapeutic value in many instances, additional rest has been obtained by varying the posture so that the patient lies on the affected side. Small bags of shot up to two pounds have been placed on each side of the chest in bilateral apical disease in order to rest the upper lobes and allow the bases to be used mainly for ventilation. When a tuberculous lung has been collapsed by pneumothorax, a considerable excursion of the lung nevertheless takes place with each respiratory cycle. Although pneumothorax frequently achieves the desirable aim of closing the cavity, it is not necessarily a substitute for natural healing since in a person with poor resistance a caseous pneumonic process may ulcerate and spread under pneumothorax as readily as if the lung were not collapsed. A person with pulmonary tuberculosis whose disease heals spontaneously is in many respects more fortunate than one who requires the help of collapse measures. The provision of a method of immobilizing the lungs and dispensing with respiratory activity rests on sound physiologic principles.

The procedure requires that the patient lie in a cylindrical chamber in which an alternating pressure is applied but with a differential pressure administered to the head as compared to that of the rest of the body. The principle of the method depends on the physical law that the number of molecules within a container varies with the pressure to which the gas is exposed, provided the volume and temperature of the gas remain constant. In normal respiration a change of the pressure in the lung of 4 mm. Hg, produced by the respiratory musculature during inspiration and the elastic recoil of the lung during expiration, is sufficient to cause an inlet and outflow of 500 cc. of air per minute, approximately one-sixth of the volume of air present in the lungs at the termination of an ordinary expiration.

Under normal circumstances excursion of the lungs takes place of sufficient extent to accommodate 500 cc. of air 16 to 18 times a minute. If the muscles of respiration are thought of as being inactive, the lungs may be conceived as gas containers with a constant volume. Under these circumstances increasing the barometric pressure one-sixth of an atmosphere would result in the passage into the lung container of an additional one-sixth number of gas molecules, in other words, one-sixth of 3,000 cc. or 500 cc. The total number of molecules after this pressure was applied would be the number contained in 3,500 cc. of air at atmospheric pressure. Since the entire body is subjected to alternating pressure, the volume of the chest does not change markedly since pressure is applied *almost* simultaneously to the outer and inner walls of the thorax (Thuneberg). However, observation of patients with chronic pulmonary tuberculosis exposed to an increase and decrease of the barometric pressure of one-sixth of an atmosphere revealed that the chest wall was slightly compressed during the positive phase, although molecules of oxygen and nitrogen were traveling into the lungs at the same time, and that the chest wall was slightly expanded at the start of the negative pressure even though air was then leaving the lung according to the mechanism referred to above (Barach). The resistance in the tracheobronchial passageway was found to account for this type of chest movement, due to slightly different pressures being applied to the outer chest wall than to its inner surface.

Experimental observations in animals revealed that the pressure in the intrapleural space was approximately 5 cm. of water less than that which was found on the outer surface of the chest wall at the beginning of the positive-pressure cycle. In patients with pathologic narrowing of the bronchi through inflammation or spasm the difference in pressure between the inner and outer surfaces of the chest wall is unquestionably much higher than this. By separating the head from the body of the patient by a soft sponge-rubber collar differential pressures may be administered of such degree as to equalize the resistance in the tracheobronchial tree. Although in most instances a pressure of 48 mm. Hg above and below the atmosphere 28 times a minute provides a respiratory exchange sufficient to make possible voluntary cessation of breathing, this alternating pressure in itself is inadequate to produce consistent freedom from chest movement and also to do away with the impulse for breathing, since the pressure on the head end of the chamber must be increased to such an extent as will completely compensate for the resistance in the tracheobronchial tree. The exact amount of pressure required must be ascertained in each case by observation of the patient. In most subjects 4 to 6 cm. of water pressure is applied as a differential pressure in the head compartment during the positive phase, although in one patient a positive pressure of 10 cm. of water was necessary to prevent the slight initial

TABLE VI

EFFECT OF ALTERNATING PRESSURE ON BLOOD GASES OF A DOG IN WHICH
RESPIRATORY ARREST HAD BEEN PRODUCED BY NEMBUTAL ANESTHESIA

Time	Equalizing Pressure	Arterial Oxygen Saturation %	Arterial CO_2 Content Vol. %
10:30 A.M.	0 cm.	71.6	51.3
1:15 P.M.	5 cm.	90.2	51.3
3:00 P.M.	0 cm.	55.0	55.6
4:20 P.M.	5 cm.	93.4	49.8
5:25 P.M.	0 cm.	77.4	53.9
6:20 P.M.	5 cm.	92.8	49.6

compression and expansion of the chest that is observed on simple alternating pressure without equalizing the chest pressure as well.

Animal experiments in which respiratory paralysis was induced by sedative drugs showed that alternating pressure was ultimately ineffective in maintaining adequate respiratory function, as demonstrated by a fall in oxygen saturation and an increase in the carbon-dioxide content of the arterial blood. However, when a suitable increase in the pressure applied to the head-end as compared to the body part of the chamber was produced, with the result that the total pressure was equal on both sides of the chest wall, an adequate respiratory exchange could be maintained in animals whose breathing was paralyzed as a result of excessive anesthesia.

In actual clinical trial it was repeatedly shown that cessation of lung movement could not be accomplished except by the provision of equalizing pressure in addition to alternating pressure. The tracheobronchial tree does not only lower the ultimate pressure that reaches the inner surface of the chest wall, but there is a slight delay in the time at which the pressure arrives within the lung as compared to the instantaneous application of pressure to the chest wall and abdomen. For these various reasons, therefore, a separation of the head from the body end of the chamber is employed to produce the differential pressure required. The most recent chamber developed for this therapy is shown in the section on method.

The effect of varying the oxygen concentration of the inhaled atmosphere has shown no decisive influence on the course of experimental pulmonary tuberculosis. Long-continued exposure to 50 per cent oxygen as well as inhalation of 10 per cent oxygen for periods of two to three months has not revealed any specific influence on the growth of the tubercle bacillus and on the extent of the pathology. Guinea pigs were used in the low-oxygen experiments. When rabbits were employed in more chronic development of pulmonary tuberculosis, the inhalation of 50 per cent oxygen was responsible for a longer duration of life but at the same time there was a progressive increase in the extent of the pulmonary tuberculosis as the animals lived longer. Interpretation of this finding was that the tuberculous process proceeded at its accustomed rate but that the animals having lived longer were in that way able to show at autopsy a larger extent of tuberculosis.

Although inhalation of low-oxygen mixtures has been considered by some to retard tuberculous inflammation or limit the extent of the tuberculous involvement, experiments of the author have not shown any decisive influence, except possibly in increased pulmonary fibrosis. However, there is an enormous enlargement in the size of the heart, with hypertrophy of the muscle, and it may be that the increased blood flow necessitated by continuous breathing of a 10 per cent oxygen mixture may be linked up with some of the chronic pulmonary fibrotic changes.[1]

The inhalation of oxygen-enriched atmospheres has been employed in the end-stage of pulmonary fibrosis in certain patients with pulmonary tuberculosis and the indications and limitations of therapy are those which have already been discussed in Chapter 13, Pulmonary Emphysema.

Inhalation of the nebulized spray of epinephrine and neosynephrin solutions is also at times of palliative value in pulmonary fibrosis of tuberculous etiology. Inhalation of the spray of promin has been shown to be effective in retarding the development of experimental pulmonary tuberculosis. Clinical application of promin by spray has also been employed in three patients but as yet sufficient opportunity has not been afforded to determine its therapeutic value.[1] Inhalation of sulfadiazine nebulin has also been tried in 2½ per cent solution in ethanolamine, to combat secondary infections.[1]

INHALATIONAL THERAPY

The patients who have been selected for immobilizing lung therapy in the equalizing-pressure chamber have been those with advanced pulmonary tuberculosis for whom no other treatment, either medical or collapse therapy, was thought to offer opportunity for further benefit. Although this treatment need in no way be confined to far-advanced cases, the selection of this type of patient was employed in order to ascertain a more conclusive answer to the question of its therapeutic efficacy in initiating a healing process.

The patient is placed in the chamber at first for periods of one-half an hour at a time, three to four times a day during the first three or four days, until cessation of voluntary movement has been thoroughly learned. In most cases this is acquired in two to three hours. The instruction consists in telling the patient to take three or four moderately deep breaths and then to stop in normal expiration. He is informed that it is not necessary for him to breathe since there will be an adequate amount of air entering and leaving his lung. When

---

[1] Unpublished experiments.

the chamber is closed and the alternating air pressure is begun, the chest wall is observed to determine whether slight compression and expansion of the chest take place in the positive and negative phase respectively, at a differential pressure of 5 cm. of water more in the head-end. If some chest movement is seen the differential pressure is changed to 4 or 7 cm. of water. It will soon become evident whether or not this differential pressure is sufficient to prevent excursion of the chest. At first the patient will breathe from time to time because a variable training period is necessary for the habit of voluntary breathing to be broken.

Movement of the surface of the abdomen may take place without necessarily indicating that the diaphragm itself is altered in its position, since some degree of compression and expansion of gases in the stomach and intestine occur. However, compression of any gas in the abdomen during the positive phase is transmitted to the under surface of the diaphragm and is counterbalanced by a similar pressure on the upper surface of the diaphragm arriving at the same time. If there is definite protrusion of the abdomen as a result of an inspiration on the part of the patient, it is evident that he has not yet learned to dispense with the ordinary breathing. The longest instance of maintenance of some degree of voluntary respiration took place in one patient in whom three days were required before he completely gave up the impulse to breathe. It is possible, however, for the patient to cough or to breathe without any feeling of hinderance, differing in this respect from the Drinker respirator in which a change in the volume of the lung is produced by a negative pressure that forcibly expands the chest wall, requiring inspiration at that time.

The patient resides in the equalizing chamber from 9 in the morning until 10 at night, except for one hour at lunch and one hour at dinner during which he is fed. In some cases the patient has been treated continuously seven days a week for a period of three and one-half to four months, but in most instances no treatment was given on Sunday. No distinct difference in response was noted if treatment was omitted in one out of seven days. Furthermore, the employment of treatment 20 hours out of 24 did not seem to be of any special value in one patient, in whom this was carried out. In this patient, pain and discharge from the ears took place after he had been exposed to variation in the pressure on the ear drum for a period of 10 days, both during the day and at night. It has now been shown that pressure on the ear drums and pain are largely preventable. A recent development in the therapy has been the application of sponge-rubber disks to the ears which in a large measure do away with the feeling of an oscillating pressure on the ear drum. Although none of the patients treated in the original series had more than temporary discomfort, except for the occurrence of pain and discharge in the patient mentioned above, the use of the sponge-rubber disk to delay the application of pressure to the external ear until it has arrived through the eustachian tube to the inner surface of the ear drum is a distinct advance in comfort and probably also in maintaining a more normal physiology in the middle ear.

One of the striking effects of respiration being taken over by the apparatus is that a state of relaxation takes place in which for hours at a time the patients have no impulse to produce movement in the voluntary musculature. There is not only local lung rest but an extraordinary form of body rest, as well as mental relaxation. Although the radio is listened to by some patients, in most instances the individual lies quietly in the chamber, in both physical and mental comfort. This is in conspicuous contrast to the state of body and mental rest that takes place on the day that he lies supposedly quietly in bed. On Sundays observation shows that complete body rest is rarely obtained, the patient reaching for a book or to turn on the radio, or simply to move from side to side to change his position. These extraneous movements take place only rarely when voluntary respiration is suspended in the equalizing-pressure chamber.

The response to local lung rest secured by this procedure is first of all a decrease in temperature and pulse rate, manifested during the first two weeks. Between four and six weeks after inauguration of therapy there is a decrease in cough and expectoration as well as a definite recognition of improvement in terms of well-being and loss of malaise. Gain in weight begins and in the majority of cases has reached as much as 20 to 35 pounds during a four-month period, even in cases in which no previous weight gain with bed rest took place. No other special treatment was provided except for a high vitamin intake and a plentiful supply of protein in the diet. It was observed that the patient was unable to eat as long as the toxemia continued but began to increase the amount of food ingested as clinical improvement itself took place.

The earliest effect on x-ray films appears to be that of an increase in infiltration, frequently observed in the second or third week, which may be in part due to the lessened desire to cough and to some pud-

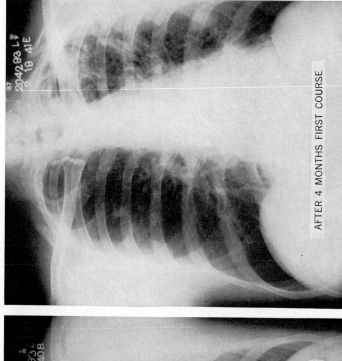

AFTER 4 MONTHS FIRST COURSE

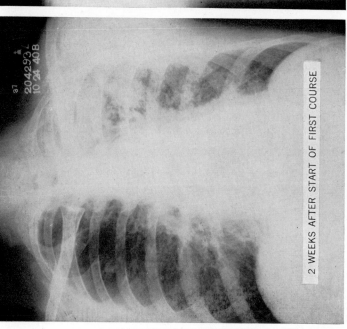

2 WEEKS AFTER START OF FIRST COURSE

Fig. 17. Patient with pulmonary tuberculosis, two weeks after start of first course and after four months, first course.

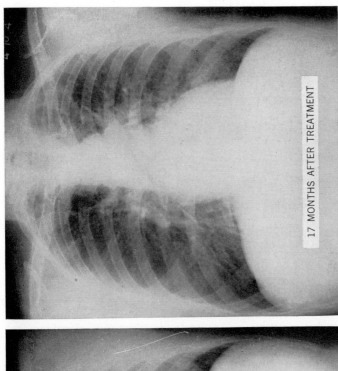

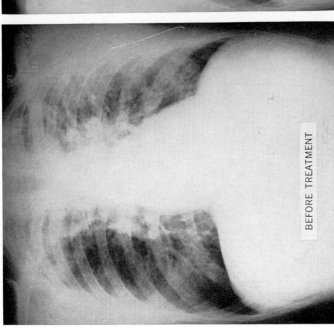

Fig. 18. Patient with pulmonary tuberculosis before treatment, and 17 months after treatment.

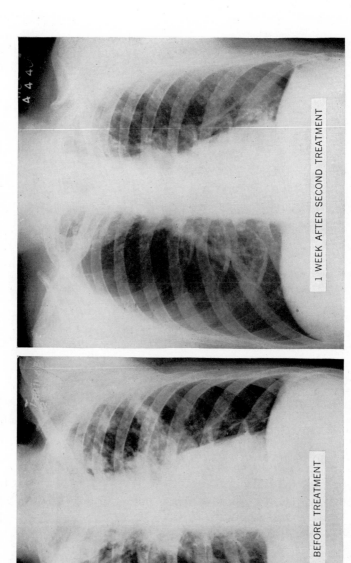

FIG. 19. Patient with pulmonary tuberculosis before treatment, and one week after second treatment.

dling of secretions in the smaller bronchioles with localized atelectasis. However, definite clearing of shadows in x-ray films begins to take place at the end of the second or third month of treatment. If an unquestionable clinical improvement has been initiated in the third or fourth month, treatment has been interrupted and the effect of convalescent care then observed. In some cases, two or three courses of therapy have been required before complete arrest of active tuber-

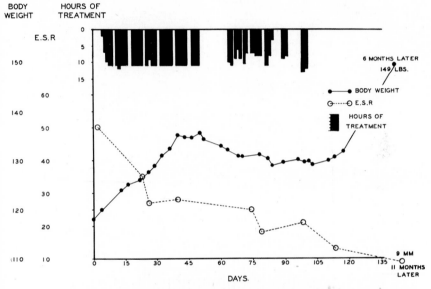

FIG. 20. Sedimentation rate and body weight of a patient during residence in an equalizing-pressure chamber.

culosis and clearing of all cavities have been obtained. This has been in part due to premature discharge from the hospital. In the accompanying roentgenograms, the effect of this type of therapy is illustrated. The clinical charts on pp. 191 and 192 show the gain in weight.

In considering the mechanism by which equalizing-pressure therapy aids the process of resolution in pulmonary tuberculosis, it has been thought that local lung rest is of value in part because the cessation of respiration takes place at the end of expiration in which the negative intrapleural pressure in the lung is at the lowest point. A view which Pinner has expressed is that a relaxation of the lung and consequently a decrease in the elastic tension of the lung favors the mechanism of healing. This is applicable to equalizing-pressure therapy since there is not only a cessation of the rhythmical increase in tension produced during the inspiratory cycle but also because breathing is stopped at the end of expiration when the elastic tension of the lung is at a low level. Amberson has pointed out that diffusion of toxins from tuberculous lesions is probably involved in the spread of inflammation and that this is increased by physical activity. Therefore, cessation of lung movement would decrease diffusion of these toxins and thereby facilitate encapsulation of caseous areas. Finally, in the

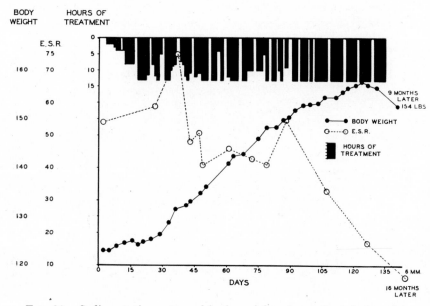

FIG. 21. Sedimentation rate and body weight of a patient during residence in an equalizing-pressure chamber.

closure and collapse of cavity the mechanism of the ball-valve no longer functions when respiration ceases. In normal inspiration enlargement of the chest sucks air into the cavity, but during expiration the small diameter of the bronchiole connected to the cavity constricts still farther and is responsible for increased pressure on the walls of the cavity, with delayed and incomplete emptying. When cessation of lung movement takes place at the end of expiration, this rhythmical distending pressure on the walls of the cavity is no longer present.

Although the total number of cases so far treated is small, the fact that five out of seven cases of advanced bilateral pulmonary tuberculosis achieved a state of complete arrest or clearing of active tuberculosis with negative gastric and concentrate sputum tests for periods in excess of one year, and with discharge from city tuberculosis institutions as ambulatory arrested cases, is evidence that immobilizing lung therapy may be of decisive value in aiding the process of healing in advanced pulmonary tuberculosis with cavity. The clinical improvement in favorable cases has been followed during convalescence by disappearance of all x-ray evidence of tuberculosis, except for changes indicative of fibrosis. In some cases this method had been used to prepare a patient with bilateral disease for thoracoplasty by achieving a stabilization of one lung, but with the unexpected result that the lesions on both sides cleared or became stabilized following immobilizing lung therapy.

Immobilization of the lung by equalizing air pressure, with maintenance of normal lung ventilation, is too recent a procedure for more than a tentative evaluation. Follow-up knowledge concerning the length of time patients remain well will be of interest in this connection. The procedure may be thought of as a measure which in some cases initiates the process of recovery from tuberculosis, with other measures, long known to be of value, to follow later. It is significant that cavities have collapsed repeatedly as a result of this mechanism of arrested lung movement, when bed rest itself did not accomplish this result, in cases that were inoperable.

Inhalation of the nebulized spray of promin may be used as a form of inhalational therapy, based on the remarkable effect of this procedure in experimental guinea-pig tuberculosis. It is possible to combine promin therapy with local lung-rest therapy as carried out in two of the patients in the series mentioned above. In carrying out the promin therapy, a 50 per cent solution diluted one-half with tap water is deposited in a large glass nebulizer which the patient holds within his mouth and breathes quietly as the spray is produced by the passage of 5 liters of oxygen per minute through the nebulizer. In this way 3 to 4 gm. of promin solution may be vaporized and inhaled during the 24-hour period.[2] In some instances it seems desirable to shrink the mucous membranes in the respiratory passageway by previous administration of 0.5 cc. of 1 per cent neosynephrin delivered into the patient's mouth in the same manner by passing a stream of 5 liters of oxygen per minute through the nebulizer with the open end held in the mouth of the patient.

In acute respiratory infection in the course of chronic pulmonary tuberculosis the inhalation of an oxygen-enriched atmosphere is indi-

[2] The nebulizer made by the Vaponefrin Company has been used for this purpose.

cated as in any other pulmonary disease in which impairment of respiratory function is present. The effect of inhalation of 50 per cent oxygen is to decrease the consequences of anoxia and excessive lung movement which would otherwise take place if the pulmonary ventilation were not lowered by adequate oxygen therapy. As indicated above, oxygen itself has no effect either in increasing or decreasing resolution of the tuberculous process. In patients who develop edema of the lung after hemorrhage, inhalation of oxygen under positive pressure has been found to clear this type of edema in a relatively short period.

BIBLIOGRAPHY

Amberson, J. B.: The process of resolution in pulmonary tuberculosis, Am. Rev. Tuberc., 33:269, 1936.

Barach, A. L.: Effects of atmospheres rich in oxygen on normal rabbits and on rabbits with pulmonary tuberculosis, Am. Rev. Tuberc., 13:292, 1926.

Barach, A. L.: The use of filtered-air chambers in pulmonary tuberculosis, Am. Rev. Tuberc., 27:508, 1933.

Barach, A. L.: Immobilization of lungs through pressure, Am. Rev. Tuberc., 42:5, 1940.

Barach, A. L.: Continuous arrest of lung movement, Am. Rev. Tuberc., 43:56, 1941.

Barach, A. L., N. Molomut, and M. Soroka: Inhalation of nebulized promin in experimental tuberculosis, Am. Rev. Tuberc., 46:268, 1942.

Feldman, W. H., H. C. Hinshaw, and H. E. Moses: The effect of promin (sodium salt of p.p'-diamino-diphenyl-sulfone-N,N'-dextrose sulfonate) on experimental tuberculosis: a preliminary report, Proc. Staff Meet., Mayo Clin., 15:695, 1940.

Pinner, M.: Mechanics of healing in collapse therapy, Ann. Int. Med., 9:501, 1935.

Richards, D. W., Jr., and A. L. Barach: Oxygen therapy in pulmonary fibrosis, Am. Rev. Tuberc., 26:254, 1932.

Thunberg, T.: The barospirator: a new machine for producing artificial respiration, Skandinav. Arch. f. Physiol., 48:80, 1926.

28

Blast Injuries of the Lungs

INTRODUCTION

The effect of bombs dropped in the vicinity of human subjects depends upon a number of factors. First of all, the heavier bombs of 500 to 8,000 pounds create powerful pressure waves, the effect of which may topple buildings at a distance of 1,000 to 3,000 feet. The results of the detonation of a two-ton bomb are as unpredictable as they are destructive. The symptoms include those arising from the lung and from the central nervous system, including cough, dyspnea, hemorrhage, pain in the chest, and also a variety of psychiatric symptoms.

PATHOLOGIC PHYSIOLOGY

The high pressure created by a bomb explosion initiates a pressure wave of enormous velocity, with the rate of movement diminishing rapidly as it proceeds, with a change in the shape of the wave. The pressure in some waves rises to a peak immediately and then falls off slowly, followed by a phase of negative pressure. The wave of positive pressure travels at a greater velocity than does the negative-pressure wave. The positive-pressure wave due to a bomb is the cause of blast injury in the lung. Some of the effects of high explosives are similar.

A pressure of 10 pounds per square inch will shatter most windows, but blast pressures may mount to 100 pounds per square inch before endangering a human being. A distance of 30 feet from a 50-kilo bomb may protect a human being from the direct effect of blast. As the bomb increases in weight the blast wave is naturally more intense and may create harmful effects at greater distances. The original studies of Hooker showed that the fatal effect of primary blast took place in animals only relatively near the explosion, a distance of three feet sometimes determining the question of life or death. The syndrome of primary shock was characterized by collapse, with progressive lowering of arterial blood pressure in some animals who were not killed by the primary blast. Hemorrhagic lesions of the lung were found in many animals subjected to the blast. Zuckerman's more recent studies have added evidence toward the view that the positive-pressure wave has effects like a blow on the chest, and is the significant factor in producing the pathology. In addition to hemorrhages in the lungs, the spleen and kidneys are often bruised or lacerated. Lesions in the central nervous systems, such as pial hemorrhages and spinal-cord hemorrhage, have been experimentally produced in rabbits. Concussion may be produced by blast, and appears to be due to movement of the brain against the skull, when the head is suddenly brought to a stop. When the head is fixed, blows that resulted in fractures of the skull may not cause concussion.

Considering the extreme pressures which are created at the center of the explosion, the blast dissipates rather rapidly in air, yet retains great shocking power because of its velocity. The change from atmospheric pressure to the blast peak occurs in from $\frac{1}{2,000}$ to $\frac{1}{10,000}$ second. It is believed that blast pressures in excess of 2.5 pounds per square inch will decrease efficiency of the victim.

The pressure wave may travel with an initial velocity of 5,000 feet per second. However, in air the pressure falls rapidly, but in water it varies directly as the distance. Thus, a pressure of 1 ton per square inch at a distance of 60 feet from the explosion would be $\frac{1}{2}$ ton at 120 feet, and so on; hence pressure effects will be experienced over greater distances in water than in air for an explosion of the same sized charge.

Internal blast injury without external marks of violence is rare, such as four cases in about 1,500 casualties. Thus usually there will be a coexisting wound of some kind or some other condition due to crushing, asphyxia, and so on.

Three main factors may be considered in estimating the consequences of the blast waves: (1) The primary increase in atmospheric pressure to 100 pounds per square inch; (2) the rate of movement of the blast wave itself; and (3) the earlier arrival of pressure to the chest as compared to the inner surface of the thorax. The positive component of blast waves exerts its damaging effect not due to sudden distention of the lungs but rather to the blast wave against the thoracic wall. Due to the constriction exercised by the tracheobronchial passageway, there is an initial increased pressure on the outer chest wall.

In experiments in an equalizing-pressure chamber in which human subjects with pulmonary tuberculosis have been treated with an alternating pressure of 55 mm. Hg 25 times a minute, it was observed that the onset of the positive phase was accompanied by a slight transient compression of the chest wall. When the wave of positive pressure to the chest was delayed and diminished by placing the body of the individual within an inner chamber, no compression of the chest wall took place during alternating pressure since the pressure had been made equal on both surfaces of the chest wall by passing the air through the inner chamber in a series of small apertures.

It has also been shown in animals that delaying the application of pressure to the chest wall by covering the chest with a sponge-rubber coat will also tend to prevent hemorrhage and other pathologic manifestations of lung blast. The suction effect of the negative component of the blast wave does not appear to exercise an important rôle in causing this condition.

A wave of moving pressure that gives acceleration of the body wall will impart an acceleration to the head and therefore will produce a type of acceleration which is an important element in the traumatic concussion syndrome. When the head is given an acceleration with the production of concussion, a transient appearance of fat droplets through the cerebral substance has been found. Since these fat emboli have been found only a few hours after the blow, the reason why fat emboli have not been previously described may be explained.

The pathology in an individual exposed to a blast wave of 100 pounds per square inch is in all probability like those reported by Zuckerman in monkeys, pulmonary hemorrhage, contusions of the thoracic and abdominal viscera, occasional areas of subdural hemorrhage, with relatively minor changes in the central nervous system. Concussion of severe degree may take place with little demonstrable pathology in the brain itself.

INHALATIONAL THERAPY

Since the picture of primary blast is frequently accompanied by shock and concussion, as well as variable signs of impairment in respiratory function, anoxia is a prominent part of the pathologic physiology of this condition. Inhalation of high concentrations of oxygen has been recommended. This is all the more indicated because the circulation through the brain has been shown to be slowed, with the production of a stagnant anoxia, when concussion is present. Judging from the effect of sponge-rubber covering of animals subjected to blast and from the demonstration of the physiology of the equalizing-pressure chamber, the prevention of lung blast might be aided if it were possible for men to know in advance that exposure may take place and to equip themselves with a sponge-rubber jacket that would fit snugly around the entire chest wall. A sponge-rubber coat of this sort has been employed in the equalizing-pressure chamber, as described in the section on treatment of pulmonary tuberculosis.

The type of inhalational-therapy equipment used depends on the severity of the injury and the presence of shock. Since it has been strongly recommended that these patients be given complete rest, comfort as well as effectiveness in the application of oxygen treatment should be stressed. If shock accompanies lung blast, either the B.L.B. or Meter mask may be employed for administration of high concentrations between 70 and 100 per cent oxygen, but the rubber bag must not be allowed to collapse at the end of inspiration, since negative pressure in the apparatus is contraindicated. A nasal catheter in the nasal or oral pharynx can be used to provide 35 to 60 per cent oxygen, and, if care is taken in its application, this method would appear to be the simplest procedure and one of considerable efficiency. If an oxygen tent is available, 50 to 60 per cent oxygen may be given continuously and comfortably, especially if a transparent canopy is provided.

BIBLIOGRAPHY

Fulton, J. F.: Blast and concussion in the present war, New England Jour. Med., **226**:1, 1942.

O'Reilly, J. N., and S. R. Gloyne: Blast injury to the lung, Lancet, **2**:423, 1941.

Williams, E. R. P.: Blast effects in warfare, Brit. Jour. Surg., **30**:38, 1942.

Zuckerman, S.: Experimental study of blast injuries to the lungs, Lancet, **2**:219 1940.

29

Aerial Transportation of Patients with Miscellaneous Diseases

INTRODUCTION

When individuals or patients are transported by airplane at altitudes of 10,000 feet or above they are subjected to two main factors which are not present at sea level: (1) Moderate anoxia, and (2) expansion of gases in body cavities in accordance with Boyle's law. Although transportation by airplane is frequently less fatiguing than by automobile or by train, there are certain clinical entities in which the effects of altitudes may produce serious disturbance.

PATHOLOGIC PHYSIOLOGY

Since the volume occupied by a given quantity of gas is inversely proportional to the absolute pressure exerted on it, a progressive expansion of a gas within a body cavity will take place on ascent to high altitudes. In the sinuses and ears, expansion of the contained air takes place, and, provided that the orifices are not closed, the pressures are adjusted without difficulty by passage of the expanded gas into the outer atmosphere.

In patients with pneumothorax, expansion of the contained gas may produce pressure disturbances on the heart and mediastinum. Furthermore, adhesions, which may be attached to a diseased lung, may be torn loose. An active pleurisy may take place which may destroy a valuable pneumothorax space or produce tuberculous empyema. In cases with pulmonary tuberculosis of moderate or advanced degree, even if quiescent, expansion of air within small cavities, provided by ascent to very high altitudes, may cause rupture of the cavity and production of a large lesion. In an investigator who had repeatedly ascended to a simulated altitude of 42,000 feet in a low-pressure cham·

ber, hemoptysis took place with a formation of a cavity which was not present prior to these experiments. In this individual it was possible to determine that a very small lesion had been present at the site of subsequent cavity formation prior to his undertaking investigations in the low-pressure chamber, but it had been overlooked.

If a patient with pneumothorax is to be transported by airplane it is desirable that the time chosen for travel should be that farthest away from the injection of air; namely, a time in which the pneumothorax contains the smallest possible amount of air. Since 1,000 cc. of air saturated with water vapor becomes 1,500 cc. of air at 10,000 feet altitude, a patient who has recently had a large pneumothorax should be warned by his physician not to attempt travel at this altitude. When an airplane is traveling at lower altitudes and in the presence of a small pneumothorax, many patients have tried air travel without ill effects. It is probable that no patient with considerable pulmonary involvement should travel at altitudes above 10,000 to 12,000 feet. The degree of expansion of a volume of gas may be calculated by the formula 760 − 47, divided by the barometric pressure at the selected altitude −47. Since spontaneous pneumothorax is more apt to occur in patients with pulmonary tuberculosis, ascent to high altitudes may make this even more likely.

Since gas in the intestine also expands at high altitude, patients with acute appendicitis may possibly develop rupture of the appendix as a result of aerial transportation. In a patient in whom gastric or intestinal distention may conceivably cause pressure on an ulcerated lesion, the selection of the site of surgery would probably be in the vicinity where he resides. However, in the case of soldiers who may not be adequately taken care of at the front, transportation by airplane in a suitably equipped airplane ambulance is generally considered better than an attempt to operate on the ground under unfavorable conditions. The importance of bearing in mind the expansion of gases will make it possible to anticipate any untoward results.

In patients with coronary artery disease, pulmonary fibrosis, emphysema, severe anemia, latent congestive heart failure, and severe hypertension, aerial transportation at altitudes above 10,000 feet should be avoided unless it is possible to provide continuous inhalation of an oxygen-enriched atmosphere of approximately 35 to 40 per cent.

INHALATIONAL THERAPY

Since inhalation of 35 per cent oxygen would compensate for altitudes of 10,000 to 12,000 feet, a mask with a collecting bag or rebreathing bag, such as the Meter mask or the B.L.B., would provide continuous oxygen therapy at this altitude with a flow of 1 liter per minute S.T.P.D. Since there is considerable resistance with such low flows of oxygen in the B.L.B., the Meter mask with an injector and with accessory inspiratory flutter valves attached to the inner surface of the oronasal mask would be more comfortable than breathing through the sponge-rubber disks in the B.L.B. mask. If a mask is not attached tightly to the patient's face, allowing slight continuous leakage between the rubber and the skin, the factor of resistance will naturally be greatly diminished.

If individual injectors were attached to each oxygen orifice alongside the seat in an airplane, a constant concentration of 35 or 40 per cent oxygen could be admitted, or, if it were so desired, a variable concentration from 40 to 100 per cent could be selected. Since low flows of oxygen are of decided advantage in airplanes because of the weight of oxygen tanks, the air admixture is more comfortably provided with the inspiratory flutter valves on the inside of the Meter oronasal mask. The oxygen which is stored in the collecting bag inevitably passes into the mask and is inhaled by the patient. Even if an injector is not used, the inspiratory flutter valve opens at a pressure of 0.2 cm. of water to admit the outside air required to complete inspiration. During expiration the light flutter valve opens at a correspondingly low pressure and makes for comfort as well as effective oxygen inhalation.

In the transportation of patients who have had air injected into the pleura or in whom distention of the intestine may be liable to cause untoward effects, a preliminary period of breathing 100 per cent oxygen might be of some value, if it were feasible to do so. The degree of abdominal distention after inhalation of pure oxygen for five hours would be a little less since intestinal gases would tend to diffuse out through the lungs. This would also apply to the nitrogen in a pneumothorax cavity but no measurements have as yet been made on the efficacy of this tentative suggestion. It should also be remembered that mediastinal hernia may be the source of dyspnea and discomfort within the chest.

Patients with asthma are not apt to be adversely affected, and in fact sometimes breathe more easily because of the lessened density of the air, which may be compared to the mechanism of relief breathing of a helium-oxygen mixture. When pulmonary emphysema is present, however, oxygen would be continuously necessary since these patients have either severe or borderline anoxia at sea level, as well as mechanically restricted chest movement.

BIBLIOGRAPHY

Bauer, L. H.: The development of commercial aeronautics and of the airplane ambulance, Mil. Surgeon, **66**:165, 1930.

Leduc, Jean: Indications et contre-indications du transport par avion dans les affections chirurgicales de l'abdomen, du thorax et du crâne, Saint-Quentin, Imprimerie Moderne, 1934.

Lovelace, W. R., and J. Hargreaves: Transportation of patients by airplane, Jour. Aviation Med., **13**:2, 1942.

Lovelace, W. R., and H. C. Hinshaw: Dangers of aerial transportation to persons with pneumothorax, Jour. Amer. Med. Asso., **118**:1275, 1942.

Simpson, R. K.: The airplane ambulance—its use in war, Mil. Surgeon, **64**:35, 1929.

30

Oxygen Poisoning

Since the question of oxygen poisoning is in a controversial state at this time, the available evidence will be reviewed and the observations of various investigators quoted. Paul Bert demonstrated that all forms of low animal life, such as plants and bacteria, were killed by oxygen at high pressures, and that higher animals who breathed pure oxygen under several atmospheres' pressure developed convulsions. That pure oxygen at atmospheric pressure would cause a state of inflammation in the lungs but yet not produce convulsions was demonstrated by Lorrain Smith. Experimenting with mice, birds, rats, guinea pigs, and pigeons, he consistently found that pathologic changes consisting of edema followed by consolidation took place in the lungs.

These observations were confirmed by Karsner, who demonstrated that rabbits exposed to 80 to 90 per cent oxygen at atmospheric pressure developed edema of the lungs within two to three days, and later bronchopneumonia. Animals exposed to 60 per cent oxygen were shown by J. A. Campbell to have a fall in red count and hemoglobin. Barach reported that rabbits could be kept in 60 per cent oxygen for one to four months without noticeable change in their general appearance, activity, and body weight, and in fact no specific alterations except that the hemoglobin and red-blood-cell count were lowered. In animals born in an atmosphere of 60 per cent oxygen the red count and hemoglobin were also about 15 per cent less than normal. Attempts to acclimatize these rabbits by keeping them in 60 per cent oxygen for an extended period and then gradually increasing the oxygen concentration to 85 per cent were unsuccessful. The animals died regularly at concentrations above 85 per cent whether or not acclimatization was previously employed. In animals the dividing line of toxicity seemed to be about 70 per cent. Although many animals may live in concentrations of oxygen of 70 per cent for periods as long as two weeks, autopsy of the lungs generally showed areas of pulmonary edema. Binger revealed similar changes in dogs and demonstrated that oxygen at 90 per cent concentration had no effect on frogs or on turtles unless they were warmed to 37.5° C., when they behaved like mammals. Paine, Keys, and Lynn have also shown that pathologic changes in the lungs of dogs take place in an atmosphere of pure oxygen in 48 hours.

Sayers showed that pure oxygen could be inhaled by animals for 16 hours a day for six weeks without fatality. Barach and Soroka confirmed this but noted that pathologic changes, such as scattered areas of edema, were frequently found in animals autopsied at the end of two or more weeks. When exposure was continued for four or five weeks, thickening of the alveolar septa and cellular infiltration were also noted. In animals continuously maintained at 70 per cent oxygen, similar changes were observed, suggesting an organizing pneumonia and fibrosis, after three to four weeks' exposure.

As a result of the reports of Evans that pure oxygen could be inhaled by a mask for periods of one to two weeks without any apparent ill effect in patients with pneumonia and other clinical illness, the stimulus for use of these high concentrations of oxygen that had been thought to be dangerous, as a result of animal experimentation, was felt by a number of investigators. Boothby has reported many patients who have been treated with 100 per cent oxygen by the B.L.B. mask for 48 hours and an increasing number who have been treated for a period of four days or more. Fine employed high oxygen concentrations, above 90 per cent, for the treatment of abdominal distention for periods of one to two days without observing ill effects. Heck, Johnson, and Barach used the Meter mask in six cardiac patients for two days and two cardiac patients for two weeks, and found that the inhalation of 100 per cent oxygen with interruptions for feeding was not followed by signs of pulmonary irritation. Measurement of the vital capacity and the venous pressure revealed no evidence that pointed toward pulmonary congestion.

On the other hand, two German experimenters who resided in an oxygen chamber at an oxygen concentration above 90 per cent reported symptoms of malaise, fever, and pulmonary irritation at the end of two to three days (Clamann and Becker-Freyseng).

It must be borne in mind that the greatest experience with inhalation of 100 per cent oxygen has been obtained from its administration by means of a mask in clinically ill patients. Under these circumstances, the mask is removed from time to time to wash the face and for eating and drinking, so that rigidly continuous use of this high concentration of oxygen is not in practice carried out. When Behnke employed 100 per cent oxygen in normal individuals he believed that certain toxic symptoms took place at the end of seven hours. He observed facial pallor and slowing of the pulse rate, with a break in respiratory compensation in certain instances, manifested by increased amplitude of breathing possibly due to accumulation of carbon dioxide in tissues; he suggested that the inhibitory action of oxygen on the chemoreceptors of the carotid body was replaced by a reaction consisting of the stimulating effect of carbon dioxide on the respiratory centers. Nausea is a common symptom when oxygen is breathed at 2.5 to 3 atmospheres, and is regarded by him as a consistent sign of oxygen toxicity. In Behnke's tests, the subject complained of substernal soreness, aggravated by deep inspiration, at the end of six hours of inhalation of 99 per cent oxygen. No objective findings were noted, however, either by auscultation or by x-ray of the chest.

Haldane believed that a high oxygen pressure slowed the circulation by a diminution of the heart rate. An additional retarding effect on the effective circulation takes place as a result of constriction of small cerebral blood vessels, when pure oxygen is breathed; this relative ischemia may protect the brain from too high an oxygen pressure.

J. A. Campbell showed that when high pressures of oxygen were inhaled in animals, the carbon-dioxide pressure in the tissues was definitely increased, in fact tremendously elevated when pressures of almost five atmospheres were employed, as a result of which the carbon-dioxide pressure in the abdominal cavity increased from 45 to 284 mm. Hg. A smaller but definite increase in carbon-dioxide pressure took place, from 50 to 66 mm. Hg, when the pressure of oxygen in the atmosphere was increased from 166 to 680 mm. Hg at sea level. This does suggest that retention of carbon dioxide in the tissues takes place, probably as a result of disturbed transport incident to inhalation of pure oxygen. It is possible that hemoglobin, being more acid when oxygen is inhaled, may not be so efficient an agent in the carrying of carbon dioxide from the tissues to the lungs. However, inhalation of 100 per cent oxygen over periods of many hours and several days has apparently shown no ill effects in a number of patients.

When patients with chronic anoxia due to cardiac or pulmonary disease were treated with inhalation of 50 per cent oxygen over a period of several weeks or months, a marked increase in the carbon-dioxide content of arterial blood was found by Barach and Richards, together with an increase in alveolar carbon dioxide. This increase in carbon-dioxide pressure in the arterial blood was due to failure to eliminate carbon dioxide when the pulmonary ventilation decreased, except under conditions of a higher carbon-dioxide tension; the high carbon-dioxide pressure in the blood flowing through the pulmonary capillaries made possible diffusion of carbon dioxide through damaged or poorly functioning lung tissue. Therefore, this elevation in blood carbon dioxide does not seem to be due to inability to transport carbon dioxide from the tissues but rather to retention associated with a lowered pulmonary ventilation; it also represents a special physiologic arrangement, described in Chapter 13, Pulmonary Emphysema, in which the high carbon-dioxide tension in the blood was part of an efficient mechanism for the elimination of carbon dioxide from the lungs. A greater molecular mass of carbon dioxide is exhaled from a smaller volume of poorly functioning lung. Some slowing of the circulation may take place in patients with cardiorespiratory illness as a result of inhaling high oxygen atmospheres, but not to the extent that would account for the relatively tremendous increases in arterial carbon-dioxide pressure in these cases.

That retention of carbon dioxide plays a significant rôle in oxygen poisoning at sea level has not been demonstrated by any of the studies so far made. In a patient of Barach and Richards', prolonged treatment with 60 per cent oxygen was accompanied by an arterial carbon-dioxide content of 132 volumes per cent, without change in pH and without signs of pulmonary edema. Other as yet undemonstrated factors may be operating, such as impairment in the enzyme responsible for tissue oxidation, but this is still a speculation for which no evidence is at present available. More work is necessary on the effect of pure oxygen in entirely normal men.

From the standpoint of safety in prescribing high oxygen concentrations, certain general formulations may be made. Inhalation of 100 per cent oxygen for periods under seven hours has shown no after effects even in the cases described by Behnke. In patients, if oxygen is administered by mask, there has been no evidence of deleterious effect when these concentrations were given for 48 hours. When inhalation of pure oxygen is maintained for periods longer than 48 hours, which may be justified by the clinical condition of the patient, careful auscultation of the lungs and examination of the patient for any signs of pulmonary edema, both subjective and objective, should be made. The value of inhaling very high concentrations of oxygen between 80 and 100 per cent may be so great in many of the conditions described in this book that an attempt should be made to administer them when the indication presents itself. There is some evidence that the lungs of the human being seem to be more resistant to the toxic effects of oxygen than are those of animals, but caution should still be exercised in the *long-continued employment of pure oxygen.* This is especially true in the use of the helmet-hood apparatus when 100 per cent oxygen is administered for long periods. It is advisable to dilute the pure oxygen with air three to four times daily, allowing a 50 per cent oxygen atmosphere for one hour at a time or even longer, before resuming 100 per cent oxygen. The difficulty in obtaining high oxygen concentrations, of 85 to 100 per cent, in tents prevents the possibility of oxygen poisoning in this method of treatment. This also applies to nasal-catheter administration of oxygen.

BIBLIOGRAPHY

Barach, A. L.: Effects of atmospheres rich in oxygen on normal rabbits and on rabbits with pulmonary tuberculosis, Am. Rev. Tuberc., **13**:292, 1926.

Bean, J. W.: Effects of high O_2 pressure on CO_2 transport, on blood and tissue acidity, and on O_2 consumption and pulmonary ventilation, Jour. Physiol., **72**: 27, 1931.

Becker-Freyseng, H., and H. G. Clamann: Oxygen poisoning from 90 per cent in 48 hours, Klin. Wchnschr., **18**:1382, 1939.

Benedict, F. G., and H. L. Higgins: Effects on men at rest of breathing oxygen-rich gas mixtures, Amer. Jour. Physiol., **28**:1, 1911.

Bert, P.: La Pression Barométrique, Recherches de Physiologie Expérimentale, Paris, Masson et Cie, 1878.

Binger, C. A. L., J. M. Faulkner, and R. L. Moore: Oxygen poisoning in mammals, Jour. Exper. Med., **45**:849, 1927.

Boothby, W. M., W. R. Lovelace, and C. W. Mayo: One hundred per cent oxygen: indications for its use and methods of its administration, Jour. Amer. Med. Asso., **113**:477, 1939.

Campbell, J. A.: Prolonged alterations of oxygen pressure in the inspired air with special reference to tissue oxygen tension, tissue carbon dioxide tension and hemoglobin, Jour. Physiol., **62**:211, 1927.

Clamann, H. G., and H. Becker-Freyseng: Einwirkung des Sauerstoffs auf den Organismus bei höherem als normalem Partialdruck unter besonderer Berücksichtigung des Menschen, Luftfahrtmedizin, **4**:1, 1939.

Cusick, P. L., O. O. Benson, Jr., and W. M. Boothby: Effect of anoxia and of high concentrations of oxygen on the retinal vessels: preliminary report, Proc. Staff Meet., Mayo Clin., **15**:500, 1940.

Evans, J. H.: A plea in behalf of the anoxemic patient, Anesth. and Analg., **14**: 209, 1939; New York State Jour. Med., **39**:709, 1939.

Karsner, H. T.: The pathological effects of atmosphere rich in oxygen, Jour. Exper. Med., **23**:149, 1916.

Keilin, D.: On cytochromes: a respiratory pigment common in animal, yeast and higher plants, Proc. Roy. Soc., **98**:312, 1925.

Paine, J. R., D. Lynn, and A. Keys: Observations on the effects of the prolonged administration of high oxygen concentration to dogs, Jour. Thoracic Surg., **11**:151, 1941.

Smith, J. L.: The pathological effects due to increase of oxygen tension in the air breathed, Jour. Physiol., **24**:19, 1899.

Stadie, W. C., B. C. Riggs, and N. Haugaard: Oxygen poisoning, Amer. Jour. Med. Sci., **207**:84, 1944.

31

Submarine Medicine and Caisson Disease

INTRODUCTION

The effect of exposure to high atmospheric pressures will be considered in this section. In divers ascending from pressures of two to four atmospheres symptoms of embolism may take place. The syndrome of compressed-air illness or caisson disease is due to the increased amount of nitrogen which goes into physical solution in the blood and tissues during exposure to air under high atmospheric pressure. When the decompression is too swift the dissolved nitrogen forms bubbles in the blood stream which may result in local blockage of a blood vessel or more severe circulatory disturbance. The symptoms of decompression sickness may take place in divers who ascend from depths under the sea of greater than two atmospheres, and similar although more severe symptoms may take place in submarine escape in which an individual may be precipitated to the sea level in a rapid manner.

PATHOLOGIC PHYSIOLOGY

For many years it has been known that air bubbles do not appear in the blood or tissues unless the pressure of the atmosphere is reduced to more than half the original pressure. For that reason decompression is more rapidly brought about by a procedure of stage decompression in which the original pressure is reduced one-half at suitable intervals. Since the bubble when originally formed consists of nitrogen, inhalation of pure oxygen has been employed to eliminate the nitrogen physically dissolved in the blood and tissues. Since pure oxygen under increased pressure is irritating to the lungs and causes convulsions when breathed for long periods, there is a definite limitation in its employment at pressures greater than three to four atmospheres. Inhalation of pure oxygen at a pressure of three atmospheres can be tolerated for a period of three hours. However, in 45 minutes of oxygen breathing at four atmospheres, severe convulsive seizures take place. These seizures are of greater intensity and longer duration than epileptic convulsions, although recovery is apparently complete when air is again breathed.

The use of oxygen in routine diving operations has been of great value because it has eliminated the necessity for stage decompression. The limits during which oxygen can be inhaled at various pressures have been now carefully outlined so that oxygen poisoning does not take place. If, for example, a diving operation is not to take longer than 30 minutes, a depth of 100 feet can be reached without symptoms provided that carbon dioxide is rigidly excluded. It has been shown that a man can breathe oxygen for a period of four hours at a pressure of 30 pounds and be removed without symptoms in a period of two minutes, whereas a man breathing air exposed to the same pressure, even when released slowly over a period of 55 minutes, nevertheless develops bends.

The symptoms of decompression sickness are very similar to those of aero-embolism referred to in that section. In so far as the problem of bubble formation is concerned, an ascent by an aviator from a pressure of one atmosphere (sea level) to 0.25 of an atmosphere (equivalent to an altitude of 34,700 feet) is equivalent to ascent by a diver from four atmospheres (100 feet below sea level) to the surface level. In each instance, nitrogen bubbles may produce pruritus, pains in the joints, or pain in the chest and coughing of frothy mucus, described as "chokes." The more serious consequences of embolism take place in the lower dorsal and upper lumbar portions of the spinal cord, which may be manifested by paralysis of the lower extremities.

Since oxygen inhalation at a pressure of four atmospheres, equivalent to a diving depth of 100 feet, cannot be tolerated for a period longer than 30 minutes because of nausea, cerebral dullness, and nervous instability, the discovery that mixtures of helium with oxygen could be employed for diving at far greater depths was of great value and made possible the rescue of the *Squalus*. It was found that at high pressures, beginning at an absolute pressure of four atmospheres, nitrogen acted as a narcotic to diminish neuromuscular function and at pressures over 10 atmospheres inhalation of ordinary air was followed by loss of consciousness. The reason for this has not been explained, but it has been related to nitrogen solubility in the lipid substances of the central nervous system. Another possibility is that carbon-dioxide elimination in the denser atmosphere in the lung may be interfered with. Although it has not been shown that any retardation in the elimination of carbon dioxide takes place under conditions of increased pressure, nitrogen narcosis is increased when there are even small pressures of carbon dioxide present in the inhaled atmosphere. Since the hemoglobin is rendered more acid by oxygen, its use in transporting carbon dioxide from the tissues may be interfered with, under conditions of high pressure.

The substitution of helium for nitrogen was found to abolish the narcotic effects of high pressures and normal divers were able to descend to a pressure of 16 atmospheres breathing helium-oxygen mixtures with full retention of their mental capacity (Behnke). It is of interest to note that argon, although chemically inert like helium, brings about the same impairment and mental depression, even greater in degree, than is caused by nitrogen. Argon has a higher specific gravity than helium.

Helium has a fat–water-solubility ratio approximately one-half that of nitrogen. The content of helium in the body in an individual breathing a helium-oxygen mixture is about 45 per cent of the nitrogen content in an individual breathing air, and the elimination rate of helium is about twice that for nitrogen. Exercise is valuable for the first 30 minutes in increasing the rate of elimination of a gas, such as nitrogen. However, exercise does not greatly influence the elimination of inert gases from the fat depots of the body.

A frequently fatal form of embolism formerly occurred during submarine escape. When a man is forced to ascend to the surface from a depth of 30 feet or less, death may take place as a result of the individual's holding his breath and rupturing his lung due to increased pressure, with air being forced into the pulmonary blood vessels. This type of air embolism from excessive lung pressure has been produced experimentally in dogs by distending their lungs. Air may be seen in the carotid arteries that has entered the blood stream through the pulmonary circulation. Death has also been recorded as a result of an ascent to the surface from a depth of only 15 feet, which illustrates the importance of a gradual release of air from the lungs when escape from a submarine is necessary. Holding one's breath during such an ascent will, therefore, cause a progressive increase in intrapulmonary pressure with the danger of lung rupture and embolism. The gradual release of air from the lung as ascent takes place relieves the increased excessive intrapulmonary pressure and prevents this type of embolism.

When an individual is wearing a mask in which too much resistance is present, great difficulty is experienced in breathing outward, and respiration under such resistance may cause fatigue of the respiratory center in susceptible individuals. This combined with fright may result in an individual shooting to the surface holding his breath and arriving dead. It is therefore evident that any breathing escape apparatus should be made in such a way as to avoid resistance whenever possible.

INHALATIONAL THERAPY

The indications for inhaling pure oxygen or helium-oxygen mixtures have been described above. Any leak-tight oxygen-mask apparatus may be employed for this purpose.

BIBLIOGRAPHY

Behnke, A. R., Jr.: High atmospheric pressures; physiological effects of increased and decreased pressure; application of these findings to clinical medicine, Ann. Int. Med., 13:2217, 1940.

Behnke, A. R., Jr., L. A. Shaw, E. C. Messer, R. M. Thomson, and E. P. Motley: Acute circulatory and respiratory disturbances of compressed air illness and administration of oxygen as a therapeutic measure, Amer. Jour. Physiol., 114: 526, 1936.

Behnke, A. R., and C. S. Stephenson: Applied physiology, Ann. Rev. Physiol., 4:575, 1942.

Behnke, A. R., and O. D. Yarbrough: Physiologic study of helium, U. S. Nav. Med. Bull., 36:542, 1938.

Behnke, A. R., and O. D. Yarbrough: Respiratory resistance, oil-water solubility and mental effects of argon, compared with helium and nitrogen, Amer. Jour. Physiol., 126:409, 1939.

Campbell, J. A.: Prolonged alterations of oxygen pressure in the inspired air with special reference to tissue oxygen tension, tissue carbon dioxide tension and hemoglobin, Jour. Physiol., 62:211, 1927.

Crosson, J. W., R. R. Jones, and R. R. Sayers: Helium-O_2 mixtures for alleviation of tubal and sinus block in compressed air workers, Pub. Health Reports, Washington, D. C., 55:1487, 1940.

End, E.: Rapid decompression following inhalation of helium-oxygen mixtures under pressure, Amer. Jour. Physiol., 120:712, 1937.

Gibbs, F. A., E. L. Gibbs, W. G. Lennox, and L. F. Nims: The value of carbon dioxide in counteracting the effects of low oxygen, Jour. Aviation Med., 14: 250, 1943.

Hilderbrand, J. H., R. R. Sayers, and W. P. Yant: Possibilities in the Use of Helium-Oxygen Mixtures as a Mitigation of Caisson Disease, U. S. Bureau of Mines, Report of Investigation No. 2670, 1925.

Sayers, R. R., and W. P. Yant: Value of helium-oxygen atmosphere in diving and caisson operations, Anesth. and Analg., 5:127, 1926.

32

Hiccough

DEFINITION

Hiccough is an intermittent chronic contraction of the diaphragm at times associated with contractions of the accessory muscles of breathing. The afferent pathway to the respiratory centers in the medulla oblongata and in the upper cervical cord may be stimulated by a variety of toxic states, indigestion, gastric dilatation, and postoperative abdominal distention, any one of which may result in continued hiccough, often severe and difficult to control, at times endangering life through its weakening effects.

TREATMENT

Pressure upon the phrenic nerve has been advocated, between the heads of the sternocleidomastoid muscle, as well as a number of other procedures such as drinking cold water and holding the breath. The inhalation of nitroglycerine has been used. Repeated traction of the tongue is tried frequently.

Inhalation of 7 to 10 per cent carbon dioxide, as recommended by Yandell Henderson, is the most satisfactory method of treatment, in the experience of the author. Henderson says that stimulation of the chief respiratory center by carbon-dioxide inhalation is effective in reducing the phrenic centers again to their normal subordination, and the hiccough is thus stopped.

The technic of application is of great importance since inefficiently treated cases of hiccough may not respond to inhalation of carbon dioxide. If the inhalation of 7 per cent carbon dioxide does not free the patient from hiccough when it has been employed for three to four minutes, 10 per cent carbon dioxide should then be used. The inhalation should be continued until the patient's consciousness is slightly clouded, at which time he may experience considerable dizziness. It is doubtful that any harm can come from inhaling high concentrations of carbon-dioxide mixtures even if consciousness is transiently lost.

In one patient treated by the author it was necessary to administer 15 per cent carbon dioxide, with the remainder oxygen, for a period of one and one-half minutes to terminate intractable hiccough. In postoperative abdominal distention or severe toxic states, the inhalation may have to be repeated at three-hour intervals, or as often as is necessary, for periods of three to seven days. Even though an individual patient may require repeated inhalation of carbon dioxide in concentrations of 10 or even 15 per cent, this procedure saves the patient the weakening effect of otherwise uncontrollable hiccough. Since the author has administered concentrations of carbon dioxide from 20 to 40 per cent to the point of creating a convulsion, daily for two to three months in the treatment of schizophrenia without any evidence of harmful effect, the physician may be reassured that the cautious inhalation of 10 per cent carbon dioxide is not harmful, and that it should be pursued until the therapeutic objective has been obtained.

In some cases the inhalation of 5 per cent carbon dioxide will terminate hiccough in three to four minutes but on subsequent days this concentration may be found ineffective. Abandonment of carbon-dioxide inhalation on this account should not be allowed, since it is entirely probable that inhalation of 10 per cent carbon dioxide will then be found effective. The physiologic factor involved in the cessation of hiccough is not the deep breathing itself but the stimulation of the respiratory center and the relaxation which carbon dioxide in high concentrations produces. It is preferable, therefore, to use concentrations of 10 per cent, or even 15 per cent if necessary, rather than to maintain deep breathing for a long period with concentrations as low as 5 per cent. In several cases observed by the author the skillful administration of carbon dioxide in sufficiently high concentrations afforded profound rest to patients who might otherwise have remained in a state of extreme fatigue, possibly with danger to life itself.

Any mask apparatus may be employed which has either a collecting bag or a rebreathing bag to permit the patient a full inhalation without undue resistance. A high flow of the carbon-dioxide mixture such as 15 to 30 liters per minute may be necessary.

BIBLIOGRAPHY

Henderson, Yandell: Resuscitation, Jour. Amer. Med. Asso., **83**:758, 1924.
Sheldon, R. F.: Control of hiccup by inhalation of carbon dioxide, Jour. Amer. Med. Asso., **89**:1118, 1927.

33

Some Considerations Concerning Research in Respiratory Function and Inhalational Therapy

Although it seems to the author that this is an appropriate time for a presentation of the principles and technic of inhalational therapy, continued controlled investigation is unquestionably necessary to confirm many of the tentative conclusions advanced in the preceding pages. The mechanics of administration of oxygen, helium, carbon dioxide, and positive pressure has made widespread application of inhalational therapy a more difficult undertaking than the prescription, for example, of the sulfonamide drugs, and a firm establishment of some of the procedures advocated must await more clinical reports than are now available. The material gathered together in this book will, it is hoped, make possible a readier approach to further studies.

Since research in respiratory function and inhalational therapy presents unusual possibilities, a discussion of future investigation may be interesting to those who will not be alienated by the admittedly speculative nature of attempts to glance at the unknown and the unproven.

Oxygen therapy was put on a physiologically sound basis with the finding of a decreased oxygen saturation in the arterial blood of patients with pneumonia and cardiac insufficiency, followed by the demonstration of elevation of the arterial oxygen saturation to or near the normal level by appropriate therapy. When it was observed some time later that the pain of coronary sclerosis and coronary occlusion was relieved by inhalation of high oxygen concentrations, in the absence of any lowering of the oxygen saturation of arterial blood, a new concept of the possibilities of oxygen therapy was developed. Some physicians still take the point of view that inhalation of oxygen cannot be of clinical benefit if the patient already has a normal pressure of oxygen in the systemic arterial blood. However, inhalation of pure oxygen results in an elevation in the oxygen concentration of the arterial blood from 95 to 100 per cent, as well as a substantial increase in the physically dissolved oxygen which makes it possible for the blood vessels bordering on a partial or totally occluded artery to furnish a considerably higher oxygen tension to tissues which otherwise might endure impaired functioning as a result of severe anoxia. J. A. Campbell has shown that inhalation of 50 per cent oxygen in a rabbit increased the oxygen pressure in the peritoneal cavity from 42 to 70 mm. Hg. This indicates that the oxygen pressure in the tissues of a normal animal may be markedly elevated, despite the presence of a previously existing normal arterial oxygen saturation.

The recognition that oxygen therapy was of value in the absence of so-called arterial anoxemia was clearly evident in patients who suffered from coronary thrombosis, in whom it has been shown to be at times a life-saving measure. In obliterative sclerosis of arteries in the lower extremities, inhalation of 50 per cent oxygen has been tried in a very limited way, and although healing of ischemic ulcers has been reported, the future of this form of treatment depends upon more research in this field. Perhaps the most significant suggestion for research in oxygen therapy emanates from the report of Poulton, who found that inhalation of high oxygen concentrations in cases of cerebral embolism and thrombosis was followed by improvement in brain function and a shorter course of invalidism.

Although it is now well known that the brain is the organ most sensitive to anoxia, both from the standpoint of impairment in function and also from the readiness with which hemorrhage and degeneration of cortical cells take place after acute oxygen-want, there is as yet only one report of the apparent value of oxygen therapy in cases of occlusion of cerebral blood vessels. It is evident that much more research is indicated in order to determine whether or not brain damage and subsequent serious invalidism may be prevented by adequate oxygen therapy.

Poulton is also responsible for a study on the preventive use of oxygen in rheumatic fever. Although the series of patients investigated was admittedly small, a far lower incidence of valvular heart disease took place in patients who were continuously treated with oxygen during the acute phase of the disease. The increased oxygen tension in the blood was considered a possible therapeutic agent in overcoming local ischemia in the heart valves due to arteritis of the small blood vessels during rheumatic fever. Further investigation of this concept is justified by the seriousness of the complication of valvular heart disease, and the tentative conclusions of Poulton.

It must be generally admitted that ischemia is followed by tissue anoxia. In many illnesses localized ischemia plays an important rôle, such as in coronary-artery disease and obliterative arterial disease of the lower extremities, and perhaps also ischemic narrowing of the blood vessels in the heart valves during rheumatic fever and cerebral thrombosis. It seems possible, furthermore, that some of the phenomena of senescence may be due to a diminishing oxygen tension in the brain as a result of narrowing of arteriosclerotic blood vessels.

Since it has been demonstrated that inhalation of pure oxygen will cause an almost immediate disappearance of coronary pain, as well as, in some cases, electrocardiographic changes in the direction of normal, it is probable that the end-products of deficient oxidation are eliminated as a result of the higher oxygen pressure in a partially occluded coronary artery and in the collateral circulation to the obstructed blood vessel. The analogy to cerebral arteriosclerotic disease permits us to suggest that ischemia and anoxia of certain areas of the brain may result in end-products of deficient oxidation accumulating in brain cells, with impairment in function comparable to the pathologic situation in coronary sclerosis. The possibility therefore presents itself that the lactic acid content of internal jugular vein blood in cerebral arteriosclerosis may be modified by oxygen inhalation and that this therapy may some day function favorably in controlling some of the pathology and symptomatology of senescence. This manifestly speculative concept seems all the more credible when it is acknowledged that the brain is an organ far more sensitive to oxygen-want than the heart itself. Intermittent inhalation of pure oxygen has lessened the incidence of cardiac pain in a series of cases of coronary sclerosis (unpublished data of Barach and Steiner), a circumstance that warrants future research concerning the relation of oxygen brain tension in senescence, in cerebral arteriosclerotic disease and in the general field of psychosomatic relationships.

The function of helium in the treatment of asthma and obstructive lesions in the respiratory passageway has been commented on fully in the text. The addition of positive pressure was of considerable value when it was used in both cycles of respiration in the treatment of obstructive dyspnea. In the treatment of edema of the lungs the employment of positive pressure is still in its infancy. Although reports have now appeared from several observers, both in the use of positive pressure in clinical pulmonary edema and in the treatment of irritant gas poisoning, much additional work needs to be done.

The inclusion in this volume of immobilizing lung therapy by means of air pressure seemed justified because it is in actual fact a form of inhalational therapy and because its presentation might stimulate others to conduct investigations on the value of local lung rest in pulmonary tuberculosis. Other uses may be made of a chamber in which immobilization of the lung takes place. Multiple fractures of the ribs with parodoxical respiration may be treated by equalizing the pressure on both sides of the chest wall, perhaps with relief of dyspnea and prevention of mediastinal shift. Whether other conditions, such as bronchiectasis, may be aided by a program of lung rest is a problem for future study.

Argyl Campbell reported that guinea pigs breathing 60 per cent oxygen were able to resist infection following injection of tetanus spores under conditions which caused tetanus in a control series. This is an example of a chemotherapeutic use of oxygen, little known and probably rarely used. The inhalation of the nebulized spray of sulfadiazine in 2.5 per cent solution for the treatment of pyogenic infections in the bronchi is a possible extension of the employment of inhalation of the nebulized sprays of epinephrine and neosynephrin. Another example of chemotherapeutic research is the inhalation of the nebulized spray of promin which has been shown in animals to prevent experimental generalized tuberculosis. Whether the inhalation of the nebulized spray of promin will be effective in the treatment of human pulmonary tuberculosis remains to be seen. However, the absorption of drugs locally in the lungs can be accomplished by the method of nebulizing solutions, either by means of a hand bulb, a stream of oxygen from a high-pressure cylinder, or by a small air pump. What the future of this form of therapy will be cannot be foretold but it is evident that the lungs offer an absorbing medium which may be utilized under certain circumstances, and that when they are themselves the site of infection or pathophysiologic change, local application of drugs by nebulization may be found more effective than systemic medication.

The future of inhalational therapy in respect to aviation medicine readily can be imagined. The importance of oxygen in conquest of the upper altitudes is well known. The use of pressure in sealed cabins was developed before the war began. Although much of the research now being intensively pursued in respect to high-altitude flying is of a secret nature, the close of the war will make this available to civil aviation. It is not difficult to be hopeful that research in this field may also have application to some of the clinical disturbances of respiration, circulation, and the central nervous system, an application that may broaden the field of inhalational therapy as well as increase its potential value.

Additional research is under way directed toward the study of the abnormal compounds of hemoglobin which interfere with the release of oxygen. Generalized cyanosis may be due to methemoglobinemia and sulfhemoglobinemia; in the former the corpuscles contain hemoglobin combined with oxygen in such a way as to form methemoglobin, in the latter hemoglobin is combined with sulfur to produce sulfhemoglobin. Drugs, such as derivatives of aniline, acetanilid and acetophenetidin, may result in either of these conditions. Constipation may be the cause of the production of certain organic sulfur compounds in the intestines which when absorbed may produce sulfhemoglobin. Methemoglobinemia may also result from inhalation of the fumes of benzene and from reducing agents and oxidizing agents such as potassium chloride. Although sulfhemoglobinemia persists for a relatively long period, methemoglobinemia will quickly disappear when the cause is removed. Further investigation may reveal other causes of the formation of these abnormal pigments and their significance in respect to limiting the oxygen supply for the individual.

Research in anesthesia includes an increasing emphasis on the provision of a normal oxygen concentration to patients who are given various anesthetic gases. Waters, Eversole, Courville, Cullen, Schreiber, Lundy, Flagg, and others have stressed the importance of preventing anoxia during the unconscious state of the individual, irrespective of the depth of anesthesia desired by the surgeon. Furthermore, the employment of higher than normal oxygen concentrations, i.e., oxygen therapy, during and after certain types of anesthesia has outlined a new field of research.

The question of the employment of carbon dioxide during and after operation is receiving intensive study. Although its value in promoting increased ventilation with consequent stretching of the bronchial walls and readier elimination of mucus is more generally acknowledged, the existence of a state of acapnea or acarbia, indicating any serious loss of carbon dioxide, is being abandoned. Additional studies are justified in elucidating the unquestionably decisive value of adequate concentrations of carbon dioxide in the relief of intractable hiccough. A state of profound relaxation occurs when a sufficiently high carbon-dioxide concentration is inhaled for this purpose. Termination of treatment with 7 to 10 per cent carbon dioxide usually should be made before loss of consciousness takes place, although little or no harm might be expected from transient unconsciousness except in hypertensive individuals, and much good may come from using carbon dioxide a sufficiently long time to achieve termination of hiccough.

The employment of carbon dioxide to produce convulsions in the treatment of schizophrenia was perhaps prematurely abandoned. Although the early investigation in which the author took part did appear to indicate that a remission in the disease followed repeated inhalations of 20 to 30 per cent carbon dioxide to the point of producing a convulsion, a further trial of the method with exposures short of the period required for production of a convulsion did not obtain favorable results. Apparently, a full convulsion is necessary for a therapeutic effect.

Loevenhart, Lorenz, and Waters had first demonstrated that periods of mental clarity took place following the inhalation of these high carbon-dioxide concentrations in patients with dementia praecox. The repeated induction of brief periods of communicability by carbon-dioxide inhalation may still turn out to be a therapeutic procedure of value if convulsions are produced. Further research in this field seems justified.

Since the various forms of shock therapy which were introduced later appeared to have a common denominator of tissue anoxia, especially in the brain, the use of nitrogen as a therapeutic gas was proposed by Himwich, Alexander, and their collaborators. Inhalation of nitrogen mixtures ending in pure nitrogen for periods of three to five minutes was followed in some cases by remission in the symptoms of the psychoses, such as dementia praecox. Further trials with this method led to less optimistic reports and at the present time the tendency is to abandon nitrogen inhalation in favor of electric-shock therapy.

Since the cells in the cortex are most sensitive to damage by anoxia, it would appear that the production of severe tissue oxygen-want was accompanied by decreased functional activity and some damage to the higher brain centers, from which arise not only the creative faculties but also excessively critical punitive influences which may be involved in both psychoneurosis and the psychoses. The treatment of psychoses by asphyxia achieved through the inhalation of nitrogen is no longer in general use, but this evidence plus that from other methods of shock therapy and the procedure of psychosurgery of Freeman and his collaborators, employing cutting nerve tissue in the frontal lobes, do nevertheless point to the concept that the brain is especially susceptible to varying oxygen tensions. Certain applications of the relation of oxygen pressure to brain function should be of interest to psychosomatic medicine.

It was pointed out in the chapter on pulmonary emphysema that patients with chronic anoxia frequently show a profound disorder in mental functioning when they are first treated with inhalation of 50 per cent oxygen. Drowsiness and mental depression may be followed by headache, stupor and a state of complete irrationality ending in coma. However, after a period of adaptation to the increased oxygen percentage in the atmosphere of two to seven days, the mind invariably clears and frequently a feeling of well-being and optimism remains as long as the oxygen concentration continues adequate for mental function. The brain is, therefore, susceptible to both low and high concentrations of oxygen under certain circumstances.

The oxygen supply to an organ regulates the functional activity of the organ in a broad way, as Barcroft and others have pointed out. Although in certain organ systems such as the circulation, the rôle of anoxia may be clearly represented, for example, by the precipitation of anginal pain during the inhalation of low oxygen mixtures, the selection of criteria for normal brain function has not been sufficiently satisfactory to record accurately what happens in anoxia. It may, however, be pointed out that depression of the activity of the higher cortical areas in the brain as a result of inhaling low oxygen mixtures, or as a result of acute exposure to moderate altitudes without oxygen, such as 15,000 feet, result in the majority of subjects in feelings of well-being, euphoria, overconfidence, and communicability. Although the later effects of altitude anoxia are those of drowsiness, sleep, headache, and if the exposure has been severe, nausea and vomiting, the initial manifestations of altered cerebral functioning are in the majority of normal human beings characterized by relief of tension and a manifestation of emotion previously repressed. The resemblance of anoxia to alcoholic intoxication has frequently been made, and seems valid. Humanity's long use of alcoholic beverages does suggest that the human being has found release from tension and excessive emotional inhibition by ingestion of alcohol, with a resultant decrease in the functional activity of certain areas of the cortex.

From observations on patients with heart disease who had undergone a complete thyroidectomy, the author was able to observe that the creative faculty in one such patient, who had been a writer and poetess, disappeared when her basal metabolism reached —40 per cent. Her writings at that time were stereotyped and sentimental, to such an extent as to result in refusal from her editors. Administration of thyroid was followed by a return of her creative capacity and acceptance of the literary contributions which she then made. However, her cardiac function was impaired by administration of thyroid and the resultant high oxygen requirement that appeared to be necessary for activity in the higher mental centers. In summary, a high oxygen pressure or oxygen consumption in the brain is the physiologic background for a critical regulation of man's faculties, which is linked up not only with his achievements and creative ability but is also responsible, in many cases, for an overintense control, a feeling of tension and burden, and an excessively severe, punitive attitude toward himself which results in some individuals in anxiety and depression.

Man may be in the process of adapting himself to an oxygen tension in the environment which is advantageously utilized by the few who can turn their surplus energies and brain functioning into scientific and artistic achievement. For many others, however, in whom the capacity or the opportunity for such accomplishment is denied, the higher centers may serve little useful purpose, being employed in wasteful, overintense self-indictment, which leads to depressed and unhappy states. The problem of dealing with excessive self-criticism, imposed apparently by an inner conscience, has not been satisfactorily solved by either the minister or the psychiatrist, nor indeed by the philosophers, psychoanalysts, or academic psychologists. A combined physiologic and psychiatric approach to brain function in respect to these matters may open a field for future research out of which new orientations may come, perhaps elucidating some of the mechanisms of personal happiness and distress.

Comparing the performance of other organs to that of the brain in respect to oxygen deficiency, there is no organ-system except the higher cortical areas in the brain that reveals even temporary benefits from a decreased oxygen supply. The feelings of elation and euphoria that occur in normal individuals during inhalation of low oxygen atmospheres are more permanent in psychotic individuals exposed to convulsions, shock therapy, and psychosurgery. Loss of mental depression is the outstanding result of shock therapy, in which repeated exposure to anoxia may be presumed.   In five of nine patients with anxiety neurosis Barach and Kagan reported that their efficiency of response was better after inhalation of 13 per cent oxygen for a period of three hours, as determined by a retention and recall memory test. It was also observed that some degree of emotional relaxation took place after exposure to lowered oxygen, and that the patients were to some degree free from their former preoccupation.   In this type of apprehensive patient, the mechanism of fear has been ascribed to over-severe conscience reactions developed in childhood.   The evidence obtained through psychoanalysis in support of this point of view is excellent.   However, a psychosomatic approach to the problem would enable us to envisage the concept that in some individuals the cerebral cells that regulate the criticizing department in a man's life, including emotional control and introspection, may be altered in their physiologic response to oxygen tension in such a way as to be an additional influence in the cause of either anxiety or depression.

It is a part of common experience to recognize that normal individuals, who have been apprehensive or depressed, are frequently relieved of their fears by drinking a sufficient amount of alcoholic beverages. For the time being their anxieties are relieved, replaced by cheerfulness or euphoria.   Since it is generally believed that alcohol produces a state of histotoxic anoxia, it is not difficult to understand that inhalation of low oxygen mixtures or exposure to altitude anoxia under suitable circumstances, especially in groups, will provoke a similar release of tension and emotional control.   The excessive development of an aggressive tendency within an individual, toward either himself or others, may therefore be not entirely a matter of psychologic conditioning, but in part related to at present unknown differences in the constitution of the higher centers of the brain.   Further study of these variations in mental function produced by varying the oxygen tension in the air may give us a new insight.

However, impairment of emotional control, beneficent as it may be in terms of doing away with self-criticism and in the development of a happy state of mind, has serious consequences when allowed to exist in circumstances that require a man's full reason and judgment.   There are many other signs of deficient functioning in the central nervous system, as a result of anoxia, which have been commented on in earlier chapters.   In fact, recurrent exposure to anoxia has been thought of as partly responsible for the development of certain symptoms in aviators, called aeroneurosis, but whether or not repeated exposure to anoxia is detrimental to the human organism or aids the development of a state of irritability and apprehension now appears doubtful to the author and still needs to be definitely confirmed.

During the First World War Haldane pointed out that soldiers who exhibited the symptoms of neurasthenia, fatigue, and breathlessness showed a shallow respiration, and suggested that military neurasthenia was a more lasting form of ordinary fatigue due to anoxia. Barcroft, Hunt, and Dufton treated patients with chronic gas poisoning who were not only physically improved but who showed definite betterment in their psychoneurotic tendencies after one week in a chamber with 50 per cent oxygen.

The possibility that acute anoxia may take place as a result of sudden alterations in permeability of the pulmonary epithelium, with production of acute anxiety, has been mentioned by Kroetz, who reported in neurotic patients showing vasomotor instability, a lowering of the arterial oxygen saturation to 88 per cent when a relatively painless arterial puncture brought about pallor and sweating. A diminished arterial oxygen saturation in psychoneurotic subjects at rest has been reported by Hicks although his findings have not been confirmed. The possibility that variation in oxygen tension may produce mental symptoms or alterations in mental functioning is substantiated by an open-minded consideration of the above findings.

In summary, it may be stated that variations in the oxygen tension of the blood both above and below that to which the organism has been accustomed may be accompanied by profound alterations in mental functioning, as well as in changes in physiologic functions. For the most part a lowering of the oxygen concentration results in a diminished efficiency of intellectual capacity with disturbances in memory, judgment, and emotional control. The effect of various forms of constriction of the cerebral arterial supply seems, therefore, a legitimate field of future research that may have considerable promise. Mention was also made of the use of low oxygen tensions in certain patients in whom a less depressed or less anxious state of mind took place as a result of anoxia. Although a decrease in the oxygen tension of the environment is not compatible with the finest type of mental work, especially creative activity, there are less fortunate individuals to whom the preservation of the critical faculty lodged in the higher nerve centers is accompanied by no achievement of either a scientific, artistic, or other nature, but rather by a persistent tendency to criticize themselves and in some instances by an overintense criticism of others. The suggestion was made that this overcritical attitude, in the absence of other capacities or sufficient opportunity to develop adequate outlets, may be a detriment rather than an advantage, and in psychotic depression the use of repeated shock therapy appears to have its beneficial results by decreasing the functional activity of these higher centers. A rich oxygen supply to the organism is especially to be valued by those who are apparently in the vanguard of human progress in respect to brain function. In respect to the other organs in the body it would appear to be a reasonable conclusion that a normal oxygen tension is apt to be accompanied by preservation of normal functioning and that a well-marked lowering of oxygen tension may be followed not only by impaired function but by pathologic changes in the organs themselves.

The author wishes to address a final word to the future student of respiratory function and its applied technic of inhalational therapy. The study of anoxia and its prevention and treatment inevitably leads to research in various organ systems in the human body. The investigator who follows this scarlet thread of oxygenated blood to the various organs whose function is maintained by it need feel no discomfiture if he is led to travel over a wide territory, since there is unity in his fundamental approach, the investigation of impairment of functioning as a consequence of potential cell anoxia.

Blake once remarked, "Woe to the generalist who is not a specialist, and woe to the specialist who is not a generalist." Additional comfort may be obtained, if it is needed, from the engaging remarks of Elmer Southard, quoted by Frederick Gay in "The Open Mind": "Among psychologists I am known as a chess player; among psychiatrists I am known as an anatomist; among philosophers I am known as a psychologist; and among clinicians as a neuropathologist." Southard reassured himself by telling his friend Gay, "No man who has stayed within the recognized boundaries of his field has contributed fundamentally to science." Whether or not this statement is true, the breadth of Southard's interest and knowledge did not hamper him, but on the contrary made it possible for him to cultivate "many different kinds of intellectual soil for the benefit that each would have on the other."

The practice of a specialty which is strictly limited to an organ system of the human body is not inevitably accompanied by increased achievement but may be employed as a method of evading the responsibility of more general knowledge. Equally valid is a specialty in which a man's dedication is toward a physiologic orientation, such as that presented by a primary interest in disturbance in respiratory function. The legend of frivolity is perhaps too easily repeated as a criticism of diversity of application, by those who feel constitutionally disinclined toward multiple interests. The aim to isolate one field of endeavor, in order to obtain more opportunity for intensive study and enlightenment, should not be considered more legitimate than the aim to cross many different fields of interest, in order to observe what contribution the application of apparently remote knowledge may have in elucidating the fundamental problem under investigation. The author intends simply to explain his own conviction that the student of impaired respiratory function and its application to disease will justifiably find himself concerned with a diversity of physiologic and clinical problems, which will encourage him to resist a too arbitrary segregation of his energy and his curiosity.

BIBLIOGRAPHY

Barach, A. L.: The Therapeutic Use of Gases: The Therapeutics of Internal Diseases. Edited by George Blumer, Vol. I, New York, D. Appleton-Century Co., 1940-1941.

Barach, A. L., and Julia Kagan: Disorders of mental functioning produced by varying the oxygen tension of the atmosphere, Psychosomatic Med., 2:1, 1940.

Barach, A. L., Alfred Steiner, Morris Eckman, and Norman Molomut: The physiologic action of oxygen and carbon dioxide on the coronary circulation, as shown by blood gas and electrocardiographic studies, Amer. Heart Jour., 22: 13, 1941.

Barcroft, J. H., G. H. Hunt, and D. Dufton: The treatment of chronic cases of gas poisoning by continuous oxygen administration in chambers, Quart. Jour. Med., 13:179, 1920.

Campbell, J. M. H., and E. P. Poulton: Oxygen and Carbon Dioxide Therapy, Oxford University Press, 1934.

Cobb, S., and F. Freemont-Smith: The cerebral circulation: XVI. Changes in the human retinal circulation and in the pressure of the cerebrospinal fluid during inhalation of a mixture of carbon dioxide and oxygen, Arch. Neurol. and Psychiat., 26:731, 1931.

Gay, F. P.: The Open Mind: Elmer E. Southard, Chicago, Normandie House, 1938.

Goldblatt, H., J. R. Kahn, F. Bayless, and M. A. Simon: Studies on experimental hypertension: XI. The effect of excision of carotid sinuses on experimental hypertension produced by renal ischemia, Jour. Exper. Med., 71:175, 1940.

Hick, F. K., A. W. Christian, and P. W. Smith: Criteria of oxygen want, with especial reference to neurocirculatory asthenia, Amer. Jour. Med. Sci., 194: 800, 1937.

Himwich, H. E., F. A. D. Alexander, and B. Lipetz: Effect of acute anoxia produced by breathing nitrogen on the course of schizophrenia, Proc. Soc. Exper. Biol. and Med., 39:367, 1938.

Hinsie, L. E., A. L. Barach, M. M. Harris, E. Brand, and R. A. McFarland: The treatment of dementia praecox by continuous oxygen administration in chambers and oxygen and carbon dioxide inhalations, Psychiat. Quart., 7:34, 1934.

Kroetz, C.: Physiologische und pathologische Schwankungen der Sauerstoffdurch-lässigkeit der Lungen, Verhandl. d. deutsch. Gesellsch. f. inn. Med., 43:105, 1931.

Leake, C. D., E. W. Leake, and A. E. Koehler: Jour. Biol. Chem., 56:319, 1923.

Leake, C. D., D. R. Wood, M. E. Botsford, and A. E. Guedel: The effects of administration of carbon dioxide and oxygen in catatonic dementia praecox, Anesth. and Analg., 9:62, 1930.

Lennox, W. G., and A. R. Behnke, Jr.: Effect of increased oxygen pressure on seizures of epilepsy, Arch. Neurol. and Psychiat., 35:782, 1936; Jour. Amer. Med. Asso., 106:2073, 1936.

Loevenhart, A. S., W. F. Lorenz, and R. M. Waters: Cerebral stimulation, Jour. Amer. Med. Asso., 92:880, 1929.

Poulton, E. P.: Local tissue anoxia and its treatment, with special reference to rheumatic myocarditis, Lancet, 2:305, 1939.

Steiner, A., D. M. Weeks, and A. L. Barach: A study of the hypothetic anoxemia factor in experimental and clinical hypertension, Amer. Heart Jour., 19:708, 1940.

Wolff, H. G., and W. G. Lennox: Cerebral circulation: effect on pial vessels of variations in oxygen and carbon dioxide content of blood, Arch. Neurol. and Psychiat., 23:1097, 1930.

34

Methods of Inhalational Therapy

OXYGEN TANK AND REGULATOR

The first requirement for effective and economical administration of oxygen for therapeutic purposes is a supply of U.S.P. oxygen in large industrial-type cylinders of 200 cubic feet or more capacity at standard industrial prices. The former provision of so-called "medical" oxygen in low-pressure cylinders exercised a deterrent influence on oxygen therapy since it was expensive, wasteful, and difficult to regulate. At the present time oxygen is available in large cylinders that contain from 5,600 to 6,900 liters under a pressure of from 1,800 to 2,200 pounds per square inch. In order to employ the oxygen in cylinders at these high pressures a dependable oxygen regulator made by a qualified company is necessary with all types of oxygen-therapy equipment.

The oxygen regulator has the function of reducing the pressure of oxygen from that in the cylinder to the relatively low pressure to which it is delivered to the rubber tubing that is connected to an oxygen tent or other form of oxygen equipment. The regulator is of the two-stage automatic reduction type which is actually two regulators in one. Oxygen from the cylinder at high pressure enters the first stage where the pressure is automatically reduced before entering the second or regulating stage. In this way the high cylinder pressure is prevented from straining the delicate mechanism of the second stage by which the ultimate purpose of the regulator, namely a constant flow in liters per minute of oxygen, is accurately controlled. Either a dial gauge or a variable orifice with float gauge may be employed to register the rate of flow. Certain rules in operating regulators are of special importance and may be listed as follows:

1. Before attaching the regulator to the cylinder of oxygen the cylinder valve should be "cracked," i.e., opened slightly, and then

quickly closed, to blow out any dust that may have lodged in the opening and prevent dust from entering the regulator. After the regulator has been attached to the cylinder the adjusting screw is released, i.e., turned counter-clockwise until it is loose. This is done in order to prevent the full tank pressure from suddenly being applied to the regulating valve mechanism. The cylinder valve is then opened slightly and slowly until the content gauge on the regulator records

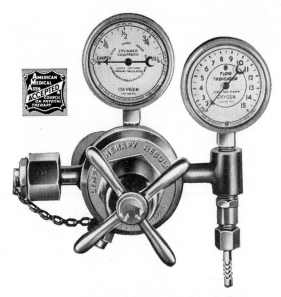

FIG. 22.   Standard two-stage hospital-type
oxygen regulator.

the total pressure; at this time the cylinder valve is opened completely.

In order to begin oxygen therapy the adjusting screw is turned clockwise until the flow gauge on the regulator indicates the desired flow in liters per minute. When oxygen therapy is stopped temporarily, the adjusting screw is turned counter-clockwise, and the cylinder valve need not be completely closed. If an efficient regulator is in use at the bedside it is sufficient simply to turn the adjusting screw counter-clockwise so that no oxygen comes through. However, if the regulator is to be set aside for a long period of time, the valve on the top of the tank should also be closed. This relieves the internal pressure in the regulator which might otherwise strain the mechanism were it to be allowed to exist over long periods of time.

2. It is of real importance never to use oil on an oxygen regulator or on any oxygen connection to the regulator. In fact, any oil or grease on the hands of the person handling a regulator should be carefully washed off. Oxygen under pressure coming in contact with oil or grease may ignite violently.

3. In considering a location for storage of oxygen cylinders it should be remembered that oil, grease, or other flammable material should not be in the vicinity. A place should be selected which will not be subjected to high temperatures, that is, away from boilers, furnaces, steam pipes, sterilizers, laundry apparatus, and hot radiators. The increase in internal pressure caused by being near a place of high temperature may open the safety device with which each cylinder is equipped and thus cause a loss of oxygen. Empty cylinders should be labeled and stored separately from full tanks.

4. In using oxygen cylinders at the bedside with any form of portable oxygen-therapy equipment, the oxygen tank should be strapped to the bedpost or placed in a truck or have some other suitable support to prevent it from being knocked over.

5. The technician in charge of oxygen therapy should have an accurate idea of how long a given cylinder will last so that adequate preparations may be made to substitute a fresh cylinder when needed. As a result of a recent modification, high-pressure cylinders are being filled to a pressure of 2,200 pounds per square inch and contain when full 244 cubic feet of oxygen. Formerly they were filled to a pressure of 2,000 pounds and contained 220 cubic feet. The contents gauges on regulators are calibrated for the old pressure levels and read "full" when the cylinder is actually only 90 per cent full. In the accompanying table the number of hours a cylinder will last with various rates of flow is shown. It will be seen that with a flow of 4 liters per minute a tank which is actually full will last 28¾ hours. When the contents gauge registers "full," indicating a content of 220 cubic feet, the cylinder will last 25 hours. At a flow of 8 liters per minute the full cylinder will last 14¼ hours, and with the contents gauge registering "½ full," 6¼ hours. It is important to know how long a tank will last that has emptied to the "¼ full" mark, in order to use it up in an economical way and at the same time not allow the patient to be left without oxygen when the tank has become empty. When the contents gauge registers 55 cubic feet or "¼ full," the cylinder will still last 12½ hours at a flow of 2 liters per minute and 6¼ hours at a flow of 4 liters per minute.

TABLE VII

HOURS OF SERVICE OF OXYGEN CYLINDER (244 CU. FT.) AT VARYING RATES
OF FLOW

Flow of Oxygen from Regulator	Gauge Reading of Contents of Cylinder			
Liters per Minute	244 Cu. Ft.: Full Cylinder	220 Cu. Ft.: "Full"	110 Cu. Ft.: "½ Full"	55 Cu. Ft.: "¼ Full"
2	57½ hrs.	50 hrs.	25 hrs.	12½ hrs.
4	28¾ "	25 "	12½ "	6¼ "
8	14¼ "	12½ "	6¼ "	3 "
12	9½ "	8¼ "	4 "	2 "

6. The fact that oxygen strongly supports combustion of flammable material makes it necessary that all operators of oxygen equipment take special precaution to avoid fires. Warning should be given both by appropriate signs and by word of mouth against the use of matches, open flames, and sparks in a room where an oxygen tent or other oxygen equipment is being used. Matches, cigarettes, and lighters should be removed from patients and visitors. Electric pads should not be employed in oxygen tents or oxygen rooms but hot-water bottles used instead. Electric call buttons should not be placed within the tent. Patients should not be rubbed with oil, alcohol, or any other ignitable substance while in an oxygen tent.

7. Regulators should be checked at frequent intervals for leaks and accuracy of flow. Leakage may be quickly discerned by shutting the regulator and then closing the tank valve. If the pointer of the contents gauge falls under these conditions a leak is present. Accuracy of flow may be checked by running gas from the regulator into a basal-metabolism apparatus. The rate of flow of the gas will be recorded on the basal-metabolism chart and may be compared to the flow-gauge reading.

OXYGEN MANIFOLDS

The installation of a central supply of oxygen for therapeutic purposes is made possible by connecting a series of cylinders to an oxygen manifold. At a convenient point in the hospital, two banks of 5 to 40 cylinders may be connected to each of two master regulators. One bank of tanks may be adjusted to flow at a pressure of 50 pounds, the other at 45 pounds. Oxygen will flow from the first bank until its gas content falls to a pressure of 45 pounds, whereupon the second bank will automatically begin to deliver oxygen. A smaller line pressure may be used. The supply of oxygen is then piped to the wards or private rooms of the hospital and in that way does away with the

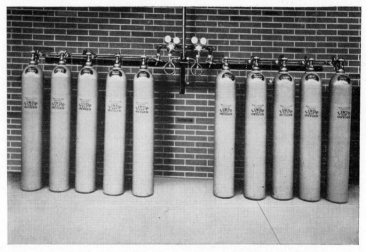

FIG. 23. Oxygen manifold.

necessity for transporting oxygen tanks throughout the hospital. Furthermore, the saving of oxygen is considerable since in many instances where manifolds are not used a tank partially full is returned to the storeroom marked empty. This practice of tanks being returned to the factory with oxygen still remaining in them is unavoidable as it is not possible to exercise constant and continuous supervision over a tank when it is almost empty.

By means of the manifold all the tanks on one bank may be almost entirely used up before the regulator on the tanks on the other side is set into action. There are also other economies such as the elimination of the cost of delivery of the tanks to and from the different wards. Furthermore, the regulators on each tank are expensive and the cost of repairing them is in itself a considerable item. With the presence of an oxygen supply at the bedside the moving in and out of cylinders is avoided, which has a good psychologic effect on the patient. The initial cost of installing a manifold oxygen supply system may be made up for in a large part during the first year of service by the economy which results.

RUBBER CATHETER IN THE NASAL PHARYNX AND ORAL PHARYNX

The nasal-catheter method of administering oxygen is inexpensive and has a very considerable degree of efficiency. The apparatus required includes a reliable oxygen regulator, a water bottle to humidify the oxygen, and a rubber urethral catheter. Water bottles of various types have been designed, including the simplest one in which a stream of oxygen is bubbled through three inches of water. In a more elaborate humidifying device, the oxygen stream is broken up into tiny bubbles and passed through water before entering into the rubber tube leading to the catheter. Either the simple water bottle or the more elaborate device may be used with both the oral pharyngeal or nasal pharyngeal administration of oxygen.

The rubber catheter should be a No. 10 French in size, never more than No. 12, because larger catheters are uncomfortable and more apt to cause mouth breathing. The terminal one inch of the catheter should be perforated by four to six small holes since a high rate of flow is better tolerated when dispersed than when a single opening is present. If the holes in the catheter become plugged by mucus, and only one small perforation remains, the stream of oxygen through it may impinge on a localized area of mucous membrane and cause a burning sensation, which may be responsible for the patient pulling the catheter out of the nose. The catheter should be cleaned every 12 hours, or more often if necessary, in order to wash away crusted mucus and prevent clogging of the apertures referred to.

The catheter when used in the nasal pharynx may be simply inserted by passing along the floor of the nose until it reaches the back of the pharynx; it is then withdrawn slightly and kept in that position by adhesive being applied to the catheter over the nose and forehead. The catheter is connected by a metal tube with a rubber hose which may be fastened to the pillow by a safety pin. Unless the catheter is withdrawn slightly from the posterior wall of the pharynx, gagging may take place. The catheter is lubricated with KY jelly or vaseline along the terminal three inches. The catheter is less apt to be loosened if it is strapped along the bridge of the nose and over the forehead rather than if it is passed laterally across the face.

Care should be taken to keep the water bottle about one-half full with tap water. This may be simply done by unscrewing the glass part of the water bottle from the metal cap. The rubber gasket should be inspected to make sure that oxygen does not escape through this connection.

The humidifier may be checked for leakage by lowering the flow of the regulator to 2 liters per minute and closing off the outlet of the humidifier with a finger. If the humidifier leaks, the gas flow, as noted by the bubbling of the water, will remain unchanged. When no leakage is present the bubbling will diminish and soon stop.

Considerable variation exists in the literature as to the concentrations obtained in the alveolar and inspired airs when nasal-catheter administration is used. These differences may in a large part be explained by variations in the quantity of ventilation. It will readily be understood that a child with a smaller volume of breathing than a large adult will obtain a relatively higher oxygen percentage with a given flow of oxygen from a cylinder. Thus, a pulmonary ventilation of 12 liters per minute mixed with 4 liters per minute of oxygen will give a far lower concentration of oxygen in the alveolar air than will be found when the pulmonary ventilation is 6 liters per minute and the oxygen flow the same. In an adult with a slightly increased pulmonary ventilation the following concentrations in the inspired air may be assumed as approximately correct for nasal-pharyngeal catheter administration: at 2 liters per minute, 28 per cent oxygen; at 4 liters, 33 per cent; at 5 liters, 36 per cent; at 6 liters, 38 per cent; and at 8 liters, 42 per cent oxygen.

When a flow of oxygen as high as 8 liters per minute is employed it may be more comfortable to insert a catheter in each nostril and connect them over the forehead with a metal Y-tube. However, when high oxygen concentrations are desired, with nasal-catheter administration, the position of the catheter is preferably changed to the oral pharyngeal placement.

ORAL-PHARYNGEAL CATHETER PLACEMENT

When it is desired to administer oxygen by the oral-pharyngeal placement of the catheter, the catheter should be inserted into the nose and into the oral pharynx until the patient begins to swallow

oxygen.   Then it is withdrawn a short distance and fastened securely
to the nose and forehead.   This method of placing the catheter, i.e.,
determining when the patient swallows oxygen in the act of deglutition, is better than looking for the catheter in the oral pharynx
through the mouth.   It will be found to be behind the uvula in most
instances, but it has been emphasized that the swallowing of oxygen
is a more reliable method of obtaining the proper position of the
catheter.   It is important that the
strapping of the catheter be very secure since a considerable amount of
oxygen may be passed into the stomach
if it slips lower in the pharynx than is
intended.

By means of the pharyngeal catheter
concentrations of oxygen in the inspired air in excess of 45 per cent can
be maintained with a flow of 6 liters
of oxygen per minute.   Because of the
relatively larger space in which oxygen
can accumulate during respiration, this
method of administration is a more
efficient one than placement in the
nasal pharynx.   Oxygen concentrations
as high as 70 per cent may be efficiently
supplied in this way.   Pharyngeal ad-

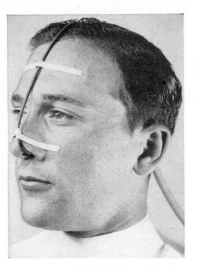

Fig. 24.   Oral-pharyngeal
catheter.

ministration of oxygen is a highly efficient and economical method.
The simple precaution of observing that if the patient swallows a
bubble of air in the act of deglutition the catheter has been inserted
too far should not be difficult to observe.   When the proper position of
the catheter is known it should be marked at the exterior of the nose in
order to expedite placement of a fresh catheter at 12-hour intervals in
the alternate nostril.   The distance of the tip of the catheter from the
external nares varies between 4½ to 5½ inches.   When viewed through
the mouth the catheter position is usually at the tip of the uvula as it
hangs quietly in breathing.   Small urethral catheters, No. 10 French,
should be used for this purpose and should also be perforated with
extra holes as indicated in administration of oxygen in the nasal
pharynx.

Due to the relatively small size of the nasal passages in infants,
and to the greater readiness for middle-ear infection, the catheter

method is less suited to them than to adults. The open-top tent, as will be described later, appears to be a serviceable method of administering oxygen to young children and infants. Either the open-top tent or the enclosed tent may be employed. The position of the catheter in the nasal pharynx and the oral pharynx is illustrated in the accompanying photographs.

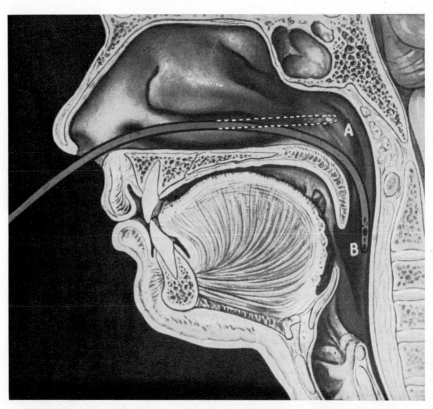

FIG. 25. Position of catheter (A) in nasopharynx; (B) in oropharynx.

Instead of catheters, nasal inhalers are sometimes employed which consist of pronged metal tubes the ends of which are inserted a short distance into the nose. The nasal inhaler is attached to a metal stem that is adjustable on a forehead plate which in turn is fastened to the forehead with adhesive plaster or a head band. The prongs are made of soft brass so that they can be molded to fit various noses. Care should be taken that the nostrils are not occluded by the metal or the patient will be forced to breathe through the mouth to supply the normal rate of pulmonary ventilation. If the prongs are too far removed from the nose the oxygen is apt to be wasted in the surrounding atmosphere. At an oxygen flow of 4 liters per minute, 30 per cent oxygen may be obtained in the alveolar air of the average adult. However, there is more reliability in obtaining a constant oxygen concentration at lower flows with the rubber catheter inserted into the oral pharynx.

Whatever the method of nasal administration of oxygen, the operation of equipment demands skillful supervision. Leaks around the top of the water bottle or humidifier are not infrequently found which result in oxygen passing into the outside atmosphere and not into the catheter itself. It is important also to check for the presence of leaks at the tube connections, especially if the rubber hose is old, and to be certain that the tubing is not pinched. The lubrication of the catheter should be performed at frequent enough intervals so that the catheter does not stick to the sides of the pharynx. Furthermore, the lubrication should not be so extensively done as to plug the holes that are made for the distribution of oxygen.

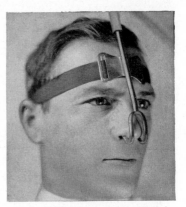

FIG. 26. Nasal inhaler.

One hour before the oxygen in the cylinder is exhausted, another cylinder should be substituted, if close supervision is not available, in order to make sure that interruption of treatment does not take place inadvertently. After the therapy is concluded the humidifier and tubing should be thoroughly cleansed with hot water and allowed to dry; the catheter should be washed and boiled for four or five minutes or sterilized in another efficient manner. The catheter is then wrapped in a clean package and put away for future use.

OXYGEN TENT

The oxygen tent is employed to administer oxygen concentrations between 40 and 60 per cent, and to provide the patient at the same time with hygienic conditions of temperature and relative humidity. The oxygen tent consists of (1) a canopy that is suspended over the bed in such a way as to enclose either the entire patient or the head

and upper portions of the patient's body, and (2) a conditioning cabinet to cool and dehumidify the oxygen-enriched atmosphere within
the tent canopy, either by a motor-blower circulation or through a
system of thermal ventilation. A suitable flow of oxygen from the
regulator is added to the tent atmosphere at a rate required to maintain the desired oxygen concentration.

Tents which enclose the body of the patient should have a capacity
of at least 12 cubic feet. A completely transparent canopy is far
preferable to a rubberized fabric with enclosed windows. Pliofilm,
transparent plastocele, or other noninflammable transparent material
furnishes a greater sense of comfort to the patient and also a better
view for the doctor and nurses than canopies that are partly transparent and partly impervious to light.

The skirts of the tent canopy are tucked under the mattress at the
head and sides of the bed. In most instances the canopy stretches
in front of the patient and lies on the sheet, and it is then necessary
to use a draw sheet over the canopy which is tucked tightly under the
mattress on each side to prevent loss of oxygen. After the canopy
has been placed over the patient the object is to make it as leakproof
as possible. A rubber sheet on that part of the mattress covered by
the canopy tends to diminish loss of oxygen, but it is generally not
necessary to employ this and it is less comfortable for the patient if
it is directly under the sheet. If it is placed under the mattress, the
task is difficult unless the patient is moved to another bed.

The ventilation of the tent may be obtained by a motor-blower
circulation in which the oxygen-enriched atmosphere is passed through
a cabinet containing chunks of ice the size of a grapefruit. In this
type of tent the ice cabinet may be of large or moderate size; the
large-size refrigerating cabinet has a very considerable advantage in
being able to provide a cool and dehumidified atmosphere for periods
as long as 12 hours without re-icing, depending on the surrounding
room temperature. Below the ice cabinet is a compartment which
contains the motor-blower unit. This is connected to the surface
of the cabinet by appropriate wiring. On the front of the conditioner
cabinet are found a motor plug, switch, pilot light, water drain, and
a rheostat for controlling the velocity of flow of the circulated atmosphere. On the support tubes that lead to and from the ice cabinet
into the tent, openings provide entrances for the thermometer, gas
inlet, and sampling pet-cock.

When the tent is about to be used, the ice cabinet is first filled with large chunks of ice. The tent is then wheeled alongside or behind the bed, the motor plug is attached to the wall socket, the switch turned to the "on" position, and the rheostat set at the midposition. The pilot light will glow when the motor is turned on. The canopy is then placed over the patient and tucked under the mattress at the head end, both sides and rear, or a draw sheet is folded over the canopy in front of the patient. The water drain is turned to the open posi-

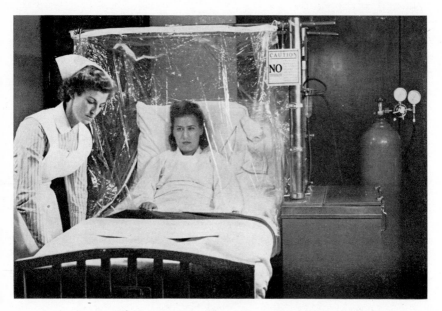

Fig. 27. Motor-blower oxygen tent.

tion so as to allow for a continuous drip of water from the melting ice. The oxygen cylinder is tied to the bed or supported on a truck. The regulator is turned to 15 liters per minute for a period of 30 minutes, which generally results in a large-sized tent in a concentration of 50 per cent oxygen, and is then turned to 10 liters per minute. When it is desired to build up a higher oxygen concentration in a shorter time, the oxygen flow from two regulators may be run into the appropriate gas inlet, in which case 30 liters per minute will produce a concentration of 50 per cent oxygen in 12 to 15 minutes. If a flush valve is present on the regulator it may be opened for a period of 2 minutes which will also produce an oxygen concentration of 50 per cent.

The rheostat is generally set at mid-position. If a higher velocity of oxygen-air movement is desired, it may be turned to the high position which will give a temperature as low as 56° F. with a relative humidity of approximately 35 per cent. If temperatures above 70° F.

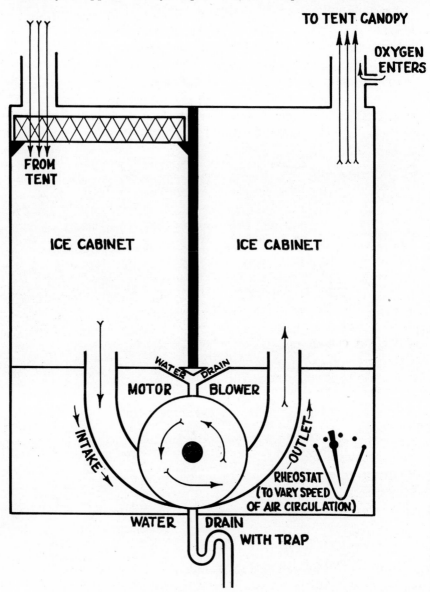

FIG. 28. Diagram of a motor-blower oxygen tent.

and relatively high humidity are desired the rheostat is turned to the low position. If this still results in a temperature that is considered colder than desired, ice may be removed until the temperature rises to the desired level. When still higher temperatures and humidities are desired, all ice may be removed from the refrigerating cabinet and the rheostat turned to the midposition or the high position. This will then provide a comfortable degree of air movement but the temperature will then rise much higher than that of the surrounding atmosphere.

To maintain a relative humidity of between 80 and 90 per cent in a cool atmosphere, a special device is being perfected for the vaporizing of a pint of water an hour. In the employment of apparatus of this type, precaution should be taken to prevent any part of the motor from coming in contact with the oxygen-enriched atmosphere.

When the initial flow of oxygen has presumably elevated the oxygen concentration to that which has been prescribed—40, 50, 60, or 70 per cent—a test of the oxygen concentration should be made by a suitable oxygen analyzer. A check of the oxygen concentration is made at least two to three times during 24 hours. If the percentage of oxygen in the atmosphere is below that prescribed, it is not sufficient simply to increase the flow of oxygen until the desired concentration has been found by subsequent oxygen test. A search should be made for the cause of the lowered oxygen concentration. If the nurse was required to open the tent canopy to feed the patient or for other nursing attention, instruction should be given to her that an additional flow of oxygen such as 15 liters per minute should be administered for 5, 10, or 15 minutes, depending upon the extent to which the canopy has been opened. However, if the tent canopy has not been opened, and the oxygen concentration was found to be lower than desired, a full inspection of sources of leak should be made, including the following: (1) The tent canopy should be inspected to see whether it is in contact with the mattress and draw sheet on all sides. (2) The top of the air-conditioning cabinet should be tightly fastened or locked to the body of the cabinet, and the sponge-rubber gasket should make contact at all points with the framework of the cabinet. (3) The flow of oxygen from the tank itself should be checked as well as all rubber tube connections. If all these sources of leaks have been inspected and no fault discovered, a new tent should be installed and the motor-blower unit of the discarded tent inspected for leaks in the shaft between the blower and the motor.

The water drain should be kept open at all times while the tent is in use for otherwise an accumulation of water may stop the flow of the oxygen-enriched atmosphere. The ice compartment in the large senior model of the Barach-Thurston motor-blower tent should be filled every eight hours; this varies between 6 and 12 hours, depending upon the speed of circulation of the motor-blower unit and the temperature of the surrounding atmosphere. In tents that have a smaller ice capacity, more frequent filling of the compartment with ice is necessary.

The testing of the oxygen concentration at least two times during the day may be increased in cases in which it is of special importance to make sure that a high oxygen concentration is continuously present in the tent. The temperature should be checked at the same time and if it is lower or higher than that desired the rheostat should be turned to a position which will give a lower or higher velocity flow respectively.

Carbon-dioxide Concentration Within the Tent. When a tent is employed which contains a motor-blower unit, with a considerable degree of air movement and a large-size canopy, it will be found necessary to maintain an oxygen flow of not less than 9, and preferably 10, liters per minute in order to keep a concentration above 50 per cent oxygen in the tent atmosphere. In most instances in which any oxygen tent is employed, the concentration of oxygen is not generally prescribed below this level. Under these circumstances the carbon dioxide produced by a heavy adult will in large measure be washed out of the tent at the connections which the canopy makes with the bed. Under most conditions the carbon-dioxide percentage will therefore be in the neighborhood of 1 per cent, and very rarely 1.5 per cent, even in large patients with an elevated metabolism. There is, therefore, no economy in the attempt to employ soda-lime to absorb carbon dioxide, as tents are generally used in clinical practice with adequate nursing attention. Although soda-lime is employed in a few well-regulated clinics, this necessitates close supervision on the part of a number of technicians who must necessarily make careful analyses for carbon dioxide as well as oxygen. In most hospitals, as well as in the use of oxygen tents in the home, the provision of a liberal flow of oxygen from the regulator not only makes it more likely that the patient will receive the benefit of an effective oxygen concentration, but it also eliminates the necessity for repeated checking for carbon-dioxide accumulation.

When it has been determined that a flow of 9 to 10 liters per minute of oxygen from the regulator prevents accumulation of carbon dioxide in the initial appraisal of a new tent, this test need not be performed in the routine management of other cases. Since higher flows of oxygen are very frequently necessary to maintain oxygen concentrations between 50 and 60 per cent, the carbon-dioxide percentage is rarely found to be above 1 per cent by actual test. If an oxygen flow of 15 liters per minute is required because of frequent openings of the tent canopy, there should be careful instruction to make proper arrangements for shifting of an empty tank in replacement of a full tank. One or two additional tanks equipped with regulators should generally be alongside the tank in use in oxygen-tent therapy. When the tank in use has very little oxygen remaining in it, it is desirable to employ a new tank. Instead, however, of discarding the tank which has not been entirely used up, it may be connected by a Y-tube to a regulator on a new tank until the old cylinder is emptied. A flow of 10 liters per minute thus enters from the new tank and a flow of 3 or 4 liters a minute admitted from the old tank, until it is exhausted. The oxygen concentration is thus built up slightly above the required level and serves as an economy and an additional insurance against undue lowering of the oxygen concentration.

Since the oxygen tent is a more expensive method of obtaining oxygen therapy than catheters or masks, it should achieve two fundamental aims: (a) To furnish an *effective* oxygen concentration by continuous administration of an oxygen percentage in the atmosphere of not less than 40, preferably 50 per cent, and, for short periods, concentrations as high as 60 or 70 per cent; (b) to provide physical and mental comfort to the patient by a hygienic atmosphere in respect to temperature, humidity, and air movement, by no appliances near to the face, and a clear view to the outside. In achieving these objectives at a *reasonable cost,* careful and intelligent operation of the tent is necessary and the following points may be emphasized even at the hazard of repetition.

Frequent analyses of the oxygen concentration in the tent, such as three times daily, prevent a diminished effectiveness of oxygen therapy and help the technician to discover mistakes in operation or management of the equipment. In an analysis of 70 technician inspections of tents in which the oxygen concentration was found lower than that prescribed by the physician, careless handling of the tent canopy was the cause of the lowered oxygen concentration in 62 instances. In five instances the oxygen cylinder was emptied and a new cylinder had not been turned on. In two instances a tear in the canopy was the cause of the leak. In one case there was a leak between the icebox door and the cabinet due to a faulty sponge-rubber gasket. In this series there was no leak in the motor-blower unit, i.e., along the shaft that connects the fan with the motor.

In ten of 100 tent inspections, the temperature was too high, due in four cases to the rheostat being turned to the low or midposition instead of the high position, in four cases to the water drain being shut off, in one case to a clogged water drain, and in one instance to lack of ice.

It is important to instruct the nurse on the case to increase the flow of oxygen each time the tent is opened, such as to 15 liters per minute for 5 minutes, or for 10 to 15 minutes if a prolonged period of contact with the outside atmosphere has taken place. The motor-blower system should always be turned off when refilling with ice or introducing a medicine or food in the tent, or when the patient is being examined for short periods. It must be remembered that the motor should be turned on immediately after closure of the tent. When sleeves are used for access to the patient the opening should be as small as possible and closed immediately after the treatment has taken place. The oxygen cylinder should be strapped to the bed so that it is not accidentally knocked over. The tent should operate quietly, almost noiselessly. If vibration of the motor is heard, it should be removed and a new one employed. Although the comfort of the patient is unmistakably enhanced by completely transparent canopies, for patients who are delirious or who tear the canopy repeatedly, a strong rubberized fabric is used with ample window space in it. When the ice is inserted into the cabinet, an attempt should be made to create as little noise as possible by inserting the ice by hand rather than letting it fall out of a large pail or letting it drop to the floor of the cabinet.

In respect to temperature and relative humidity within the tent, the individual patient may frequently be consulted. In the average adult febrile patient, a temperature of between 60° and 68° F. is more comfortable and allows a more efficient heat elimination than temperatures above 70°. In some cases with high fever, a tent temperature of 58° F. and plentiful air movement are desirable, and may easily be obtained with motor-blower circulation.

The relative humidity does not become unduly elevated in the use of tents that have motor-blower circulation of the contained atmosphere over chunks of ice, and it need not be tested routinely. Under these circumstances, even with the rheostat at low position, the relative humidity is never above 60 per cent. It will be found by actual tests generally in the neighborhood of 40 per cent. In very old patients in whom a higher temperature is desired, with at the same time air movement for comfort, the ice may be entirely or partly removed and the rheostat set at high position.

THERMAL-CIRCULATION TENT

In thermal-circulation tents the principle of warm air rising and cool air falling is responsible for a gradual movement of the tent atmosphere to the top of the tent as a result of the heat given off by the patient, and, after entrance to the cabinet containing ice and soda-lime, a downward movement of the oxygen-air mixture which is cooled, dried, and deprived of carbon dioxide. The cool atmosphere enters the canopy at the side of the patient in the Oxygenaire Tent. There is a slow air movement with a relatively cold atmosphere on the side of the patient that is exposed to the ice cabinet. An oxygen flow of 5 to 6 liters a minute will maintain a concentration above 50 per cent oxygen but at the cost of an excessive carbon-dioxide concentration in the tent atmosphere unless soda-lime is employed and periodic test-ing of carbon-dioxide concentration pursued. When oxygen flows of 9 to 10 liters per minute are used, soda-lime may be dispensed with, provided sufficient leakage is created or an injector is used to main-tain concentrations of 50 or 60 per cent. When an injector is at-tached to the regulator, as will be fully explained in describing the Meter-mask apparatus, the oxygen passing through a fine orifice in an enclosed cylinder draws a varying proportion of air into the stream of oxygen that enters the tent. The oxygen percentage on the dial of the injector tells the concentration of the mixture entering the tent but oxygen testing of the contained tent atmosphere is still necessary, since a leak in any part of the canopy may be followed by a lowering of the oxygen concentration.

The use of the injector with a small flow of oxygen will not lower the carbon-dioxide concentration of the tent if a 50 or 60 per cent oxygen concentration is maintained. With an oxygen flow of 6 liters per minute and a concentration of 60 per cent in the tent the total flow of oxygen and air entering the tent is 12 liters per minute, since 6 liters of oxygen mixed with 6 liters of air yield this percentage. If the patient is eliminating carbon dioxide at the rate of 275 cc. per minute the concentration of carbon dioxide might reach a level of

$275/12,000 \times 100$, or 2.3 per cent, which is too high for the patient's comfort. With a 10-liter flow under the same conditions the carbon-dioxide concentration will be 1.3 per cent or less. Use of the injector

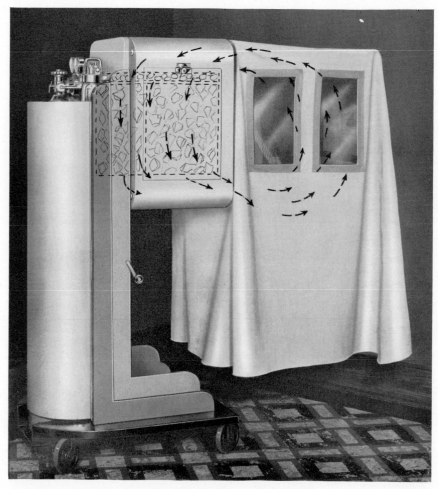

FIG. 29. Thermal-circulation tent.

is preferable to soda-lime if economy is sought in this type of tent. A thermometer should be placed inside the tent within clear view of the observer; the relative humidity should be tested in the initial appraisal of the tent with the ice container full and half full. Due to the relatively small size of the compartment containing ice, special care should be taken to prevent the temperature from increasing to undesirable levels. This applies to dehumidification to an even greater extent since there is no provision except through thermal circulation of air over ice to remove the moisture given off by the patient.

Thermal-circulation tents have the advantage of being able to provide high oxygen concentrations in the neighborhood of 70 per cent with greater ease than in the motor-driven types. Furthermore, the tent does not require electricity and, therefore, may be used in regions where this is not available. However, air movement is limited.

In operating tents of this kind oxygen is admitted at first at a flow of 15 liters per minute until the desired concentration of oxygen is obtained by test and the regulator then turned to a maintenance flow which varies depending upon whether or not soda-lime is to be used. If soda-lime is to be dispensed with, flows of 9 to 10 liters per minute or above are indicated. With the use of soda-lime these flows can be lowered to the neighborhood of 5 liters per minute, provided that determination of carbon-dioxide percentage in the tent atmosphere does not rise above 1.5 per cent. The extent of thermal circulation can be varied by opening or closing the shutter control, which increases or decreases the aperture to which the tent atmosphere may enter the air-conditioning cabinet. Although a wide range of air-movement, temperature and humidity control is not available, as in the motor-blower circulation tent, the atmosphere in the tent canopy is sufficiently cool and does not contain excessive humidity when its operation is carefully supervised. Many patients, however, complain of the cold temperature on the side nearest the refrigerating cabinet. Provision for adequate elimination of carbon dioxide must be made.

DRY-ICE OXYGEN TENT

The dry-ice oxygen tent utilizes solidified carbon dioxide as the refrigerant. A block of this material has three times the cooling power of a block of ordinary ice of equal size. A cylindrical container 7.5 inches in diameter and 20 inches long contains 25 pounds of the refrigerant which is sufficient for approximately 12 hours of use. The container is placed directly over the bed, and the cooling fins with dry ice evaporating at $-109.6°$ F. efficiently cool the oxygen-air mixture. The cool and therefore heavier air circulates downward, being directed to the front of the tent by a baffle, and warm air given off by the patient rises toward the back of the tent to enter into the container above. Excess moisture from the patient's lung condenses on the fin and a satisfactory temperature and relative humidity are obtained. By rotating the tray in which the dry ice is placed, a greater or lesser degree of cooling may be obtained.

The dry ice is furnished in neat easily handled blocks which fit into the tray and as it evaporates directly into the gaseous form it leaves no residue to be disposed of. None of the carbon-dioxide gas evolved

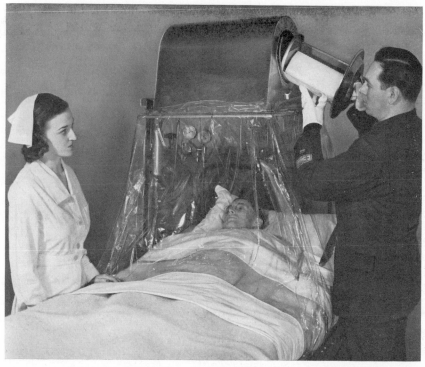

FIG. 30. Dry-ice oxygen tent.

enters into the tent canopy. . The carbon dioxide given off by the patient is eliminated from the tent largely by passing into the tent a flow of 9 liters per minute of oxygen. Low oxygen flows cannot be employed for the reason outlined under thermal circulation; namely, provision for adequate elimination of carbon dioxide. The advantage of this unit is that the stand and container weigh about 30 pounds and may be readily carried about. Dry ice should be placed in the conditioning unit 15 to 20 minutes before use to avoid the noise due to the contracting action of the dry ice on the conditioning compartment (D. J. Cohn).

Since dry ice evaporates steadily it must be obtained when needed and cannot be stored. In hospitals that have ordinary ice available to them, the use of dry ice is apt to be more expensive. However, the comfort of the patient in this type of thermal-circulation tent is generally maintained and effective oxygen therapy may be provided.

OPEN-BOX TENT

In this apparatus the top of the tent is completely open, and closure is made at the neck. When a flow of oxygen of 6 to 7 liters per

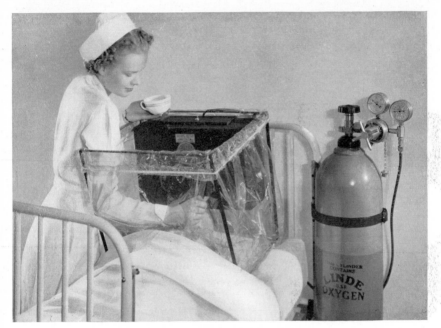

Fig. 31. Open-box tent.

minute is maintained, oxygen concentrations of 50 per cent can be secured at the level of the patient's nose without undue accumulation of carbon dioxide. The principle is that a moderate rate of flow will result in a therapeutic concentration of oxygen at the lower end of the box because the rate of diffusion of oxygen is less than the rate of inflow. This simple arrangement has been used with very considerable success in the treatment of infants but has also been employed for oxygen therapy in adults. It appears to be especially desirable in infants and young children who do not give off as much heat and moisture as large adults. Furthermore, masks and catheters are not suitable for infants. Frequent tests of the atmosphere should be made at the level of the patient's nose. It is important to avoid placing the tent in a draught or near an open window in which case the high oxygen atmosphere might be blown out through the open top. A small ice cabinet may or may not be used; it is set in the rear of the hood and achieves a thermal circulation of the oxygen-enriched

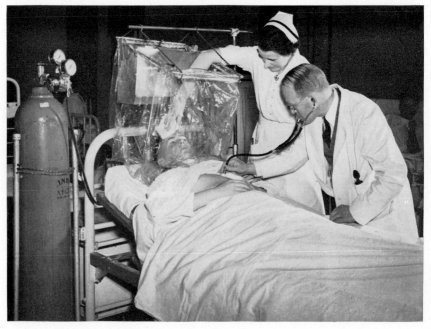

FIG. 32.   Open-box tent (adult).

atmosphere. This type of tent is the simplest and least expensive in manufacture (A. M. Burgess).

Measurement of the carbon-dioxide concentration is not necessary because the open top allows a free diffusion of carbon dioxide.

In reviewing closed-circulation tents it should be understood that low oxygen flows (4 liters per minute) may maintain effective oxygen concentrations if the patient is not examined, nurses not allowed to open the canopy, the patient kept well tucked in, and the mattress rubberized. Under these circumstances the carbon-dioxide concentration will rise to 3 to 4 per cent with toxic manifestations unless continuous care is taken to apply fresh soda-lime in the tent. In thermal-circulation tents this is necessary two or three times a day, and the trays should be only thinly covered with soda-lime in order not to interfere with the circulation within the tent. When the tent is frequently opened, higher flows of oxygen are obviously required. When in continuous operation, the ice basket needs an additional supply of ice every three to four hours to insure maximum efficiency. With a full supply of 55 pounds, even with a room temperature of 78° F., sufficient cooling may be obtained with a thermal-circulation tent. The most important consideration is the question of elimination of carbon dioxide if low oxygen flows are employed. This requires an initial careful appraisal of the tent in terms of varying oxygen flows and carbon-dioxide percentage, with soda-lime, and subsequent frequent testing of the tent in operation, both in respect to carbon dioxide as well as to oxygen concentrations. If an injector is employed which seems more suitable to this type of tent and a more liberal maintenance flow of oxygen is used, sufficient washing out of carbon dioxide will take place so as not to require soda-lime, thus avoiding the fear of excessive accumulation of carbon dioxide, as well as the necessity for frequent determinations of the carbon-dioxide percentage in the atmosphere. The total inflow of oxygen should then be not less than 9 liters per minute when oxygen concentrations below 60 per cent are maintained.

OXYGEN TENTS FOR INFANTS

Since oxygen therapy in infants does not make use of all the general principles that apply to oxygen-tent therapy in adults, the points of difference may be emphasized. First of all, infants may be rapidly deprived of heat by circulation of a cold atmosphere over them, with an abrupt fall in body temperature. In the second place, infants produce so little heat, water, and carbon dioxide that the special measures for the removal of these constituents are not necessary. The open-top tent may be used effectively and inexpensively in the treatment of all conditions requiring simple oxygen therapy. Neither the mask nor the nasal catheter is as satisfactory in the treatment of anoxia in infants. A small box tent may be used with a transparent window in front, or, preferably, transparent canopy throughout. This allows an accurate inspection of the condition of the patient and frees the infant from feelings of claustrophobia. Small oxygen flows such as 6 liters per minute will generally maintain an oxygen percentage of 50 per cent, without undue increase in carbon dioxide, temperature, or humidity. The mechanism of the increase in oxygen concentration, as described above, is simply the instillation into the enclosed box of a flow of oxygen which is higher than that which leaves the tent through diffusion.

AN OXYGEN TENT WITH MECHANICAL REFRIGERATION

In this tent the cooling and drying of the oxygen-enriched atmosphere is accomplished by a frigidaire conditioning unit which uses a

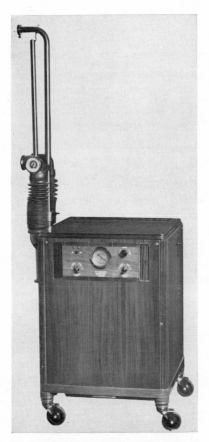

FIG. 33. The refrigeration unit of
the Electri-Cool oxygen tent.

nontoxic, noninflammable refrigerant which has been developed for air-conditioning application. A master switch is on the front of the panel for the control, there is an oxygen-flow meter and a mechanism for regulating the degree of ventilation. When the proper temperature has been established in the tent the cold control may be set so that the unit will automatically provide an even temperature. The humidity in the tent can be varied by changing the cold control to operate the cooling coils at various temperatures. The colder the coils the lower the relative humidity. The drain box which is provided to collect condensation moisture is of large capacity and needs very little attention. The electrical consumption is said to be 8 kilowatts for 24-hour use; at 2.5 cents per kilowatt-hour there is a daily operating expense of approximately 20 cents.

AN OXYGEN TENT WITH THE EMPLOYMENT OF LIQUID OXYGEN

Liquid oxygen has been used both as a supply for oxygen and for cooling by Hartman. Special care must be observed to prevent a spark from coming in contact with liquid oxygen and flammable material, for in that event very rapid combustion would be initiated. Liquid oxygen is subject to constant evaporation and would be more expensive to operate in most communities. Since there are hazards in handling liquid oxygen which are not present in operating cylinders of high-pressure oxygen, this tent will not be discussed in detail but interested readers may refer to it in the accompanying illustration and reference.

STERILIZATION OF THE OXYGEN TENT

After the termination of each case tents should first be washed with soap and water, both inside and outside. This procedure should be relied upon mainly for cleaning and removal of infected secretions. After this is thoroughly performed, the method of choice is to rub down the pliofilm or rubberized canopy with a 70 per cent alcohol solution. The tent canopy may also be allowed to remain for ten minutes in 70 per cent alcohol if provision is made for a suitable container. Any alternative method of effective sterilization may be pursued, such as dipping the canopy in a solution of 1:10,000 of bichloride of mercury for five minutes. If this is done the mercury solution should be carefully washed off with water. If a plastocele window is present in the tent, alcohol should not be used since it clouds the surface of the window. In patients on the private side of the hospital, a new pliofilm canopy can be employed and charged to the patient. If the patient suffered from a disease as infectious as tuberculosis, the pliofilm canopy should be destroyed and the rubberized canopy sterilized with special care. In the treatment of cardiac patients, routine precautions are used.

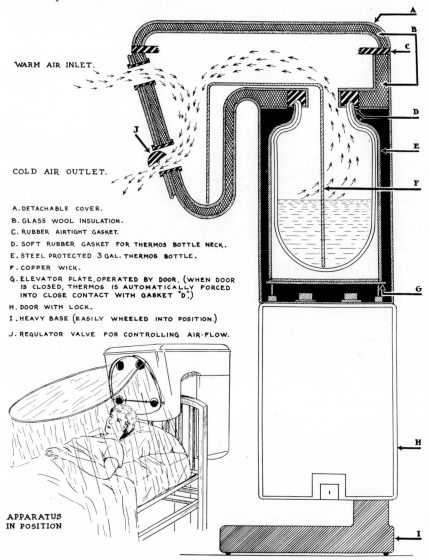

WARM AIR INLET.

COLD AIR OUTLET.

A. DETACHABLE COVER.

B. GLASS WOOL INSULATION.

C. RUBBER AIRTIGHT GASKET.

D. SOFT RUBBER GASKET FOR THERMOS BOTTLE NECK.

E. STEEL PROTECTED 3 GAL. THERMOS BOTTLE.

F. COPPER WICK.

G. ELEVATOR PLATE, OPERATED BY DOOR. (WHEN DOOR IS CLOSED, THERMOS IS AUTOMATICALLY FORCED INTO CLOSE CONTACT WITH GASKET "D".)

H. DOOR WITH LOCK.

I. HEAVY BASE (EASILY WHEELED INTO POSITION.)

J. REGULATOR VALVE FOR CONTROLLING AIR·FLOW.

APPARATUS IN POSITION

FIG. 34. Tent with employment of liquid oxygen (Hartman).

Particular care should be exercised to remove accumulation of débris, such as lint, from the water drain of the ice cabinet at the termination of the case. It dries and hardens on standing and frequently clogs the drain.

OXYGEN CHAMBERS AND OXYGEN ROOMS

Among the methods for administration of oxygen, the oxygen room is the most comfortable to the patient. Although the large-sized oxygen tent ventilated by motor-blower circulation, with a canopy that stretches over the entire bed, provides adequate comfort for most cases, as well as an effective concentration of oxygen and a cool, dry atmosphere, there are patients who appreciate long-continued oxygen

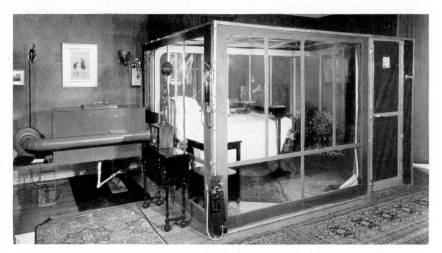

FIG. 35.   Portable oxygen chamber.

therapy in a room in which no mechanical appliance is seen. The oxygen concentration may be accurately regulated, and nursing and medical attention carried out with minimal variation in the concentration prescribed. The expense of upkeep is greater than that of other forms of therapy, since four to five tanks of oxygen are required daily instead of two to two and one-half cylinders for a large bed tent. The two simplest types of oxygen chambers will be described: (1) Conversion of a room in the hospital into an oxygen room, (2) erection of a portable oxygen chamber.

Past experience in the development of oxygen chambers indicates that thermal circulation of the atmosphere is better in many ways than motor-driven ventilation in an oxygen room to be used in a hospital. In private residences, however, the portable oxygen chamber is desirable since it can be erected in a short space of time, and consists in essence simply of an enlarged oxygen tent.

The Oxygen Room. In converting an ordinary hospital room into an oxygen room, the various fixtures in the room and, if present, the adjoining bathroom are made leak-tight; the walls are re-covered with several coats of leak-tight paint or enamel. The door at the entrance of the room is lined with a rubber gasket so as to be air-tight when closed. This requires the employment of a special door-frame with suitable fittings. A long handle on the door is employed in order to exert greater pressure on the rubber gasket and for easy access to and from the oxygen room. A rubberized curtain is suspended inside the door from the margins of the frame in order to prevent rapid diffusion of oxygen when the door is opened. If the curtain is not pushed to one side when entering but allowed to remain in place until after the door is closed, frequent entrances and exits from the room may be made with small loss of oxygen. This curtain device is superior to an air lock in the saving of oxygen. The lock which was formerly used was not so efficient as it first appeared to be, since opening of the door into the lock allowed free passage of oxygen from the room into the lock, and the subsequent opening of the inner door permitted the air in the lock to enter the oxygen room. The window in the room is made leak-tight by placing over its margins a double window which is fastened to the window frame with an intervening soft rubber gasket.

Installed along one wall of the room are two horizontal banks of brine coils of one-inch brass pipe, spaced four inches apart, beginning two feet from the ceiling and extending downward to two feet from the floor. These coils are equipped with a thermostatic control valve which turns off the brine when the temperature falls below 35° F. Ice water was first employed with a circulating water pump. Under the coils a metal trough catches the condensed water. At the opposite side of the chamber a hot-water or steam radiator is placed and to it is connected a thermostatic control valve, which regulates the room temperature. A panel is placed in front of the brine pipes so that the patient is not aware of any apparatus in the room. Indirect lighting may be used with a suitable glass shield at the upper extremity of one wall for a width of one foot for the entire length of the room. An alternative procedure is to put a glass window in a dropped ceiling with the lighting fixtures outside. All electrical connections should be arranged in such a way that electrical contact is made outside of the room in order to avoid any sparks in the oxygen-enriched atmosphere. This is done by transmitting the mechanical pull of a light cord through a gas-tight piston imbedded in the wall or ceiling, the outside end of which is connected by cord or rod to the switch of the electrical fixture. The patient may pull on a string above the bed which will produce an appropriate signal, both a light and a bell, at the nurse's desk, but in each instance the electrical contact is made in the space above the dropped ceiling of the oxygen room.

The oxygen-enriched atmosphere in contact with the brine pipes is deprived of its moisture and passes downward behind the panel across

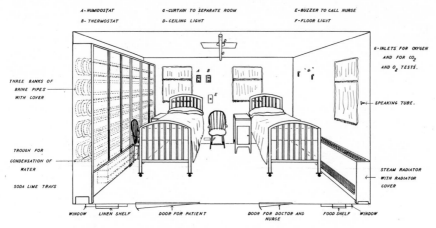

FIG. 36.   Oxygen room with thermal circulation.

the room to the other side where heating of the atmosphere takes place by means of the radiator, resulting in an upward movement of the oxygen-air mixture to the ceiling and thence across the top of the room to enter the space behind the panel. In this way a range of temperature of between 50° and 90° F. may be obtained simply by setting the thermostatic regulator to the temperature desired. The relative humidity is generally in a low range between 35 and 40 per cent.

Oxygen is admitted from the adjoining room through a silencer so that even during the raising of the concentration to 60 per cent the rush of oxygen from the cylinders is not disturbing. The actual operation of the chamber is noiseless. A concentration of 50 per cent oxygen is maintained by admitting oxygen from a cylinder manifold. One bank of tanks is in use at a time, adjusted at a pressure of 50 pounds. When the pressure falls below 50 pounds the oxygen from the other bank is automatically admitted into the chamber at a liter flow which is pre-set at 12 to 15 liters per minute. No special apparatus for absorbing carbon dioxide is necessary since a flow of 15 to

20 liters into the room washes out the carbon dioxide given off by the patient and nurse. The cost of four to five cylinders to a hospital which uses much oxygen is generally not greater than eight to ten dollars a day, which is the total expense of providing both the oxygen-enriched atmosphere and elimination of carbon dioxide. If brine is present in the hospital there is no additional cost from this source. If the hospital is not near a producing plant, the cost of oxygen is higher than that mentioned above.

Special precautions must be observed in order that no sparks or source of flame be admitted into the room. As mentioned in connection with oxygen-tent therapy, electric pads should not be employed. All matches and cigarette lighters are removed from visitors before entrance. Spark-proof flashlights are employed, such as are used in mine operations. When blood cultures are performed the alcohol lamp is taken off the tray. Sparks which may be produced sometimes by the hand passing over a woolen blanket have never resulted in ignition. In 18 years' experience with this type of chamber at the Presbyterian Hospital, New York, no fire of any kind has ever been encountered.

The Portable Oxygen Chamber. The portable oxygen chamber may be visualized as an extension of a large tent; it is less expensive to build and install, and may be used both in hospitals and private residences. A convenient size is 10 feet long, 9 feet wide, and 8 feet high, although this may be varied as desired. An angle-iron framework supports a rubberized fabric or, in later models, a transparent plastocele covering. As is seen in Fig. 35, the walls may be made almost entirely of transparent material. A leak-tight door is made out of an angle-iron frame the body of which may be made out of rubberized fabric or transparent plastic material. Outside the chamber a large metal refrigerating tank capable of holding 300 pounds of ice and fitted with a four-inch opening at the top and at the bottom constitutes the mechanism for cooling and dehumidifying the atmosphere. Drain water from the melting ice leaves a tap attached to the bottom of the tank. A silent motor-blower unit capable of circulating 400 cubic feet of air per minute is placed on a small movable truck along with the refrigerating tank. A small thermostatically controlled radiator may be added to maintain a constant temperature, although this has been dispensed with in practice to conserve ice. The temperature within the chamber may be lowered 10 degrees below the outside temperature when the motor-blower unit is operating at full speed. If additional cooling is desired, salt may be added to the ice. Four cylinders of high-pressure oxygen per day are adequate both to provide a concentration of 50 per cent oxygen and to wash out the carbon dioxide produced by the patient.

THE POSITIVE-PRESSURE HELMET APPARATUS

This is also called the helium-oxygen hood. The apparatus is designed essentially for the administration of positive pressure either with a helium-oxygen mixture or with 100 per cent oxygen. It consists of a conditioning cabinet and a hood with a removable rubber collar that makes contact at the neck. The conditioning cabinet contains two cans for chemical absorption of carbon dioxide, a motor-blower unit, a motor switch, and a pilot light. A rheostat is present for varying the velocity of the atmosphere passing through the conditioning cabinet. The hood is attached to the conditioning cabinet by means of two lengths of one-inch rubber tubing. At the top of the hood is an outlet to which is attached a rubber hose that leads to a water bottle which constitutes the pressure control valve. The length to which the glass tubing at the end of the rubber hose is inserted into the water bottle determines the pressure existing within the helmet. If the glass tube is 4 cm. below the surface of the water, the atmosphere will bubble off at this pressure and not be present within the hood at a higher pressure. If 100 per cent oxygen is employed, the regulator of the oxygen cylinder is connected to the hood by appropriate rubber tubing. If helium is to be used a tank of 80 per cent helium-20 per cent oxygen is placed alongside a cylinder of pure oxygen and the two connected through a Y-tube to the inlet petcock on the hood.[1]

Directions for Use. The two carbon-dioxide absorbing cans are filled with baralime. This chemical is selected because it absorbs carbon dioxide in a cold atmosphere and does not remove excessive amounts of moisture. If a dry atmosphere is desired shell natron is used. However, in most cases of asthma and tracheobronchitis a relative humidity of 50 to 70 per cent is preferred to one of 35 to 40 per cent. Under these circumstances baralime is preferred. After the baralime has been placed in the carbon-dioxide absorbers, the lids are

[1] Pure helium should not be employed since asphyxia would result if the oxygen supply ran out. Cylinders of helium mixed with oxygen are therefore universally necessary, such as 80 per cent helium, 20 per cent oxygen.

screwed down tightly and placed in the ice compartment, clamping them securely so that they will not float. The ice compartment is then filled with cracked ice and sufficient water to keep the cans completely submerged. The hood is then attached to the conditioning cabinet by means of the one-inch tubing. The collar is adjusted to the hood so that the neck opening is nearest the bottom of the collar

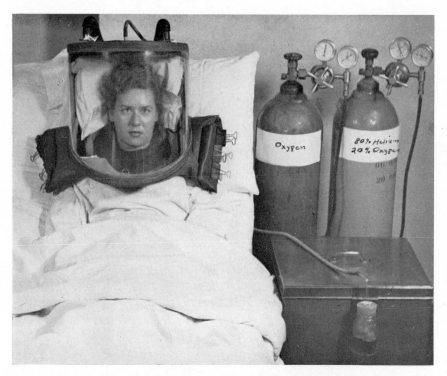

FIG. 37.   Positive-pressure helmet apparatus.

ring. The collar is firmly attached to the ring by means of heavy rubber bands. Before placing the hood over the patient's head, the motor switch should be snapped to the "on" position and the rheostat adjusted to the midposition. The pilot light on the switch panel of the conditioning cabinet will glow while the motor is in operation.

A small pillow is placed in the hood before it is adjusted over the patient's head and neck. It is then tied to the bed with straps provided for this purpose. One sleeve of the hood is open and oxygen is admitted into the hood with a needle valve or a flush valve to wash out all air in the hood, conditioning cabinet, and connections. Approximately 500 liters of oxygen, i.e., 150 pounds' pressure, will result in 100 per cent oxygen in the hood. If this is the gas to be administered the sleeve may be closed and the oxygen flow lowered to 2 or 3 liters per minute. If a helium-oxygen mixture is desired a similar quantity of the helium-oxygen mixture may be admitted in this way, or, as is more common and economical, the hood is first flushed with pure oxygen and then a flow of 15 liters per minute of the helium-oxygen mixture is admitted for 20 minutes, which will generally provide a concentration of 20 per cent oxygen and 80 per cent helium within the hood. In most cases a somewhat higher oxygen concentration, from 25 to 35 per cent, is desired in helium-oxygen therapy, since anoxia is present if there is involvement of the lungs. It is only in localized tracheal or laryngeal obstruction in adults in which a mixture of 20 per cent oxygen and 80 per cent helium is employed.

A higher concentration of oxygen in the hood atmosphere is obtained by running 1 to 2 liters of oxygen with a flow of 3 to 5 liters of the helium-oxygen mixture from the standard regulator. (The flow of an 80 per cent helium–20 per cent oxygen mixture is actually 1.7 times that registered on the oxygen dial gauge, due to its swifter rate of effusion, as described in the chapters on its clinical use.) If the hood is carefully supervised a flow of 2.5 liters of the helium-oxygen mixture and 1 liter of oxygen will provide a concentration of approximately 30 per cent oxygen and 70 per cent helium. The inlet of 1 liter of oxygen will take care of the oxygen consumption of the patient, between 300 and 400 cc. per minute, and in addition increase slightly the concentration of the combined mixture. When the helium-oxygen concentration is obtained, the sleeve of the hood is closed by appropriate clamps and the pressure-control water valve is submerged to a depth equal to a pressure desired; namely, from 2 to 6 cm. of water. The rheostat position may be varied depending upon whether a cool or warmer atmosphere is used. In the helmet apparatus, in which only the head is enclosed, a cooler temperature is generally preferred.

One can of the carbon-dioxide absorbent is generally changed after 12 to 16 hours of continuous or total service. It is unnecessary to interrupt the treatment to carry out this procedure; by clamping with large clamps the rubber connection to and from a single can, it may be removed without causing any leaks in the circuit. After the can has been filled with baralime the rubber tubing should be connected to the arms of the cans before removing the clamps. The ice cabinet should be filled with ice at six-hour intervals. Sufficient water is run off to make room for the added ice, but at all times the absorbent cans should be submerged under the ice water, and, therefore, leak-tight.

If the pressure-control valve is not bubbling on expiration, a leak is present and should be searched for around the collar or at the can lids. If the hood sleeve is opened for any reason the flow of either oxygen or the helium-oxygen mixture is increased to 10 liters per minute during this period. If the oxygen or helium-oxygen mixture is first set at 10 liters per minute before the sleeve is opened, it is generally not necessary to flush the apparatus afterwards since a positive pressure within the helmet will force leakage of gas outward and prevent an inward leak. The concentration of oxygen and carbon dioxide should be tested within the hood one-half hour after the treatment has been initiated to determine that the atmosphere breathed by the patient is that prescribed by the physician. In most instances helium-oxygen therapy is carried out for periods of two hours and a test may be made at the end of this time. When continuous administration of either 100 per cent oxygen or the helium-oxygen mixture is employed the testing of the contained atmosphere should be performed at least three times during the 24 hours.

When the apparatus is used at a flow of 2 to 3 liters from a cylinder containing 20 per cent oxygen and 80 per cent helium, the concentration of oxygen may be from 2 to 5 per cent lower than the tank mixture because of the oxygen consumed by the patient. For this reason it is always desirable to have an oxygen tank connected with the helium-oxygen cylinder through a Y-tube and a flow of at least one-half a liter of oxygen per minute, preferably 1 liter per minute, admitted together with a flow of 2 to 3 liters of the helium-oxygen mixture.[2] When 100 per cent oxygen is employed a total flow of 5 to 7 liters per minute is useful in retaining a continuous pressure in the hood and also washing out carbon dioxide, thus extending the period of usefulness of the carbon-dioxide absorber, but smaller flows of 2 to 3 liters per minute are permitted if the pressure in the hood is maintained.

In the management of obstructive dyspnea high pressures may be required to overcome urgent inspiratory difficulty in breathing. In most instances, however, pressures of 4 to 5 cm. of water are adequate. As the clinical condition of the patient improves the pressure may be gradually lowered by raising the glass tube to a depth of 1 or 2 cm.

---

[2] A cylinder of 25 per cent oxygen and 75 per cent helium may also be employed.

of water.   In edema of the lungs, pressures such as 3 to 4 cm. of water are usually adequate to cause clearing of râles.   When the lungs have become clear the pressure is gradually lowered 1 cm. of water at intervals of two to four hours, depending upon the condition of the patient.   It may be remarked here, as emphasized in the clinical section, that the systolic pressure should be observed, especially in cases of peripheral circulatory failure or shock, and the pressure should not be employed if a fall of systolic pressure greater than 10 to 15 mm. Hg takes place after application of the hood.   Under these circumstances a smaller pressure such as 1 to 2 cm. of water may be found useful without causing a decrease in the return of the flow of blood into the right heart.

In patients with congestive heart failure the decrease in the return of blood into the cardiac circulation is not a disadvantage since the heart is able to work more effectively on a smaller volume of blood. In patients with paroxysmal cardiac dyspnea, the length of treatment may be brief, as the condition may clear after 5 to 10 minutes of treatment.   It should be remembered that the pulmonary capillaries filter serum through their walls into the alveolar spaces, depending upon the permeability of the vessel wall and the internal capillary pressure.   The pressure in the pulmonary capillaries is undoubtedly small, and even if high positive pressures may not be administered except at the cost of a fall in systolic blood pressure, a therapeutic result may nevertheless be achieved with as little as 1 cm. of water pressure applied to the outside of the capillary wall.   In cases of obstructive dyspnea, relatively higher pressures, such as 6 cm. of water, may be safely used since the intrapleural and intrapulmonary negative pressures at the height of inspiration are excessively elevated and the provision of a positive pressure forcing air inward to the respiratory passageway lowers the pathologically elevated negative pressure during inspiration.

OXYGEN FACE TENTS AND LOOSE-FITTING MASKS

Loose-fitting oxygen masks or so-called face tents were introduced by Campbell and later employed by Barach, Taylor, and Lombard. In general they consist of plastocele or cardboard coverings which may be molded over the bridge of the nose to include the mouth and nasal openings.   In the accompanying illustrations, a light plastocele loose-fitting mask is illustrated; it is attached to the face by an elastic band or by earpieces. Oxygen is admitted through a rubber tubing that is placed horizontally on the upper part of the mask. When 6 liters per minute of oxygen is admitted into the face tent a concentration of approximately 40 per cent oxygen is generally present in the inspired air and 8 liters per minute will provide a 50 per cent oxygen percentage in the inspired air. Flows of less than 6 liters per minute will result in accumulation of carbon dioxide in concentrations higher than is generally desired; namely, 1.5 per cent. It is therefore useful to employ an injector attached to the regulator, such as the one used in the Meter-mask apparatus. Under these circumstances a flow of 5 liters

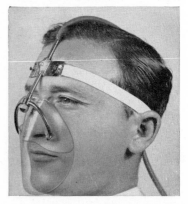

FIG. 38.   Face tent, Lombard inhaler.

per minute of oxygen, with the meter set at 50 per cent, will result in a high total flow of an air-oxygen mixture sufficient to wash out carbon dioxide given off in the expired air and to provide a sensation of air movement that is refreshing.

In some patients the face tent is found more comfortable than is a tight-fitting rubber mask. Although it is not so efficient as masks which contain either a collecting bag or rebreathing bag for oxygen, the device is inexpensive and useful in the treatment of many types of anoxemic dyspnea. A flow of oxygen of less than 6 liters per minute should not be used unless an injector is also employed.

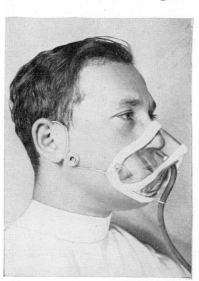

FIG. 39.   Plastocele face tent.

In the Lombard inhaler a plastocele covering encloses the nose and mouth and is attached to the forehead by a metal inhaler through which the oxygen enters into the mask. The concentration of oxygen obtained in this apparatus is approximately similar to that in the face tent described above. Higher total flows of an air-oxygen mixture provided by an injector attached to the regulator will furnish 50 to 60 per cent oxygen and promptly wash out the exhaled atmosphere, as described above. At low oxygen flows the sensation of hot moist air being reflected back from the inner surface of the inhaler to the face is apt to promote discomfort.

OXYGEN-MASK APPARATUS

Oxygen masks may be used for administration of any concentration of oxygen from 40 to 100 per cent, but they are especially effective in providing the very high oxygen concentrations, such as from 70 to 100 per cent, which are difficult to obtain with other methods. In recent years it has been demonstrated that pure oxygen is not irritating to human pulmonary epithelium when administered by a mask for as much as two days and probably for four days as well. Since the mask is removed from time to time in order to wash the face, give nourishment, and for other reasons, the exceptional tolerance of patients for 100 per cent oxygen may perhaps be explained by the fact that oxygen-mask therapy is to some extent interrupted. At any rate, it may be pointed out here that previous warnings against the danger of pulmonary edema on inhalation of these very high oxygen atmospheres were based on experiments in animals that were kept in leak-tight chambers continuously for three to five days. Satisfactory clinical evidence has been obtained from a number of hospitals which indicates that oxygen may be inhaled from a mask in concentrations of 70 to 100 per cent from two to four days without evident damage to the lung. This is of considerable importance since the large increase in physically dissolved oxygen is often of crucial value in shock, hemorrhage, and cardiorespiratory failure. Two types of oxygen-mask apparatus are considered both comfortable and effective in providing high oxygen concentrations: (1) The B.L.B. apparatus devised by Boothby, Lovelace, and Bulbulian, and (2) the Meter mask devised by Barach and Eckman.

There are two essential differences in these masks which should be recognized in order to carry out skillful oxygen-mask therapy; one is concerned with carbon-dioxide accumulation and the other with resistance in the mask.

The B.L.B. Mask. In the B.L.B. mask a well-fitting rubber nasal or oral-nasal mask is attached to the face and a small bag is suspended from it in which a moderate amount of rebreathing takes place. Two sponge-rubber disks on each side of the mask serve as inspiratory and expiratory valves. During inspiration at low oxygen flows, such as from 2 to 4 liters per minute, the gas in the bag is first inspired and after the bag is collapsed air is drawn through the sponge-rubber disk to complete the tidal volume. The air that is first inhaled consists of the first part of the previous expiration and contains a lower percentage of carbon dioxide than that which is expired at the end of expiration. During expiration the rebreathing bag is filled with the first portion of exhaled air and the remainder then passes through the sponge-rubber disks. The resistance imposed by the sponge-rubber disks serves, therefore, as a combination inspiratory and expiratory valve. The oxygen concentration in the inspired air is approximately estimated by the liter flow from the tank. Thus, in a large adult without dyspnea 4 liters per minute may provide 50 per cent oxygen, 5 liters per minute 65 per cent oxygen, 8 liters 95 per cent oxygen. For oxygen concentrations of 95 to 100 per cent the liter flow should be adjusted to a sufficiently high rate so that the rebreathing bag does not generally collapse at the end of inspiration. Obviously, the full collapse of the rebreathing bag will necessitate the drawing of air through the sponge-rubber disk. The administration of 100 per cent oxygen depends on the volume of breathing; in an individual who is breathing at 12 to 15 liters per minute, the liter flow in order to provide the highest oxygen concentration should be at least 10 to 12 liters per minute. In the administration of moderate concentrations of oxygen, such as 50 per cent, 4 liters would not be sufficient if the

TABLE VIII

Oxygen Concentrations with B.L.B. Mask at Various Liter Flows

Liters Per Minute	Small Person (Per Cent)	Medium-sized Person (Per Cent)	Large Person (Per Cent)
3	45–60	40–55	35–50
4	60–75	55–70	50–65
5	75–90	70–80	65–75
6	90–100	80–90	75–85
7		90–100	85–92
8			92–100

respiratory volume was elevated. A high minute volume of respiration would dilute the 4 liters to such an extent as to lower the oxygen concentration of the inspired air considerably. Conversely, in a small child a low pulmonary ventilation would give a correspondingly higher oxygen concentration at a liter flow of 4 liters per minute. The con-

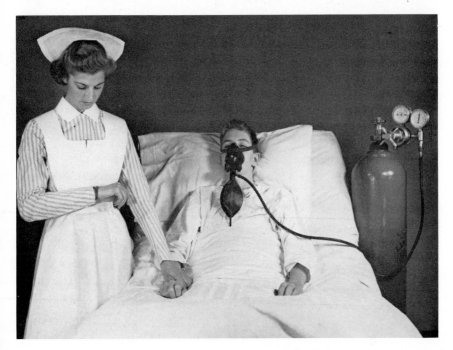

FIG. 40. B.L.B. mask, oronasal type.

centrations given in the table are higher than would be found in dyspneic subjects, as explained above.

The carbon-dioxide concentration in the inspired air is definitely elevated at low oxygen flows, such as 3 or 4 liters per minute, generally reported to be between 2.0 and 2.5 per cent. When 2 per cent carbon dioxide is inspired the breathing is stimulated between 40 to 50 per cent above the range existing prior to inhalation of this concentration of carbon dioxide. In most cases of cardiorespiratory illness this augmentation of breathing increases the dyspnea. Low flows of oxygen should not therefore be employed in this mask unless stimulation of the respiratory center with 2 per cent carbon dioxide is desired. A liter flow from the regulator above 6 liters per minute will result in an adequate washing out of carbon dioxide from the mask in most cases.

Resistance in this mask is also present when *low* oxygen flows are used, due to the necessity of inhaling through the sponge-rubber disks when the oxygen mixture in the bag has been exhausted. The resistance during expiration is not considered harmful; this has been fully discussed in the section on the pathologic physiology of obstructive dyspnea. However, the resistance during inspiration is of considerable importance as the patient is required to suck the additional component of air through the inspiratory valves, which consist of sponge-rubber disks. In quiet breathing the negative pressure which builds up in the mask at the end of inspiration is of small degree and of little significance.

However, in patients with dyspnea or in normal human beings whose ventilation is increased by exercise, exposure to negative pressure of 1 to 2 cm. of water during inspiration exerts a suction action on the pulmonary epithelium and from a physiologic point of view would increase the tendency of serum to ooze out of the pulmonary capillaries. Breathing against a negative pressure during inspiration has consistently produced edema of the lungs in animals and therefore inspiratory resistance should be avoided, especially in patients with obstructive dyspnea, pneumonia, heart failure, and in any patient in whom a tendency toward edema of the lungs might develop. This includes the large range of cardiorespiratory dyspnea and is an indication that *low flows of oxygen* should not be employed with this mask. It is therefore recommended that the regulator should be set at 6 to 8 liters per minute even when moderate concentrations of oxygen such as 40 to 50 per cent are prescribed. It is true that if the mask is fitted to the face loosely so that leakage may occur, the negative pressure within the mask will not develop during inspiration. Even though this amounts to leakage of air inward during inspiration, thus diluting the oxygen mixture, it is far preferable to arrange the mask on the face so that leakage of air takes place rather than to have a tight-fitting mask when a liter flow of 3, 4, or even 5 liters per minute of oxygen is employed. These comments are restricted to the operation of the clinical B.L.B. nasal or oronasal mask, since the type designed for aviators will not be discussed.

Two sizes of the B.L.B. mask are available; it may be employed in the oronasal mask form which surrounds the nose and mouth or in the nasal type which encloses the nose only. If high concentrations such as 95 to 100 per cent are prescribed, the oronasal type is indicated; otherwise the preference of the patient may be allowed to make the decision between the nasal or oronasal mask. The oronasal mask is more reliable in providing a high or moderate oxygen concentration. A plug in the bottom of the mask can be removed for insertion of the Miller-Abbott or Wangensteen tube. In summary, the B.L.B. mask is an effective and comfortable method of administering high concentrations of oxygen. Its use as a tight-fitting mask with low liter flows such as 3, 4, and 5 liters per minute is accompanied by undesirable negative pressures during inspiration in patients with dyspnea, or in exercising adults. If low flows are necessary for the sake of economy, the B.L.B. mask should be fitted sufficiently loosely to permit a definite leak so that patients are not required to breathe through the sponge-rubber disks. This leakage should not be at the top of the mask, for the air will then blow into the patient's eyes and become irritating, but at the bottom, and may be obtained by placing absorbent cotton over the chin.

The Meter Mask. In this mask no rebreathing is permitted except that which inevitably takes place in the small volume of the mask itself. However, the percentage of carbon dioxide in the inspired air does not arise above 0.2 per cent even with low flows of 2 liters per minute. This is made possible by a delicate disk inspiratory valve placed at the bottom of the mask which prevents the exhaled atmosphere from entering the large light latex bag which serves to collect oxygen during expiration and offer it to the patient during inspiration. The latex bag acts as a reservoir, collecting inflowing oxygen during expiration. A light rubber flutter expiratory valve, placed in front of the mask for exit of the exhaled atmosphere, operates under a minimal resistance.

An injector is attached to the regulator which consists of a leak-tight metal device from which oxygen passes into the rubber hose connection to the mask. As the oxygen stream passes through the injector it creates a negative pressure which draws in a varying amount of outside air or no outside air, depending upon whether the injector is open to the atmosphere by one of a series of orifices which gradually increase in diameter. When all orifices are closed the mask provides 100 per cent oxygen. When the largest aperture is opened there is sufficient introduction of air into the injector to create an oxygen concentration of 40 per cent. Calibration of these varying-sized orifices makes possible the instantaneous provision of an oxygen concentration from 40 to 100 per cent with an error of not greater than ±3 per cent. This constancy of the oxygen percentage in the atmosphere inspired by the patient is maintained regardless of the size of the patient or the volume of ventilation, provided that the oxygen flow is sufficient to prevent the collecting bag from completely collapsing at the end of inspiration. If 100 per cent oxygen is desired the liter flow from the regulator will correspond to the volume of breathing of the patient, such as 10, 12, or 15 liters per minute.[3]

A concentration of 40 per cent oxygen may frequently be obtained with a liter flow of 2, 3, or 4 per minute if the volume of breathing is not excessive. When 2.4 liters per minute pass through the injector with the orifice set at 40 per cent, 7.2 liters of air are drawn into the oxygen stream and the patient is thus offered 9.6 liters per minute of a 40 per cent oxygen mixture in the collecting bag, which opens during inspiration with a minimal resistance. However, when a flow of 2 liters per minute enters the B.L.B. mask, it is inhaled by the patient

TABLE IX

Oxygen Concentrations with the Meter Mask

Oxygen Flow: Liters Per Min.	Total Intake Oxygen and Air: Liters Per Min.	Oxygen % at Dial	Oxygen % by Test	CO_2 % by Test
8.4	8.4	95+	97.5	0.2
7.2	8.2	90	89.5	0.15
6.0	8.0	80	78.0	0.25
5.1	8.2	70	68.0	0.2
4.3	8.6	60	58.0	0.2
3.4	9.1	50	51.0	0.2
2.8	8.9	45	45.0	0.2
2.4	9.6	40	40.5	0.15

[3] When the Meter mask is used for helium-oxygen therapy, a flow of 8 to 10 liters per minute of the helium-oxygen mixture will wash out the exhaled carbon dioxide; it is, therefore, suggested that the inspiratory disk be removed to eliminate even the minimal pressure required to open this valve when patients with asthma or obstructive dyspnea are being treated. A cylinder of 25 per cent oxygen and 75 per cent helium is more convenient than the 80 per cent helium-20 per cent oxygen mixture, since the latter requires an additional oxygen cylinder to administer 0.5 to 1.0 liter per minute of oxygen, i.e., to take care of the patient's oxygen consumption and raise slightly the oxygen concentration of the inspired atmosphere.

together with the residual expired air in the rebreathing bag and when the bag is collapsed the additional quantity of air required by the pulmonary ventilation of the patient is obtained by a negative pressure which pulls air through the sponge-rubber disks.

In the management of the injector Meter mask the flow of oxygen from the regulator is determined by observation of the collecting bag.

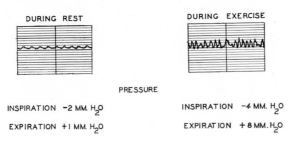

FIG. 41. Resistance during rest and dyspnea with minimal oxygen flows with Meter mask.

If it is collapsed at the end of inspiration a higher flow is employed. It is important to observe the operation of the mask for a minute or two since in many instances the pulmonary ventilation is higher than that which obtains after the patient has breathed an oxygen-enriched atmosphere for several minutes. An emergency inlet valve is present

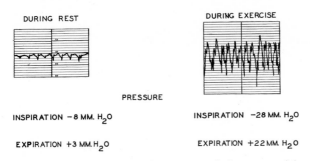

FIG. 42. Resistance during rest and dyspnea with minimal oxygen flows with B.L.B. clinical mask.

in order to provide additional air if the collecting bag is inadvertently collapsed. This has recently been made of light rubber, serving as an inspiratory flutter valve. If two are placed in the oronasal mask, the apparatus can operate comfortably with oxygen flows as low as 1 liter per minute, although the flow will not yield a concentration much above 30 per cent in the inspired air. Furthermore, if there is a desire to dispense with the injector, which offers instantaneous and accurate provision of the oxygen concentration desired at low resistance, the oronasal mask with two inspiratory flutter valves may be employed with less resistance than that found in other masks. The accompanying charts reveal the lessened resistance of breathing in the Meter mask with the accessory flutter valves, even without the injector, as compared to the B.L.B. clinical oronasal mask under conditions of low flows of oxygen and exercise dyspnea. In addition, the accessory inspiratory and the expiratory flutter valves are interchangeable and may easily be removed.

The nasal mask is also equipped with a new rubber flutter emergency inspiratory valve in the metal tube that houses the inspiratory valve in front of the collecting bag and may be employed without the injector if it is desired. However, it is believed that the injector is of unquestionable value to both patient and physician when low or moderate oxygen flows are used, since it does decrease the necessity for mixing air with the oxygen stream at the cost of the patient's own effort and since it supplies a continuous oxygen concentration which is within 3 per cent of that prescribed for him. Care should be taken in the operation of the injector that the tube leading to the mask is not kinked since therefore the oxygen which would otherwise be admitted through it would leave through an intake vent in the injector. The application of positive pressure can be made with any concentration between 40 and 100 per cent oxygen, since the orifices through which air enters are protected from excessive back pressure by the inspiratory valve, as will be discussed in the next section.

Although these newer types of oxygen masks are comfortable for a large number of patients, they become objectionable to a good many others on continuous use. When discomfort is manifested by the patient a shift should be made to the oxygen tent if it is feasible, or, if not, to the oxygen catheter inserted into the nasal pharynx for relatively low concentration or into the oral pharynx for high concentrations in the inspired air. Comfort may be increased if the mask is removed from time to time and the patient's face washed, dried, and powdered. The rubber parts of the mask should be washed with soap and water and boiled for five minutes after using, preferably wrapping in a double thickness of gauze before boiling. Metal parts should not be boiled but washed with soap and water and then allowed to dry. In a patient who is thought to be infectious the steel or plastic parts may be sterilized by a suitable antiseptic solution. The equipment should be dried and then packed away neatly. The sponge-rubber disk should be thoroughly dried.

The Oxygen-injector Mask Metered for Positive Pressure. This mask is designed solely for the treatment of pulmonary edema due to cardiorespiratory illness or gas poisoning. It should be em-

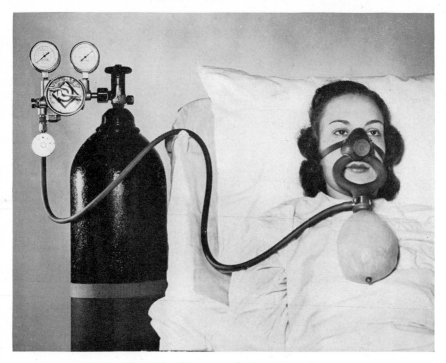

FIG. 43. Meter mask (nasal type).

ployed cautiously in patients with shock according to the instructions given previously.

The injector mask has been equipped with a metal disk that surrounds the expiratory flutter valve and contains on its surface five orifices of varying diameters. Expiration proceeds naturally without pressure when the largest orifice is employed. When the disk is turned to progressively smaller orifices the patient exhales under a positive pressure which is 1, 2, 3, or 4 cm. of water depending upon the size of the orifice. These pressures have been recorded during quiet breathing, and would be higher in dyspneic patients. It will be found that expiration at a pressure of 4 cm. of water is uncomfortable and can be used for short periods only. However, a swifter clearance of pulmonary edema, especially in chlorine and nitric-acid gas poisoning, may be obtained when the higher pressures are used for short periods. In pulmonary edema taking place during the course of clinical illness, 3 cm. of water may be adequate to result in a disappearance of the signs of moisture in the lungs and a smaller pressure of 1 to 2 cm. of water may then be used for periods of one to three

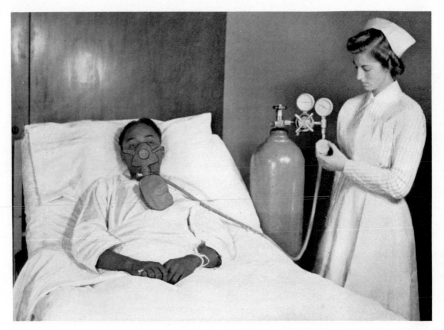

FIG. 44.   Meter mask (oronasal type).

hours as may be required. Return of signs of moisture in the lungs indicates re-application of positive-pressure breathing.

In order to employ 100 per cent oxygen a high liter flow such as 12 to 15 liters per minute is necessary to prevent collapse of the collecting bag. Under these circumstances it is desirable for the injector to be one-third full of water so that the oxygen may pick up some moisture as it passes through. Test of the relative humidity of 100 per cent oxygen passing over the water surface in the injector has shown a relative humidity of 20 per cent of the air entering the mask. However, it has also been demonstrated that additional moisture is contributed to the inspired air because the inner surface of the mask is itself wet with moisture which has condensed on it from the expired air and the actual relative humidity of air entering the mask under these circumstances is 40 per cent. If a higher relative humidity is desired during the inhalation of 100 per cent oxygen, either with or without positive pressure, the injector may be removed and a water bottle attached to the regulator. The oxygen then passes through 2 or 3 inches of water and possesses a higher relative humidity.

The patient may be treated with 50 or 60 per cent oxygen, and the positive pressure desired, by setting the injector and pressure dials at

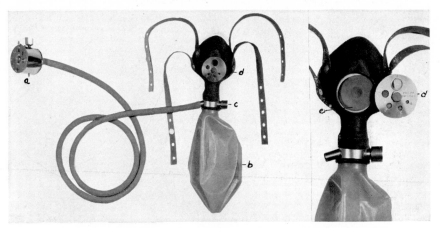

Fig. 45. Meter mask (oronasal, positive-pressure type).

    a. Oxygen concentration meter.
    b. Collecting bag.
    c. Accessory inlet valve.
    d. Disk metered for positive pressure.
    e. Expiratory flutter valve.

the appropriate orifices. This results in considerable saving of oxygen and is a therapeutically effective, efficient, and practical procedure. Although a swifter clearance of edema of the lungs may be obtained by expiration at high pressures, it is frequently desirable to employ lower pressures, such as 2 to 3 cm. of water, even though a longer time is necessary for complete clearance of the signs of edema. This is in part because of lessened discomfort to the patient but also because low pressures do not significantly retard the entrance of blood into the right heart. In patients with cardiac illness, such as congestive heart failure, the retardation of blood is comparable to tourniquetting the extremity and facilitates the recovery of the heart muscle by making it possible for the heart to work on a smaller volume of blood.

However, in patients with peripheral circulatory failure, pressures of 1 cm. of water may be employed in the attempt to eliminate pulmonary edema without causing any significant decrease in return of blood from the right heart. As mentioned previously, the systolic blood pressure should be carefully recorded at 10-minute intervals in all patients with shock. When pulmonary edema has cleared the patient may breathe 60 to 100 per cent oxygen without pressure. If no recurrence of edema takes place and the patient is clinically better, the injector may be turned to 50 per cent oxygen and then to 40 per cent and the mask may be finally removed when the clinical condition of the patient indicates that he is out of danger. If pulmonary edema recurs after termination of positive pressure, the pressure should be applied again at 3 cm. of water and then gradually lowered at longer intervals.

THE ADMINISTRATION OF 5 TO 10 PER CENT CARBON DIOXIDE WITH OXYGEN

The administration of 5 to 10 per cent carbon dioxide with the remainder oxygen is indicated primarily in carbon-monoxide poisoning and other forms of accidental asphyxia, and in the treatment of hiccough and postoperative atelectasis. In carbon-monoxide poisoning the H.H. inhalator is commonly employed by rescue squads. In hospital and private practice the Meter mask or the B.L.B. mask or an anesthesia mask may be used with a tank of 90 per cent oxygen and 10 per cent carbon dioxide. The inhalation of high carbon-dioxide concentrations is continued until the specific objective is attained. In carbon-monoxide poisoning the inhalation of 93 per cent oxygen and 7 per cent carbon dioxide may have to be continued for 15 or 20 minutes before normal breathing is established.

The employment of carbon dioxide and oxygen in the treatment of hiccough is of greater importance than is commonly recognized. In a few cases 10 to 15 per cent carbon dioxide with the remainder oxygen may be required in order to terminate a persistent spasm. If the patient inhales these high mixtures for one and a half to two minutes, consciousness may become clouded and at that time the hiccough will cease. Even exceedingly severe cases of hiccough have been terminated if sufficiently high concentrations of carbon dioxide have been given. Although toxic symptoms may be produced by prolonged administration of carbon dioxide, the severity of the hiccough syndrome is such as to indicate the inhalation of carbon dioxide even if moderate symptoms of carbon-dioxide toxicity do take place. In any event, even if a convulsion should be produced by carbon dioxide, there will probably be no harm done since repeated convulsions have been used in the treatment of dementia praecox. Convulsions do not take place until consciousness is first lost, and need not worry the physician carrying out this therapy for intractable hiccough.

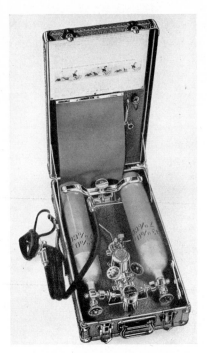

FIG. 46.   H.H. inhalator.

The use of carbon dioxide and oxygen in postoperative atelectasis is generally for the purpose of expanding the lung and freeing the mucus from the sides of the bronchial wall as well as to promote coughing and to expel these secretions. Inhalations of carbon-dioxide–oxygen mixtures for two to three minutes may be adequate. An anesthesia mask is commonly used for this purpose.

THE ADMINISTRATION OF THE NEBULIZED SOLUTIONS OF THERAPEUTIC DRUGS

It has been found convenient to use a nebulizer with a hand bulb to vaporize 1 : 100 epinephrine in the treatment of asthma, and 1 per

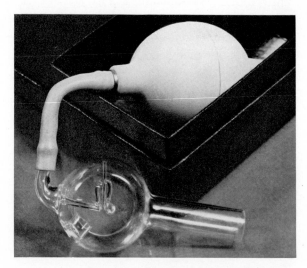

FIG. 47. Glass nebulizer.

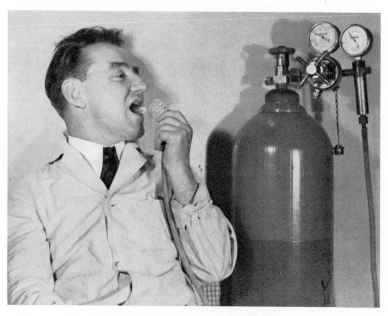

FIG. 48. Glass nebulizer, in use.

cent neosynephrin in pulmonary emphysema. Since it has been shown that additional therapeutic effects may be obtained by inhaling larger amounts of these solutions than can be vaporized with a hand bulb, a tube from an oxygen tank is connected to the small glass outlet instead of the hand nebulizer, and the regulator turned to 5 liters per

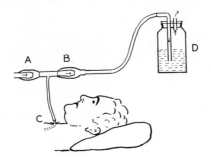

A-INSPIRATORY VALVE   C-TRACHEOTOMY TUBE

B-EXPIRATORY VALVE   D-PRESSURE BOTTLE

Fig. 49. The tracheotomy positive-pressure apparatus. The application of positive pressure after tracheotomy, to prevent oozing of mucus from the intrathoracic bronchioles and serum from the pulmonary capillaries, requires a tracheotomy tube with an extension beyond the surface of the larynx. To this is connected a T-tube by which the patient may inhale through an inspiratory valve and exhale through the expiratory flutter valve, the latter connected to a tube submerged in water to the depth desired, generally 4 to 5 cm. Another apparatus is that which maintains a positive pressure during inspiration and expiration by means of a motor-blower unit (Pilling & Sons, Philadelphia, Pa.).

minute, to accomplish continuous vaporization of the solutions used. In the treatment of pulmonary edema and obstructive lesions in the larynx and trachea, in tracheobronchitis and in other conditions in which shrinking of the mucous membrane in the respiratory passage-way is indicated, 1 to 2 cc. of 1 per cent neosynephrin may be inserted into a glass nebulizer and the solution inhaled through the mouth over a period of 10 to 15 minutes.

Other solutions may be nebulized and employed for therapeutic purposes at intervals of two to three hours, such as a 25 per cent solution of promin, and also 2.5 per cent sulfadiazine in an ethanolamine solution. One to 2 cc. of these solutions may be inhaled at intervals prescribed by the physician for a local application of these chemicals to the bronchi and alveoli.

After the nebulizer has been used it is better to rinse it with hot water to prevent clogging. When epinephrine or neosynephrin is used, it may be desirable to use a warm mouth wash and gargle after the spray in order to prevent drying of the throat.

Various types of nebulizers are employed which vary in their effectiveness. The glass hand-made nebulizer appears to be superior to others although the plastic variety is less apt to break.[4]

---

[4] The glass nebulizers are made by the Vaponefrin Company, Parke Davis, DeVilbiss and other concerns; the plastic model is manufactured by Stearns Co. In the Vaponefrin nebulizer the nebulin is directed against a glass target before passing into the outer atmosphere. This results in the larger droplets being precipitated within the nebulizer, and, therefore, less apt to lodge in the mucous membrane of the pharynx.

35

Care of Inhalational-therapy Equipment

Inhalational therapy conducted in a hospital or in private homes depends not only upon skillful management of the apparatus employed and an understanding of the need for which it is used, but also on the maintenance in good condition of the original equipment. Inspection of the equipment should be made at intervals depending upon the use to which it has been subjected; the following procedures should be performed.

The oxygen-flow gauge or regulator should be checked in order to determine whether the rate of flow indicated on the dial is correct or not. A spirometer may be employed with a stopwatch, the oxygen flow being set at a predetermined rate, such as 2 liters per minute, and the time recorded in which the spirometer rises to the prescribed volume. If the pointer on the meter gauge is stuck at any liter flow the regulator should be returned and overhauled by the company from which it was purchased.

Inspection of the oxygen tent includes the ice cabinet, and its capacity to drain water freely from the cabinet into a suitable container. The commutator of the motor and the brushes should be checked and cleaned. All movable parts in the motor should be oiled but no oil should be applied to the regulator. The speed of the motor should be checked, and the efficiency of the rheostat in regulating velocity of air flow. The metal of the ice container should be polished at intervals and painted when necessary. Inspection of the hood should be made to determine whether or not any holes are present that would make for leakage. The rubber gasket that makes a leak-tight closure between the ice cabinet and the cabinet door may become torn and leaks therefore may occur. It is of very considerable importance to check this rubber gasket frequently. The plug at the ends of the electric cords that connect to the wall socket may show an undue separation of the prongs or loose wiring, and a new outfit should be installed so that short circuit does not take place. Water bottles used to humidify oxygen should be checked for leaks by running a stream of oxygen into them and by closing the outgoing rubber tube. In many instances the rubber gasket gets worn, and a leak may take place. At times the cap is not screwed on as tightly as is necessary or the screw fitting itself becomes worn and leaky.

The oxygen mask should be inspected for operation of the air injector and for the efficiency of the inspiratory and expiratory valves. The sponge-rubber disks should be cleaned from time to time since the accumulation of dust in them will clog the small pores and may thus cause excessive resistance to breathing, both on inspiration and expiration.

Catheters should be carefully inspected after use since the holes may become clogged with dried mucus. In other instances the catheter may be so worn as to make it possible that the tip of the catheter may fall off.

Soda-lime trays in thermal-circulation tents should also be inspected and testing of the contained atmosphere with the use of the amount of soda-lime employed should also be made to determine the efficiency of carbon-dioxide absorption and the rate of thermal circulation.

36

Respirators

The Drinker respirator, as shown in the accompanying illustration, consists of a cylindrical chamber in which a negative pressure is produced by the movement of an electrically operated bellows underneath the chamber. When the rubber bellows expands the air pressure in the chamber is lowered. The mild negative pressure produced around the chest and abdomen of the patient causes an expansion similar to that produced by normal inspiration. The head of the patient is in the outer atmosphere, closure being made at the neck with a soft sponge-rubber collar separating the head from the body. When the bellows contract the pressure in the chamber rises to that of the atmosphere and the lifting action on the chest disappears. The chest and diaphragm then return to their former position in passive expiration. The negative pressure employed is generally about 15 cm. of water and the rate of chest expansion is between 20 and 30 times per minute. The bellows is operated by an electric motor of a heavy-duty type designed for 24-hour continuous service for months on end. In recent years the noise of the power plant has been considerably reduced. Suitable portholes are present in the chamber so that nursing attention may be provided without interruption of artificial respiration. Regulation of this respirator is extremely simple. As a result of experience the rate of expansion of the chest as well as the extent of negative pressure employed is adjusted to meet the needs of the patient. Dangers of hyperventilation are far less than those which would be present if the respirator were not employed.[1]

[1] The two manufacturers of respirators of this general type are Warren E. Collins and John H. Emerson & Co.

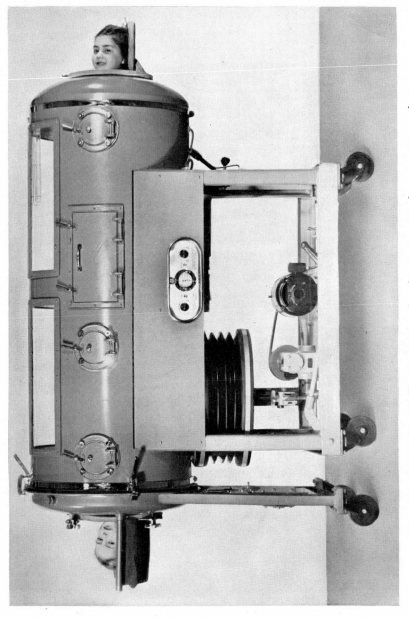

Fig. 50. A Drinker-Collins respirator for the treatment of one or two patients.

A COMBINATION EQUALIZING-PRESSURE CHAMBER AND RESPIRATOR [2]

An apparatus is herewith illustrated which may be employed as a respirator when the head compartment is opened (as seen in the picture), or as an equalizing-pressure chamber when the head compartment is closed. A motor-blower and valve system alternate the pressure in the chamber above and below atmospheric pressure when the chamber is used for respiration with immobilized lungs. The same motor-blower and valve arrangement with minor adjustment will vary the pressure between atmospheric and —15 to —25 cm. of water when the chamber is utilized as a conventional respirator. In this instance the head end of the chamber is turned back, exposing the face to the outer atmosphere.

When the head and body compartments are attached the patient is completely enclosed and an alternating pressure of 70 cm. of water above and below the atmosphere is produced 25 to 28 times per minute. In operating the equalizing-pressure chamber the air is first admitted to the head compartment and thence to the body part of the chamber. The reason for this is to bring about an earlier arrival of pressure to the nose and mouth in order to compensate for the very slight time delay in the arrival of pressure to the tracheobronchial tree and to the inner surface of the lung. The collar which separates the head from the chest interposes variable resistance to the passage of air, which is aimed to equal the resistance interposed by the tracheobronchial tree to the transmission of pressure to the inner surface of the chest wall. By regulating the distance between the neck and the collar a differential pressure on the head end may be obtained which will completely equalize the pressure on both sides of the chest wall. A water manometer attached to the head and the body compartment reveals the extent of differential pressure on the head end. In most instances a pressure of 5 cm. of water higher in the head compartment during the positive phase and 5 cm. of water lower during the negative phase is sufficient to compensate for the tracheobronchial resistance interposed in the lung. In some cases in which more extensive narrowing of the bronchi is present differential pressures of 7 cm. of

[2] The combination equalizing-pressure chamber is made by John H. Emerson & Co.; the original heavier duty chamber is built by special manufacturing contract by the Plaza Welding Co., N. Y. The details of construction are described in the reference in this section.

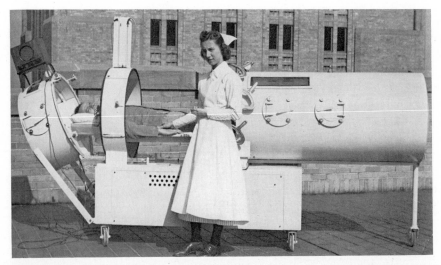

FIG. 51. Combination equalizing-pressure chamber and respirator.

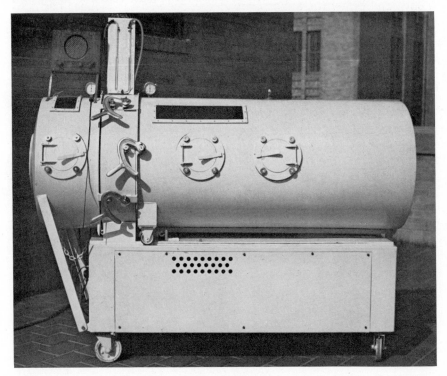

FIG. 52. Combination equalizing-pressure chamber and respirator
(closed).

water in the head end of the chamber are required.   An alternating pressure of 46 mm. Hg with a rate of 28 or 30 times per minutes is generally preferable to a pressure of 50 to 55 mm. Hg 25 times per minute.

There is a sensation on the eardrum of the oscillating pressure which is not uncomfortable to most patients.   This can be minimized

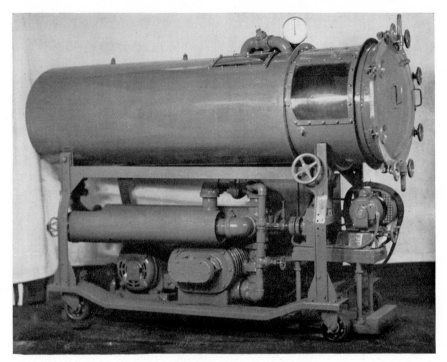

FIG. 53.   Equalizing-pressure chamber.

by application of sponge rubber to both ears which delays the application of pressure to the outer eardrum without interfering with hearing.   The head end of the chamber contains a compartment for insertion of ice.   The air which goes in and out of the chamber is first directed toward the cool surface of the ice container and thus provides the patient with a comfortable air atmosphere.

An equalizing chamber of sturdier construction was originally employed, utilizing a larger motor and compressor unit and a four-way valve for the production of alternating pressure.   The construction of this chamber was made of heavier metal than was required for the pressure used, and the mechanism of achieving alternating pressure is different from that employed in the combination respiratory and equalizing-pressure chamber.[3]

THE RESUSCITATOR [4]

The resuscitator illustrated herewith operates on the energy of compressed oxygen in oxygen cylinders. A rubber-cushioned face mask is applied to the patient and oxygen is blown into the patient's lungs until a pressure of 14 mm. Hg is reached, when it automatically reverses and breathes out to a negative pressure of 9 mm. Hg. The rate of respiration is determined by the volume of the patient's lungs and the time at which the pressure arrives at the blow-off level. In this way the apparatus is adjusted to the rhythm of the natural breathing rate of the individual, whether adult or child.

If obstruction is present in the airway a rapid clicking signal constitutes a warning to the operator. Under these circumstances aspiration may be employed with the same apparatus by turning a control lever to the mark set at aspiration. The apparatus then produces a continuous negative pressure which sucks mucus into a bottle or a trap through a rubber catheter. The aspirating part of the apparatus is entirely separate from the resuscitator. The control level may be turned to a mark set for inhalation, in which case the patient may breathe oxygen or oxygen–carbon-dioxide mixture from a rebreathing bag in the apparatus. The patient then breathes under his own effort either oxygen or an oxygen–carbon-dioxide mixture in the bag during inspiration and exhales through a release valve into the outer atmosphere. The apparatus employs a two-stage reducing regulator.

THE OXYGEN INCUBATOR

The oxygen incubator is a small chamber which has been developed to provide a safe administration of increased temperatures and humidities as well as an oxygen-enriched atmosphere, for the continuous care and isolation of premature infants, and also for the treatment of the full-term infant with either a subnormal temperature or with symp-

---

[3] The combination equalizing-pressure chamber is made by John H. Emerson & Co.; the original heavier duty chamber is built by special manufacturing contract by the Plaza Welding Co., N. Y. The details of construction are described in the reference in this section.

[4] This apparatus is called the Emerson Resuscitator and may be obtained from the John H. Emerson Co., 22 Cottage Park Ave., Cambridge, Mass.

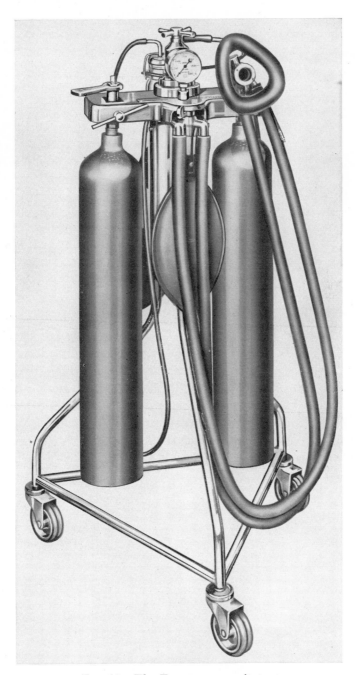

FIG. 54. The Emerson resuscitator.

toms of anoxia due to atelectasis of the lungs or to other disturbances in cardiac and respiratory function. With the modern incubators, an infant may live for an almost indefinite period with a temperature and at a relative humidity prescribed by the physician. When oxygen therapy is desired, a low flow of oxygen will provide 50 to 60 per cent oxygen continuously. When premature infants show a disturbance in respiratory function it is generally desirable to place them in a warm, humidified, oxygen-enriched atmosphere as soon as possible after delivery, and to keep them there without interruption of treatment for a prolonged period of time, such as ten days or even longer. Infants weighing as little as $17\frac{1}{4}$ ounces have lived in an incubator for 41 days and then developed into a normal healthy infant.

The Davidson Incubator. The Davidson incubator is a unit made of metal and bakelite 38 inches long, 41 inches high, and 17.5 inches wide. This unit operates by means of a slow-speed quiet motor blower which draws air from the bassinet compartment through a filter to remove bed lint and dust, and a tray of soda-lime to absorb carbon dioxide. After passing through the blower it may be connected to an ultraviolet-ray compartment where air-borne bacteria are presumably killed. In the ultraviolet-light tube developed by the General Electric Company for this particular use, the rays do not come into contact with the infant and the production of ozone is eliminated. The ultraviolet-ray tube is optional. The air then passes over the primary humidifying tray and then to the secondary humidifying tray and heater where the temperature and humidity are stabilized. From here the air is returned to the bassinet compartment and slowly flows over the infant without a direct draught. If oxygen is used the air circuit is closed and no room air enters. When oxygen is no longer necessary the air passes out through the vent and room air is drawn in to replace it.

The air and mattress temperatures are automatically controlled by two thermostats, one of which may be adjusted to provide and maintain the desired temperature while the second thermostat acts as a sentinel to shut off the heaters if the temperature should ever go as high as 102° F. This eliminates the possibility of the temperature ever rising above this degree. A buzzer and an indicating light are automatically turned on to sound an alarm if the air-vent door is closed before a flow of oxygen is started or if the oxygen cylinder is empty, or if the flow is interrupted from any other cause.

The humidity of the air in this incubator ranges from 60 to 65 per

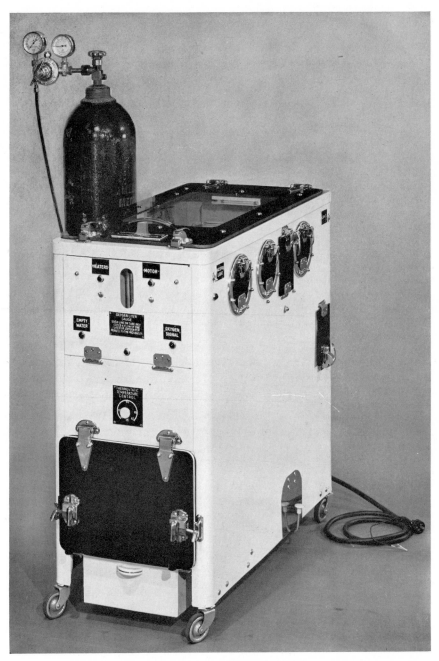

Fig. 55. The Davidson incubator.

cent saturation depending upon the temperature maintained. It is controlled by the area of water surface over which the air flows. This degree of relative humidity has been found to be ample to prevent dehydration of the infant, and has become recognized as a safe standard. Indirect lighting for the interior of the incubator is done with a fluorescent daylight-type lamp. The light rays do not come in line with the infant's vision.

Portholes are available by which nursing may be accomplished on each side. All hand ports are equipped with rubber cuffs to prevent loss of oxygen and drafts. The pediatrician may examine the patient without taking the infant out of the warm, humidified, oxygen-enriched atmosphere by means of a stethoscope which is standard equipment in this apparatus. The detailed directions for the use of this incubator are as follows:

1. Have the crib made up ready to receive the infant.

2. Place at least 2 quarts of water in the tray in the top of the compartment for ice and at least 4 quarts in the bottom of this compartment.

3. If oxygen is to be used, place a large piece of ice (not crushed ice) in the space provided for same; do not put water in the bottom of this compartment as this will be provided by the melting ice. Have a large cylinder of oxygen and gauge ready and attached.

4. Turn on the heater switch and set temperature for the degree prescribed, if possible ½ hour or more before the infant is placed in it, so sufficient time will be allowed for the heat to come up.

5. When the infant is placed in the crib, start the motor. If oxygen is necessary, close the air-vent door at the side and start the flow of oxygen at 10 liters and maintain this for 20 minutes, and then reduce it to 3 liters or as prescribed.

6. If no oxygen is used the air-vent door must remain open.

7. A buzzer sounds if the air-vent door is closed before oxygen is turned on or if the cylinder goes empty or the flow is interrupted from any cause. Be guided by the bell float oxygen meter on the gauge.

8. Empty waste water pan when light in front shows it is full.

9. Keep water in bottle on the wet bulb and refer to the humidity tables to determine humidity.

10. Do not lift the cover for any reason. Every nursing service can be done through the hand and utility ports.

The Hess Electric-heated Incubator Bed and Oxygen-therapy Unit. The Hess electric-heated incubator bed and oxygen-therapy unit is used for purposes identical with that of the Davidson oxygen incubator. It is a somewhat simpler unit which provides a relatively high temperature with small fluctuations and an increased amount of humidity in the atmosphere. It is equipped with interchangeable covers. One cover is employed when the outfit is used as an incubator with air and the other cover converts the incubator into an oxygen-therapy chamber. Detailed instructions in the operation of this apparatus are supplied with each unit.

37

Oxygen Analyzers

The effective and economic administration of oxygen in tents and chambers can be accomplished only with routine use of oxygen analyzers. The principle of oxygen analysis consists of taking a known quantity of the atmosphere to be tested, usually 10 cc., and injecting it into a burette in which the oxygen will be absorbed from the test sample. Measurement of the gas that remains is then read off and the difference in volume between the original sample and the remainder represents the percentage of oxygen in the sample. The measuring burettes or syringes employed are calibrated so that the reading is directly in terms of the percentage of oxygen. Carbon-dioxide analyzers are employed according to the same principle with a different absorbing medium.

THE ORSAT-BINGER OXYGEN ANALYZER

This method of oxygen analysis is the best of the simple methods. It consists of a 10-cc. burette containing three petcocks. The burette is connected to a glass absorption chamber which contains a tightly wound roll of 50-mesh copper screening. The chamber is inserted in a reservoir containing a solution of equal parts of saturated ammonium chloride and concentrated ammonium hydroxide. A layer of mineral oil is placed over the solution to prevent evaporation of the ammonium hydroxide. A leveling bulb which is connected to the lower end of the burette is filled with slightly acidulated water.

At the beginning of an analysis the solution in the absorption chamber must be brought into the neck at the level marked (H). This is accomplished by opening petcock "D" and turning petcock "C" to the III position. By raising or lowering the leveling bulb the liquid level in the absorption chamber may be adjusted to the desired height. Petcock "C" is then turned to the IV position, and petcock "B" to the I position.   By raising the leveling bulb the gases in the burette will be expelled to the outside air.   A sample of gas is then drawn from the tent by turning petcock "C" to the II position and lowering the leveling bulb.   The first two or three samples of gas drawn into

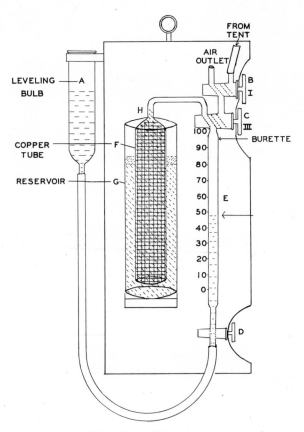

Fig. 56.   The Orsat-Binger oxygen analyzer.
The arrow at the right indicates the reading of
the oxygen concentration.

the burette should be expelled through the open arm of the upper petcock to insure thorough washing out of the sampling tube connecting the burette to the tent.   On the fourth drawing of the gas sample, the liquid level in the burette is brought to the zero mark and petcock "D" is closed.   With petcock "C" turned to the III position and petcock "D" reopened, the gas sample in the burette may be forced into the absorption chamber by raising the level bulb.   Care should be exercised to prevent the acidified water in the burette from rising above the middle petcock and entering the absorption chamber. The gas sample is left in contact with the copper screening for a minute and a half, during which time the oxygen is absorbed. At the end of this period the leveling bulb is lowered until the solution in the absorption chamber is brought to level "H." Close petcock "D" and determine the percentage of oxygen by reading the liquid level in the burette.

The test board should be checked daily for accuracy by analyzing room air which should record a reading of 21 per cent oxygen ± 1 per cent. With continued use the copper screening in the absorption tube dissolves at the top and the solutions become opaque. These should be changed when the test board becomes inaccurate.

THE RISEMAN-LESNICK OXYGEN ANALYZER

This simple analyzer makes use of the method previously described of absorbing oxygen from a known volume of gas by displacing the sample from the tent atmosphere into a reservoir which contains copper gauze in an ammoniacal solution. Subtracting the absorbed oxygen from the known volume of gas permits a correct reading of the oxygen percentage. The apparatus consists of a syringe, a reservoir solution, and a calibrated scale. A stop built in the box which contains the analyzing apparatus limits the withdrawal of the plunger of the glass syringe so that 10 cc. of the sample may be obtained consistently without inspecting the 10-cc. mark.

A three-way petcock is labeled I, II, and III, representing positions of the valve handle. In position I, withdrawal of the syringe obtains air from the tent atmosphere. By turning the handle to position II, the gas sample is then passed into the absorption chamber by compressing the plunger. The sample will force solution up into the burette. As the oxygen is absorbed the liquid level in the burette will continue to fall. When it comes to rest the oxygen percentage can be read on the scale along the side of the burette. The petcock is then turned to position III, which resets the apparatus for the next analysis.

When the handle is turned to the I position for taking a gas sample from the tent, the syringe plunger should be raised and lowered full length five times in order to wash out any atmosphere remaining in the rubber tube that is connected to the tent. The procedure is then continued as described—namely, forcing the gas in the syringe into the absorbing chamber and allowing the liquid level in the burette to fall gradually, while oxygen absorption is taking place, until it comes to rest, whereupon the oxygen percentage may be read.

The efficiency of the apparatus should be frequently tested by analyzing room air which would be found to yield approximately 21 per cent oxygen if the analyzer is in good condition.

The absorbing fluid may be made by dissolving 65 Gm. of ammonium nitrate in 45 cc. of water, adding 15 cc. of ammonium hydroxide. The apparatus is then filled with this solution, 30 cc. being able to absorb about 400 cc. of oxygen before a sediment forms which may clog the pores of the copper gauze and coat the burette. In testing for oxygen concentrations above 90 per cent, an absorbing solution is used containing equal parts of water and concentrated ammonium hydroxide and saturating this mixture with ammonium chloride. Although 30 cc. of this solution will absorb 400 cc. of oxygen before a precipitate forms, it does not yield as accurate analyses with low oxygen concentrations and is more apt to form a troublesome precipitate on the copper gauze.

When a precipitate has formed on the copper screening or in the burette, it should be promptly removed as follows: Connect the burette to an empty bottle with a length of rubber tubing, and the side arm of the valve to a bottle of unused absorbing solution. A 20 per cent solution of ammonia

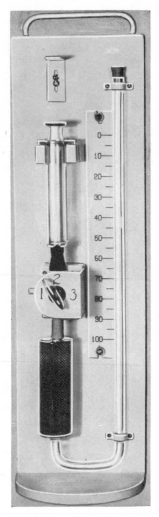

Fig. 57. The Riseman-Lesnick oxygen analyzer.

may be used for cleaning. It is less expensive but works more slowly. Direct the unused absorbing solution into the absorption chamber until the old blue fluid has been removed. The entrapped air is eliminated by turning the valve to the No. II position and raising the plunger of the syringe. The solution is allowed to remain in the absorbing chamber until all visible precipitate is dissolved, which takes about five minutes. Fresh solution is then added until the blue color disappears. Rubber tubing from the burette is then disconnected and with the valve at No. II position the plunger is raised in order to empty the

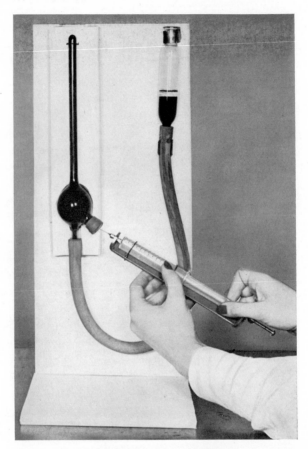

FIG. 58.   Pyrogallic-acid absorber for oxygen
analysis (Sholander-Hall).

burette to the 100 mark. The syringe is cleaned and dried and the barrel lubricated with a small amount of liquid petrolatum. It is important to take special care in cleaning the apparatus in order that accurate determinations may be obtained. The simplicity of the analyzer is a strong point in its favor and its operation readily can be learned if proper precautions are observed to keep it in condition. It is satisfactory as an analyzer for oxygen-tent therapy.

PYROGALLIC-ACID ABSORBER FOR OXYGEN ANALYSIS
(SHOLANDER-HALL)

A glass burette is herewith shown filled with concentrated alkaline pyrogallate solution and containing a rubber stopper through which the sample to be analyzed for oxygen is inserted. The burette is connected to a leveling bulb which serves as a reservoir for absorbent solution displaced by the gas sample during a test. A layer of mineral oil is poured over the pyrogallate in the leveling bulb to help prevent continuous absorption of oxygen from the atmosphere. A 10-cc. sample is drawn into a syringe from a mask or other apparatus and inserted with a fine hypodermic needle through the rubber stopper. The calibrated burette is then removed from the stand and rotated gently upward and downward so that the gas sample is in contact with the pyrogallate solution in the bulb. At the end of one minute the burette is placed next to the leveling bulb with the liquid levels in each at an equal height. The gas remaining in the apparatus after absorption of oxygen may be expelled by turning the burette bottom end up and permitting the gas to escape through the rubber tube and leveling bulb. Caution must be exercised to make a tight closure of the rubber cap or stopper through which the gas sample is inserted in order to avoid leakage of the strong caustic absorbent solution.

38

An Accurate Method for Obtaining the Oxygen and Carbon-dioxide Concentration of the Inspired Air in Oxygen Masks and Other Oxygen-therapy Equipment

It is important to determine the percentage of oxygen and carbon dioxide in the inspired air in appraising the efficiency of a mask. If air is drawn from the mask itself during inspiration at a point near the nose, the sample may show a different oxygen concentration depending upon whether it was taken at the beginning or end of inspiration. The same criticism would apply to determination of carbon-dioxide percentages. A true guide to the concentrations of both oxygen and carbon dioxide should include the total inspired air, which is obtained in the apparatus herewith illustrated.

It should be emphasized that alveolar air samples are in no sense an accurate guide of the carbon-dioxide percentage in the inspired air since the volume of ventilation is designed to keep the alveolar carbon-dioxide concentration constant. In fact, carbon-dioxide accumulation in oxygen masks has been found when the alveolar air samples failed to reveal a significant increase in carbon dioxide in the inspired air. As pointed out many years ago by Haldane, the alveolar carbon-dioxide percentage tends to be maintained at a constant level by variations in the minute volume of breathing. A test of the carbon-dioxide concentration in the alveolar air does not, therefore, tell whether carbon dioxide accumulates in the mask itself since augmented breathing might have lowered the alveolar carbon dioxide even though as much as 2.5 per cent carbon dioxide may have been present in the inspired air.

In order to obtain a gas sample from the mask equal in volume and at a rate equivalent to a normal inspiration, a sample is collected in a calibrated collecting bottle connected to a reservoir placed at a lower level. By simply regulating the volume and rate of flow of acidified water from the full sampling bottle to the reservoir, a quantity of gas is drawn into the former which is equivalent to that which would normally be inspired. The individual holds his breath at the end of

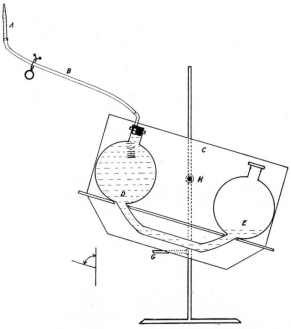

FIG. 59. Apparatus for obtaining oxygen and carbon-dioxide concentrations of the inspired air.

expiration and the gas sample is drawn at the rate of a normal inspiration. The apparatus consists of two bottles of 2-liter capacity each connected by a glass tube of 1-inch diameter and mounted on a wooden support frame, secured to a large ring stand. With an axle arrangement the support frame may be tilted so that the sample bottle may be brought to any desired level above the reservoir bottle. Connected to the sampling bottle by means of a rubber stopper is a rubber tube of 0.5-inch inside diameter fitted with a pinch clamp. Attached to the open end of the rubber tube is a glass connecting tube. In calibrating the sampling bottle it is important to include the volume of the rubber tube.

In making the test 3 liters of acidified water are added to the bottle.

The support frame is tilted to lower the sampling bottle and the pinch clamp on the rubber tube is opened to allow the gas in the bottle, the rubber tube, and the glass connecting tube to be expelled. The tube is then reclamped and the sampling bottle is raised by tilting the support frame until it is well above the water level in the reservoir. The tip of the glass connecting tube is then fitted into the mask, or other apparatus to be tested, at a point near the nose. At the end of a normal expiration the subject is told to hold his breath and the pinch clamp is opened long enough to permit a sample equal in volume to the tidal air to be drawn into the sampling bottle. The size of the sample may be determined from the calibration on the sampling bottle and the speed of intake can be varied by the height of the sampling bottle above the reservoir so as to conform to the velocity of inspiration of the subject. In this way an accurate sample of the mixed total inspired air is obtained from which one may determine by analysis the percentage of oxygen and carbon dioxide that would have been inspired by the subject. The large sample of gas obtained by this method is of value in determining accurately the content of inspired gas in masks which are being tested at very high altitudes. Alveolar samples obtained under very low pressures decrease in volume when brought to sea-level pressures, to such an extent that insufficient gas remains for accurate analysis. A 500- or 600-cc. sample of inspired air, however, when brought to sea level, will leave sufficient volume of gas for many analyses.

BIBLIOGRAPHY

Andrews, A. H., Jr.: Oxygen Therapy Techniques Including Carbon Dioxide Helium and Water Vapor, Chicago, Year Book Publishers, 1943.

Banash, J. I., and G. O. Carter: Researches in oxygen therapy equipment: some aspects of the mechanical phases of oxygen therapy apparatus, Anesth. and Analg., 12:52, 1933.

Barach, A. L.: Simple apparatus for administering oxygen, Jour. Amer. Med. Asso., 78:334, 1922.

Barach, A. L.: Methods and results of oxygen treatment in pneumonia, Arch. Int. Med., 37:186, 1926; M. Clin. N. Amer., 9:471, 1925.

Barach, A. L.: New oxygen tent, Jour. Amer. Med. Asso., 87:1213, 1926.

Barach, A. L.: A new type oxygen chamber, Jour. Clin. Invest., 2:463, 1926.

Barach, A. L.: Acute disturbance of lung function in pneumonia; methods of oxygen treatment, Jour. Amer. Med. Asso., 89:1865-1868, 1927.

Barach, A. L.: The administration of oxygen by the nasal catheter, Jour. Amer. Med. Asso., 93:1550, 1929.

Barach, A. L.: A new type oxygen chamber ventilated by thermal circulation of air, Modern Hosp., 32:144, 1929.

Barach, A. L.: The importance of ventilation in oxygen tent and oxygen chamber therapy; with a description of an improved oxygen tent, N. Y. State Jour. Med., 31:1263, 1931.

Barach, A. L.: Analysis of 376 consecutive oxygen-treated cases from a study made at the Presbyterian Hospital, New York City, from 1929 to 1932, N. Y State Jour. Med., 34:41, 1934.

Barach, A. L.: An oxygen chamber simplified in design and operation, Jour. Amer. Med. Asso., 97:390, 1931.

Barach, A. L.: The use of helium in the treatment of asthma and obstructive lesions in the larynx and trachea, Ann. Int. Med., 9:739, 1935.

Barach, A. L.: Oxygen treatment, Jour. Amer. Med. Asso., 106:725, 1936.

Barach, A. L.: "Pilot error" and oxygen want; with a description of a new oxygen face tent, Jour. Amer. Med. Asso., 108:1868, 1937.

Barach, A. L.: Recent advances in inhalation therapy in the treatment of cardiac and respiratory disease, New York State Jour. Med., 37:1095-1110, 1937

Barach, A. L.: Immobilization of lungs through pressure, Amer. Rev. Tuberc., 42:586, 1940.

Barach, A. L.: The therapeutic uses of gases, Modern Medical Therapy in General Practice, 1:199-143, 1940.

Barach, A. L.: Alternating equalizing pressure chamber and control pressure panel, Amer. Rev. Tuberc., 43:91, 1941.

Barach, A. L., and Binger, C. A. L.: Portable oxygen tent, Jour. Amer. Med. Asso. 85:190, 1925.

Barach, A. L., and M. Eckman: Use of a photo-electric cell in respiration apparatus, Proc. Soc. Exper. Biol. and Med., 35:295, 1936.

Barach, A. L., and M. Eckman: A mask apparatus which provides high oxygen concentrations with accurate control of the percentage of oxygen in the inspired air and without accumulation of carbon dioxide, Jour. Aviation Med., 12:39, 1941.

Barach, A. L., and M. Eckman: Physiologically controlled oxygen mask apparatus, Anesthesiol., 2:421, 1941.

Barach, A. L., and N. Molomut: An oxygen mask metered for positive pressure, Ann. Int. Med., 17:820, 1942.

Barker, K. H., D. M. Parker, and G. Wassel: Nasal catheter administration of oxygen—with observations on alveolar saturation, Jour. Amer. Med. Asso., 103:244, 1934.

Binger, C. A. L.: Construction and management of oxygen chamber, Mod. Hosp., 24:186, 1925.

Birnbaum, G. L., and S. A. Thompson: Resuscitation in advanced asphyxia, Jour. Amer. Med. Asso., 118:1364, 1942.

Boothby, W. M.: Miniature oxygen chamber for infants: a modification of the Hess incubator, Proc. Staff Meet., Mayo Clin., 9:129, 1934.

Boothby, W. M., and W. R. Lovelace, II: Oxygen in aviation: the necessity for the use of oxygen and a practical apparatus for its administration to both pilots and passengers, Jour. Aviation Med., 9:172-198, 1938.

Boothby, W. M., W. R. Lovelace, and A. H. Bulbulian: Oxygen administration and therapeutic use: I. Value of high concentration of oxygen for therapy; II Oxygen for therapy and aviation and an apparatus for the administration of oxygen and oxygen-helium by inhalation; III. Design and construction of the masks for oxygen inhalation apparatus, Proc. Staff Meet., Mayo Clin., 13:641, 646, 654, 1938.

Boothby, W. M., W. R. Lovelace, II, and A. Uihlein: The B.L.B. oxygen inhalation apparatus: I. Improvements in design; II. Efficiency as determined by studies on oxygen percentages in alveolar air, Proc. Staff Meet., Mayo Clin., 15:195, 1940.

Buerki, R. C.: A method of reducing the cost of oxygen for therapeutic purposes, Mod. Hosp., 43:88, 1934.

Bullowa, J. G. M.: A simple method for the calibration of clinical oxygen regulators, Jour. Lab. and Clin. Med., 20:526, 1935.

Bullowa, J. G. M., and G. Lubin: New York City studies performance of different oxygen tents, Mod. Hosp., 40:83, 1933.

Burgess, A. M., A. S. Briggs, and A. M. Burgess, Jr.: Oxygen therapy by the open box method, New England Jour. Med., 210:254, 1934.

Campbell, J. A.: Box type face mask for oxygen administration, Brit. Med. Jour., 1:1245, 1936.

Campbell, J. M. H., and E. P. Poulton: Oxygen and Carbon Dioxide Therapy, Oxford University Press, 1934.

Christie, R. V., and M. McGill: Oxygen therapy—with a note on a new nasal mask, Lancet, 2:876, 1938.

Cohn, D. J.: Dry ice oxygen tent, Mod. Hosp., 52:76, 1939.

Cowan, S. L., and J. V. Mitchell: Improved equipment for oxygen therapy, Brit. Med. Jour., 1:118, 1942.

Davison, Francis W.: Some observations on the control of temperature and humidity in oxygen tents. Ann. Otol., Rhinol., and Laryngol., 49:1083-1090, 1940.

Drinker, P., and C. F. McKhann: The use of a new apparatus for the prolonged administration of artificial respiration: 1. A fatal case of poliomyelitis, Jour. Amer. Med. Asso., 92: 1658, 1929.

Eckman, M., and A. L. Barach: Inhalational therapy equipment, Mod. Hosp., 52: 78, 1939.

Eckman, M., and A. L. Barach: A method for obtaining gas samples of the total inspired air, Proc. Soc. Exper. Biol. and Med., 48:346, 1941.

Erikson, C. A.: Designing and building an oxygen therapy unit, Mod. Hosp., 37:81, 1931.

Hartman, F. W.: New oxygen tents are electrically air conditioned, Mod. Hosp., 42:96, 1934.

Hashagen, J. B.: Temperature and humidity control of an oxygen chamber, Heating, Piping and Air Conditioning, 2:122, 1930.

Henderson, Yandell: Adventures in Respiration: Modes of Asphyxiation and Methods of Resuscitation, Baltimore, Williams & Wilkins Co., 1938.

Henderson, Y., and J. McC. Turner: Artificial respiration and inhalation: the principle determining the efficiency of various methods, Jour. Amer. Med. Asso., 116:1508, 1941.

Hill, L.: A simple oxygen bed tent and its use in a case of edema and chronic ulcer of the leg, Jour. Physiol., Proc. Physiol. Soc., 55:20, 1921

Lombard, A. B., and C. Nelson: A new apparatus for oxygen therapy, Jour. Lab. and Clin. Med., 24:724, 1939.

Lovelace, W. R., II: Technique of treatment with helium-oxygen using B.L.B. inhalation apparatus, Proc. Staff Meet., Mayo Clin., 13:790, 1938.

Lubin, G., and J. G. M. Bullowa: A thermal conductivity recorder for oxygen and carbon dioxide for clinical atmosphere control, Proc. Soc. Exper. Biol. and Med., 27:568, 1930.

Martinez, D. B.: The mechanical resuscitation of the new-born, Jour. Amer. Med. Asso., **109**:489, 1937.

McSwiney, B. A., and B. Savage: B.L.B. (Boothby, Lovelace, and Bulbulian) mask for administering oxygen, Lancet, **1**:398, 1940

Poulton, E. P., and T. W. Adams: Oxygen tents and nasal catheters, Brit. Med. Jour., **1**:567, 1936.

Richards, D. W., Jr., A. L. Barach, and H. A. Cromwell: Use of vaporized bronchodilator solutions in asthma and emphysema; a continuous inhalation method for severe asthmatic states, Amer. Jour. Med. Sci., **199**:225, 1940.

Riseman, J. E. F., and G. Lesnick: A simple method of oxygen analysis for use in oxygen tent therapy, New England Jour. Med., **215**:65, 1936.

Rosenbluth, M. B., and M. Block: Oxygen therapy without soda lime, Jour. Amer. Med. Asso., **98**:386, 1932.

Roth, P.: Improved apparatus for therapeutic administration, Mod. Hosp., **22**:404, 1924.

Rovenstine, E. A., I. B. Taylor, and K. E. Lemmer: Oropharyngeal insufflation of oxygen: gas tensions in the bronchus, Anesth. and Analg., **15**:1, 1936.

Ryle, J.: The therapeutic administration of oxygen, Lancet, **1**:1269, 1922.

Schwentker, F. F., and H. K. Fallin: Simple method for analysis of helium, Bull. Johns Hopkins Hosp., **61**:210, 1937.

Stadie, W. C.: Construction of an oxygen chamber for treatment of pneumonia, Jour. Exper. Med., **35**:323, 1922

Taylor, T. A., and W. H. Taylor: Oxygen therapy: with an improved motorless apparatus, the "Oxygenaire," American Hospital Supply Corporation, Internat. Jour. Med. and Surg., **46**:596, 1933.

Thalhimer, W.: Oxygen therapy in hospitals, equipment and management of service: with a discussion on its postoperative use by Dr. George W. Crile, Bull. Am. Coll. Surgeons, **16**:15, 1932.

Thunberg, T.: The barospirator: a new machine for producing artificial respiration, Skandinav. Arch. f. Physiol., **48**:80, 1926.

Waters, R. M., R. C. Buerki, and H. R. Hathaway: Oxygen therapy at the Wisconsin General Hospital: Technic, Hospitals, **10**:1, 1936.

Waters, R. M., and J. W. Harris: Anesth. and Analg., **10**:59, 1931.

Wineland, A. J., and R. M. Waters: Oxygen therapy; insufflation into oral pharynx Arch. Surg., **22**:67, 1931.

INDEX

A

Abdominal distention, *see* Distension, abdominal

Acapnia, 8

Acarbia, 8

Acclimatization to altitude, 20, 27, 35

Acid-base equilibrium, in anesthesia, 8
in anoxia, 26-27
in low oxygen inhalation, 71
in obstructive dyspnea, 106
in oxygen therapy for heart failure, 63
in pneumonia, 40
in pulmonary emphysema, 117, 129
in shock, 76

Acidosis, in anesthesia, 8
in anoxia, 26

Adrenal glands, effect of anoxia on, 32
heat therapy on, 170

Adrenalin, 95, 96, 101, 102

Aero-embolism, 2, 20, 156-158
etiology, 156
pathologic physiology, 156-158
prevention, 157-158
See also Caisson disease

Aeroneurosis, 223

Air, 1-2, 3, 10-11

Air-ambulances, dangers in pathologic states, 199-201

Alcoholism, 136-137

Alkalosis, caused by fever therapy, 170
high altitudes, 26
effect on capillaries, 29, 71-72
in cardiac pain, 71-72

Altitude, effect of, 4, 20-29
on arterial and alveolar carbon dioxide, 21, 23, 24-28
on arterial and alveolar oxygen, 20-25, 28
on water vapor in lungs, 21-25
tolerance tests for aviators, 33
See also Aero-embolism; Altitude sickness

Altitude sickness, 20-36, 221
etiology, 20
oxygen therapy, 33-36
pathologic physiology, 21-29
signs and symptoms, 25-26, 29-33

Alveolar carbon dioxide, effect of altitude, 21, 23, 24-28
in heart failure, 61

Alveolar oxygen, effect of altitude, 20-25, 28

Aminophyllin, 97, 100, 101, 102, 103

Ammonia poisoning, 165

Analysis of inspired air, 300-302

Anemia, effect of air transportation on, 200

Anemic anoxia, *see* Anoxia, in hemorrhage

Anesthesia, 8, 151-154
effect in anemia, 153
on breathing, 8
in coronary disease, 152, 153
in shock, 153
oxygen therapy, 153-154, 219
pathologic physiology, 151-152

Angina pectoris, *see* Coronary disease

Anoxemia, *see* Anoxia

Anoxia, adaptation to, 27
in aeroneurosis, 223
in alcoholism, 136
in anesthesia, 151-154, 219
in asthma, 88
in barbiturate medication, 151
in brain disorders, 179-180
in dyspnea, 106-107
effect on brain, 32, 33, 35, 179, 216, 217, 220-225
fetal, 139-141
in fever therapy, 170-171
in head injuries, 172
in heart disease, 70-71
in heart failure, 60-62
in hemorrhage, 145-146
in morphine medication, 151
in neurasthenia, 224
neuromuscular control in, 32, 33